The Spirit of the Place

Literature and Medicine
MARTIN KOHN AND CAROL DONLEY, EDITORS

The Spirit of the Place

◊ ◊ ◊ *A Novel* ◊ ◊ ◊

Samuel Shem

The Kent State University Press   *Kent, Ohio*

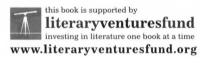
this book is supported by
literaryventuresfund
investing in literature one book at a time
www.literaryventuresfund.org

Library of Congress Cataloging-in-Publication Data
Shem, Samuel.
The spirit of the place : a novel / Samuel Shem.
p.   cm. — (Literature and medicine series ; 14)
ISBN 978-0-87338-942-6 (alk. paper) ∞
1. Physicians—Fiction.   2. New York (State)—Fiction.   I. Title.
PS3569.H39374S66 2008
813'.54—dc22   2008001526

British Library Cataloging-in-Publication data are available.

12 11 10 09 08   5 4 3 2 1

For three generations:
Rose Fuchs Bergman
Janet Lynn Surrey
Katie Chun Surrey-Bergman

For some years
I have been afflicted
With the belief that
Flight is possible to man.

—Wilbur Wright, letter,
May 13, 1900

Part One

◊ ◊ ◊

Beware of foreign entanglements . . .

—*George Washington (apocryphal)*

1

Even a shy American can be happy in Italy, and Orville Rose was about as happy as a childless man can be. From a low point two years ago when, in a test tube in New Jersey his sperm had failed to impregnate a hamster egg and medical science had declared him sterile, he felt that his life had gotten a whole lot better.

Now, the summer of 1983, he was steadying the oars of a red rowboat as Celestina Polo was pushing away from a dock. With that sweet sense of gliding over ice, they were off. Orville always felt great when setting out, running off, and he sighed happily. He took a first pull against the weight of the water.

As her hand pushed against the rough wood of the dock and she sensed the rowboat ease out onto the lake, Celestina felt a hit of apprehension. Leaving land made her nervous. She settled uneasily onto the plank seat.

"Two bad things will happen today."

"What?"

"This will be a bad day, *caro*. Two bad things will happen today."

Orville laughed. In her years of Buddhist study in India, Celestina claimed to have seen things that he, a doctor, saw as outrageous. A man who was 132 years old. A yogi who could transmit and read thought. Another who could levitate, however briefly. A woman who could predict the future. Lately, Celestina herself had been trying to predict the future. She had ventured several predictions, none of which had happened.

"So far, kid," Orville said, "you've been wrong every time."

"Of course I am being wrong every time," she answered. "I am *learning*. I know it is hard for you to believe, *dottore,* but I am not yet totally enlightened." She smiled. "Two bad things will happen today."

"Are you talking about money? I mean, if you're talking about money, I agree. We're almost broke. We can't keep staying at these expensive hotels and—"

"Do not talk to me about money! Never to talk to me about money! I don't care about money, and if you—"

"But you don't care about money! You don't seem to understand that if you put it on that little plastic card now, you have to actually pay for it later. With interest. With Mafia-type interest. You're overdrawn, I'm in debt, deep in debt. We're almost broke."

"In our very brokenness," she said mischievously, "is our wealth."

"Oh boy!"

"And in our very wealth is our brokenness."

"Terrific."

"The two bad things are not about money, no." She closed her eyes and pointedly took a meditative breath. "Not about American Express." Another. "Not even about the Diner's Club." And another.

He chuckled. She opened her eyes and smiled at him. The gap between her two front teeth was suddenly endearing to him. He shook his head.

"You're nuts."

"*Si, caro,* nuts enough to love you."

"Yeah, well, try it from my side. You are *insano. Discumbobulo!*" Laughing, Orville grasped the worn handles of the wooden oars. He glanced over his shoulder toward the tiny island of San Guilio, set like a child's sandcastle, off center, in Lake Orta, the smallest of the northern Italian lakes. He pulled at the oars.

It was past noon. The August sun was hot. The water, still as air, gave off that subtle lake scent that reminds you of wet earth. The day so far had been smooth, suffused with all the glossy luminescence of summer.

Soon they were far out from shore. Back across the water the ancient resort town of Orta San Guilio had diminished to a colorfully painted toy. Above it, amid the grave green cypress, Orville could see the occasional spires of the twenty chapels of the celebrated pilgrimage site on top of the Sacre Monte. He lowered his eyes from the tiny mountain to Celestina's long face, a Modigliani face framed by silky black hair cut smartly short, to her walnut eyes, to her white gauzy dress molding transparently to her breasts, to her browned toes that during their lovemaking that morning had intertwined with such strength with his—she was tall for a woman, he short for a man—and felt a rush of love.

She felt it, too, and smiled. Smiled at his short chestnut hair with the bald spot; at his tanned face with substantial forehead, Sephardic hawk's nose, fine lips, close-cropped beard, eyes the color of the Mediterranean set off by his rose-toned shirt and at his browned toes. She smiled at all this and at their passion.

"This is getting serious," he said.

"*Allora,* we are laughing." She reached over, the hollow of her breasts distracting him so that when she suddenly squeezed his toes hard, he squeaked in pain. "So serious, *tesoro,* we must keep on laughing."

4

"Tesoro?"

"Treasure." The word hit him hard. He blushed.

Had he ever been loved like this before? Been loving like this before? Sure, there had been a non-Jewish first love back in high school in Columbia, New York, which had been destroyed by his parents, and in med school a Jewish practical kind of love that had led to marriage. In those loves, like in this one, there had been that same astonishing feeling when your heart seems made of feathers and diamonds and floats up sparkling in your chest when you even think of her or see her hairbrush or her car or her toes.

But this was different. This love was surprising and familiar all at once. The things she said were so outrageous—sometimes seeming totally kooky and sometimes totally wise, as if she really had understood a few secrets of life. So outrageous that they seemed to expand the usual things that rolled around his head day and night. This love seemed always fresh—maybe because she was so different, and yet so known. Or maybe fresh because she seemed so known, and then took his hand and led him someplace so unknown; led him not only into it, kicking and screaming, but through it to a strangely peaceful place. Nothing like this ever before, no.

This is it, Orville thought. You've really found something here. Something lasting, something of real depth. Please, God, don't let me screw it up!

"You know," he said, his voice wobbling like a dying top, "that—that *tesoro*—it's the most beautiful thing anyone has ever said to me."

Celestina blushed, smiled shyly, and said nothing.

"I love you so much!"

They embraced, holding each other close, losing track of time.

Shouts!

Their rowboat had drifted into the path of another rowboat. He picked up the oars. There were tears in her eyes, too.

They docked and walked around the tiny island, hand in hand. She opened a small tin of licorice. They popped the tiny flecks into each other's mouths. The sharp violet taste was a comfort.

◊ ◊ ◊

It had started a few months ago in Woudschoten, Holland. Orville was working as the *Sportsdoktor* at Camp Zeist, a center where athletes from all over Europe came to train. He had spent years dealing with injured, diseased, and dead bodies, first in suburban New Jersey and then, after his divorce, in the worst trouble spots around the world with *Médecins Sans Frontières*.

Being a doctor in the thick of horrific situations had taken its toll. In the past, finding himself up to his elbows in blood and gore and trying to put noses back in the approximate middles of faces and make bones as straight as a five iron, he had come to wonder about the stupidity and viciousness of men toward other men, women, and children. He had discovered that he did not like disease and that he had a particularly hard time with handicaps. He shied away from deformities of all kinds. Hollowed out, he had drifted to Holland to heal. He chanced on a job dealing with healthy bodies. As the *Sportsdoktor,* for almost a year he'd had a practice of the best bodies in Europe. He had many opportunities to engage a woman member of a team during its stay at Zeist, but he resisted. Somehow it seemed pointless. He still hurt too much, from the vicious end of his marriage, and from what he had seen out in the world and could not forget.

Celestina Polo had arrived at Zeist as the yoga teacher and motivator of the Italian women's swim team. His first sight of her had been one morning at dawn as he walked up the graveled pathway between the soaring pines and had seen, in a place in the woods cleared of trees, her leading a class in meditation and yoga. Several young women sat in a circle with her, their eyes closed. She was the only one all in white, and the only one sitting in a full lotus. Shafts of sunlight lit up the limpid mist of the low-country morning. The pine scent was flecked with burning incense. Smoke spiraled up along the trunk of a pine. The sight of this woman sitting there so still, a forest spirit in white amid the deep green of these ancient trees took his breath away. He stopped and stared, taken with the moment, reluctant to keep walking lest his shoes on the loose gravel disturb the silence. It wasn't just the beauty or the quiet; it was something to do with the stillness. The word that came to his mind was a strange one for him: serenity.

As he stood still and watched, the other women fidgeted. She did not. After awhile she reached for a small brass cup that she held carefully in the palm of one hand. In the other she picked up a small mallet. She tapped the cup with the mallet, leaving the mallet against it so there was a dull clunky sound. Then she hit it fully. The little cup rang out, a bell to signal the end of the meditation. The clear, bright sound seemed to awaken the air, the pines, and ferns, seemed to awaken him. She held the bell until the ringing stopped. She put it down and placed both hands together, palm-to-palm, under her lips and bowed slightly to each of the other women, as they did to her.

Then she saw him. Without surprise—as if expecting him to be there— she held his gaze. The moment was riveting.

6

She bowed to him. He didn't know what to do. And then, smiling, feeling terribly awkward, he hastily put his palms together under his chin and bowed back to her.

With a certain grace she unwrapped herself from her lotus and stood up. She said something in Italian to the others and they too stood. As they began their yoga on the mat of pine needles in the glen, he walked away. Something else had happened. That's all he knew, right then, that something else had happened, and that he had to find out what. Their attraction was magnetic.

To him she was white linen and dark secrets, alive in a world different than he had ever experienced—a world he had learned, on the conveyer belt of American medicine, to discount. To her he was Western science and American optimism, hiding under a cynical edge that prompted her to see his potential. In each conversation she said things that at first seemed preposterous but which, as they went deeper, made more and more sense. One day he realized that her worldview seemed to encompass his but not vice-versa. He was enticed and challenged by this idea. He didn't understand what she was saying a lot of the time and understood even less about her meditative practices. But in it all there was a surprising glimmer of possibility for him, which he sensed was a possible end to his hurt, his cynicism, his suffering.

Their lovemaking sealed it. He was exuberant and boyish, she explosive and tantric. Here, too, at first, she was surprising and exotic. But as they got to know each other, the tantric peeled away, and they were left with the ordinary sensual pleasure and playfulness of two people daring to hope—as if some of Celestina's Indian stuff was a protection against being at the mercy of love.

Like all the rest of us, he said to himself at the time, yes.

After two weeks together in May at the sports center, they were crazed with each other. During their first month apart they called each other at least twice a day and sent flowers and silly gifts.

In June Celestina returned to Amsterdam for a retreat led by an Indian teacher, a woman whom she had studied with in Mount Abu, India. Orville attended a few lectures. He was impressed with the power of the teacher and the depth of Celestina's understanding, but it wasn't for him. Each talk was preceded by a thirty-minute meditation, a sitting in silence "following the breath." He sat there, knees aching, back sore, going bananas. It seemed like forever. Celestina asked him what it was like.

"Garbage," he said. "My mind is full of garbage."

"Good."

"Good? How is that good?"

"It is true. It is your karma."

"The karma of garbage?"

"For you, it is a gift."

Orville groaned. "I don't think so. You do it. I'll watch."

"Just come to her last lecture tomorrow. For *our* sake, okay?"

The last lecture was on psychological suffering. The root of psychological suffering, so said the Indian guru, lay in comparing yourself to others. The trap is in the process of becoming rather than being. "The flowering of being," she said, "puts an end to all psychological suffering."

Afterward, as they walked arm in arm back to The Canal House, their hotel, both were quiet. Neither spoke about the lecture until they were at the hotel. Sitting in their room overlooking the Keizersgracht, Orville said, "You know, I have to admit it made some sense, what she said. I mean, in terms of my life."

"Good," she said, casually. "What shall we do for dinner?"

"I mean, there's something there, something new. My whole life I've been into comparing, competing, being someone special. She made sense to me."

"I know."

"How do you know?"

"I watch you listen to her. Your ears get bigger."

"You mean I heard what she was saying."

"No, I mean as you listened to her talk, your ears really did get bigger. You understood something, *si?*"

"Yeah."

"*Bene.* Now let it go."

"Can't we talk about it?"

"No."

"Why not?"

"It is not about the words. The word is not the thing. If something happened, it will last. Can we have fish?"

He was surprised at this, that she didn't want to talk about it. But then he realized how he loved that in her, her being always surprising. With her that night, he felt light of heart, happy. It was a wonderful night. They did eat at a fish place. They walked the humpbacked bridges over the canals, dodged the bicycles, walked the cobblestones, stared longingly at the lights in the waters. It was as close to her as he had ever felt, as if their love was lightening up the whole damn world.

8

The next morning he put her on the train back to Rome with plans for him to come to Italy for a holiday in a few weeks.

After she'd gone he couldn't forget what she had said, about the garbage of his mind being his gift, his way to be free. When he called her a few days later and said he was trying to meditate for short periods, she screeched with delight.

"*Si, si,*" she said, "you never forget what you understand."

◊ ◊ ◊

In July Orville went to Italy. They had arranged to take a long holiday together. He had decided on a surprise of his own. He had quit his job at Camp Zeist. At the end of their holiday he would tell Celestina that he was moving to Rome to be with her.

They met up in Venice, rented a car, and drove through the Dolomites, doing the lakes east to west: the ominous Garda nestled up under the Swiss Alps, the terrific Lugano and calm Como, the seedy Maggiore, and, finally, the tiny gem of Orta, an afterthought which, like so many afterthoughts, was the most exquisite of all. But for the conflict around Celestina's insistence on staying at the finest hotels and eating at expensive restaurants, this time together had deepened and broadened their love.

They discovered that their birthdays were only two days apart: on July 22 she was thirty-four, and on July 24 he was thirty-nine. He asked if she believed in astrology.

"No way! You think I am some kind of lightweight? Astrology is the New Age fluff, for those seeking a spiritual shortcut. The real path is hard. The Eight-Fold Path is made of *rock.*"

For her birthday he gave her a smooth oval of black marble that fit into her palm, a stone on which was etched

NOTHING IS ETCHED IN STONE

She gave him a watch, on whose face, in the place of each of the twelve numbers, was the word

NOW

◊ ◊ ◊

Now, having strolled around the tiny island, they sat outdoors for an afternoon wine at a *trattoria* shaded by a pleached arbor of Muscat grapes. Members of a large Italian family sat nearby, a family in which, to Orville's doctor's eye, obesity ran, if not raced. The family members were eating, laughing, sometimes singing. The wine went to Orville's head. The scene began to float and fuzz, as if all the elements—humans, chairs, wine-glasses, forks, pasta, and grapes were levitating, a little. He closed his eyes, feeling the heat on his lids, as if the sun were sunning herself there.

There was a stir. The bufalo mozzarella had arrived, shipped fresh all the way from Napoli. The Italian family went wild, falling on it like chubby bears on a honey pot. Great white chunks flopped in the sunlight, floated, disappeared into mouths, muffling the peals of laughter.

Orville watched the Pappa Bear of the family laughing and waving his arms around and sounding as if he were singing the *Aria to the Bufalo Mozzarella* when suddenly the sound stopped, and he started waving his arms in toward his chest—at first frantically and soon dyingly. He was choking. His eyes started to bulge. People started to scream. Someone pounded him on the back. No luck. The pounding, Orville knew, merely sealed the mozzarella more tightly in the trachea. Orville and Celestina rushed over, she clearing a path and shouting over the chaos that he was a doctor.

Panic in others provoked calm in Orville. He had even come to enjoy the way time slowed at such moments, like before a car crash. It almost makes you believe in eternity, he thought. Even more calm for the rosy glow of the Chianti, he grabbed the bulky Pappa for a Heimlich maneuver. Barely getting his arms around him, fist over diaphragm, he pushed. *Niente.* Again. *Niente.* Orville stuck his finger in the man's mouth, fishing the pharynx for food. Nope. The man was slumping, turning blue, no longer gesturing.

"A straw!" he called out to Celestina. "Tell them to get me a straw."

"*Cannucia!*" she shouted to a waiter. "*Per favore una cannucia!*"

Lying the man down on a table, he took out his Swiss Army knife and opened the fine blade. The anatomy clicked in. His fingers started at the chin and walked down the tracheal rings over the Adam's apple to the cricohyoid cartilage and down another notch—otherwise, he knew, you hit bad shit like the parathyroids and the tracheael artery. Holding a napkin to either side, he popped the knife edge into the trachea. Bright-red blood spurted out. Over his shoulder there was the sound of someone vomiting. He felt a whoosh of steamy air from the lungs.

"*Cannucia!*" he sang out like a tough surgeon making his grand entrance, announcing the *Aria to the Hopefully Plastic Straw.* He held out his hand for it, as if for a scalpel. Celestina handed it to him. It was plastic, not paper. *Bene.* Orville rotated the knife point against the ring of tracheal cartilage until, as when you carve down through the turkey leg-joint and feel the gristle give, the aperture widened enough to insert the straw. Immediately the air whistled in and out through the clear plastic and the fat guy went pink and tried to talk but couldn't, because no air could get above to his vocal chords, still paralyzed by the gob of bufalo mozzarella shipped fresh all the way from Napoli. Some lucky Italian doc, he mused, cutting the straw to size and taping it in place, will have the tricky job of coaxing the cheese back up from above.

Pappa Bear again started waving his arms around comically, a sure sign of resurrection. There were *bravos* and thrown kisses, and, as they waited for the *vaporetto,* Chianti and mozzarella all around.

Celestina and Orville sped back to the mainland with the smiling Pappa, helped the snappily uniformed ambulance attendants stuff the fat man into one of those thin ambulances, and then floated hand in hand up the hill to their hotel. At the door, as he put his arm around her, Orville was surprised to find Celestina trembling.

"What's wrong?" he asked.

"Now that I predicted it, it scares me." She turned to face him, her eyes alive with fear. "It can come at any moment, that tap on the shoulder. Especially, my dear one, at the moment of great love."

"Well, we're safe now, for the day."

"Not yet. That was just the first."

"Beginner's luck."

At the desk was a telegram for Orville from his sister.

MOTHER DIED TODAY AUG 1 TRIED TO CALL YOU
FUNERAL AUG 3 TO GIVE YOU TIME TO COME HOME
CALL COLLECT LOVE PENNY

He felt the shock. The blood drained out. He sat down.

Celestina stared at him.

"My mother's dead."

"Oh God!" she said, crossing herself.

Orville saw his shock mirrored in her eyes. "Yeah. God."

Celestina knelt down to him, cradling his head between her palms. "I am with you, dearest. I am with you."

"Yeah . . . yeah, thanks. . . ." With a sinking feeling Orville realized that the telegram must have arrived at the sports center in Holland late on August the first, almost two weeks ago. "Shit. What the hell do I do now?"

"Breathe," she said. "I love you and I am here. Find the breath."

2

"Columbia! Next stop Columbia!"

It was late the next afternoon. With an iron inevitability, the Hudson Highlander, northbound out of Grand Central Station, was veering from a trestle out over the Hudson River back onto land. Orville glanced out the right-hand window. At the top of a hill he saw Olana, the Persian-turreted mansion built by the nineteenth-century landscape painter Frederick Church. Its limestone face was a creamy gold against the lowering sun, and he felt the bite of nostalgia. Grabbing his backpack from the overhead rack, he walked to the space between the cars. He would be home in a couple of minutes.

No he would not. The train screeched, slowed, re-screeched with a lot more oomph, shuddered, and fought itself to a stop.

Orville and the other passengers waited. No information was forthcoming. The air conditioning clicked off. Figures, Orville thought, I come 4,000 miles from Orta to Milan to Zurich to Kennedy to Grand Central and then up the Hudson 128 miles—a whole day's journey—and as soon as we poke up into the southern tip of this shit hole of a town, things break.

Columbia, he knew all too well, was a town of breakage. At public events things would unerringly break. School microphones would consistently give out just after someone said, "Testing, testing." On Memorial Days in Columbian cemeteries, just as the Gettysburg began, viewing stands would collapse. In deep summer at public tennis courts, water fountains were always going dry so that if, after a hot game of tennis on the asphalt courts, when your feet felt like grill-side-down burgers and your tongue like a bun, you went to the water fountain and turned the handle, the one thing you could be sure would not come out was water. Columbians learned to talk affectionately about past breakages, such as "the Great Breakage of '37," when, in the Thanksgiving Day parade a massive five-axle Universal Atlas cement truck disguised as a turkey exploded in front of the Niagara Mohawk power station, knocking out lights and heat for weeks. Or "the Dinosaur Breakage of '52," when the Paul Jonas life-sized sculpture of the brontosaurus bound for the New York World's Fair broke the back of its barge and sank, its neck poking up out of the Hudson River in the most lifelike way.

After another fifteen minutes Orville had had enough of the sweltering Amtrak car. Figuring it was only a mile or so to town, he decided to walk. He opened the door and jumped down from the car. The wet heat smacked him in the face like a big sweaty hand. Shouldering his backpack, he walked along the cinders to the front of the train. There were two tracks.

"Hey pal, you can't do that," said the engineer. "It's illegal."

"So sue me. *Ciao.*" He walked away a few steps before being jolted by a tremendous blast—the engineer had blown his horn. Orville picked up an empty can of Budweiser and threw it. It hit the engine with a pitiful *plink,* and he walked on.

Feeling good out in the unconditioned world, his Nikes striking the cross ties with soft, firm thunks, Orville stretched his arms out to the dome of sky and let his eyes skate the innermost layer from the light blue at its apex, west along its thickening blue to where it met the light-purple cutouts that, so high that at first he thought them clouds, as his eyes followed their smooth undulations north toward Albany and south toward Rhinebeck, he realized were the peaks of the Catskills. Taking a deep breath, he let his eyes ease down the slopes of the mountains through the green, shadowed foothills to the inlet at Catskill Creek with its oil tanks and red neon sign for Mikes Pizza and to the river itself, at eye level all silvery, tidal even a hundred miles north of its mouth, running hard in its straight glacial trough to the sea.

He passed under the mile-long Rip Van Winkle Bridge, its belly arched and ribbed like the roof of a yawning cat's mouth. Orville had worked summers as a toll collector up there, the graveyard shift from midnight to eight so that he could play golf during the day and read all night long. Looking down into cars in those dark hours, he learned a lot about life, like what goes on in cars and how short the night really is.

He heard a whistle, a train coming toward him, southbound from Columbia. He moved off the inside track to the track next to the river and watched it approach. The engineer was waving at him in what at first seemed a greeting, but as the train screamed past he realized it was a warning. He jerked around. The northbound train he'd just left was bearing down on him, its own whistle masked by the other's. Orville jumped feet first into the river. The train thundered past, shrieking like a lunatic.

Orville found his footing in the rocky shallows, feeling the beats of hot air on his face. The train whistles echoed back off the mountains. He looked down, seeing in an oily slick around his knees the inevitable river plastic: a Valvoline bottle and a Tampax applicator. His elbow was skinned and bleeding. He was sore but okay. As he hauled himself up onto the tracks, he caught the acrid scent of creosote.

Creosote. The harsh scent stunned him. All at once he saw himself as a six-year-old, one summer's day, lying on his back in a neglected grassy field down the street from his house on Ten Broek Lane. The scent of creosote was strong from the railroad tracks running nearby. Alone, he stared up at the clouds passing across the sky and suddenly had the sense that the world as he was seeing it was only a part of something else. For the first time in his life he saw himself as part of some whole, some whole world to which his own being was seamlessly connected. He felt lighter, more alive, as if something else had clicked on—or in. He leapt to his feet, making his fat legs go as fast as they could, and ran home to tell his mother. He burst into the kitchen and blurted out his discovery as the screen door slammed—bam!—behind him.

Selma Ariel Fleischer Rose, a large, aproned shape looming over the stove, didn't respond.

He persisted, dragging a chair over, climbing up, and telling her again, slowly and loudly, as if trying to get through to a foreigner.

"Something else! Mom, I'm part of something else!"

Selma, startled to find her little boy at eye level, stared at him. He saw a cloud pass across her gaze. She sighed. "Orville-doll, there's nothing else but this. Go get dressed for the Catskill Game Farm."

The boy felt a rough, twisting pain in his chest. He clenched down on it, trying to make it go away. He fought back tears.

"What's wrong, honey-bunny?"

Dread was rising, the pain was going. He felt himself numbing up, like his mouth did when he was at Basch the dentist's. He broke eye contact. Feeling her fearful concern, he said, "Nothing." He turned and ran back out the door.

Now, standing on the tracks, he realized how that moment had been one end of the thread that had unspooled all these years in a life spent running, a life restless with questions. And now she's dead? he asked himself. What the hell does that mean?

Realizing that now there would be a breakage—the train arriving, Penny and Amy meeting it and not finding him on it—he hurried on. As he passed the rotting two-story brick lighthouse and rounded Mount Pecora, the vista north opened up. There across the rust and purple wash of wildflowers and golden cattails that furred the skin of the marsh, starting at Parade Hill—a high cliff over the river—and then riding down and up a ridge eastward to the heights of Cemetery Hill, was his hometown, Columbia.

A shiver swept over him. How beautiful, the muted pallet of the summer marshland and the shifting reflections from the town. How tiny Columbia looked, no more than a few glitters of the lowering sun off the church spires and metal roofs and the green copper dome of the Courthouse and the glass windows of the abandoned factories and the nine-story housing project and, nicely adjacent to the cemetery, Kinderhook Memorial Hospital. So small, so innocent and needy, as if you could cup it in the palm of your hand and hold it there happily, a live thing, say a kitten, it and you safe there for the rest of your life. With a stab of excitement, he walked toward it.

But then the day attacked. Not having been back in Columbia for over two years, Orville had misjudged the distance badly, imagining things to be closer than they actually were, as if he were seeing his past in a passenger-side rearview mirror. He had miles yet to go. The sun, sinking behind the soggy clouds snagged on the peaks of the Catskills, was soon a reddish ulceration. The marsh turned to swamp, and mosquitoes began to work his flesh, even through his shirt. Tumorous red lumps appeared and itched wildly. To smoke them off, Orville lit a cheap, stumpy Italian cigar, a Parodi, which had the virtue of not staying lit, so it lasted forever. He put on Celestina's going-away gift to him, an Italian women's swim team sweatshirt in the red, white, and green of Italy that to him always signified the tomato, cheese, and basil of a pizza. He flipped the hood over his head and drew the string tight, leaving just an opening for his eyes. Soon he was roasting. His pants clung wetly to his thighs, rubbing together as he walked. Sweat oozed down from the hollow of his throat onto his chest and belly and pooled in his crotch. It was now past midnight in Italy. His adrenals were depleted for the day, and waves of fatigue swept over him.

Cursing, panting, hooded, puffing smoke like a steam locomotive, Orville at last rounded a turn and saw the old train station. A rusted crane rose close by the tracks, a forgotten sentry, its hook dangling down. The station was in shambles, paint peeling, brick crumbling. A sign read

OLU B A

Some pestilential Caribbean outpost, perhaps? In the murky dusk, the shapes seemed spectral. Orville looked around, hoping someone had stayed to meet him.

No. No one was there to meet him.

In the waiting room he found a water fountain. Thirsty, he stared at it, at first hopefully, then superstitiously, and then, with each slow, stalking step he took toward it, accusingly. He pulled the handle. Nothing.

He walked out of the station and up the hill to the main street, Washington. How small everything seems, he thought, as if it's a toy town for a child. A banner spanning the mouth of the town featured a spouting grinning whale and the message

WELCOME TO COLUMBIA

A WHALE OF A TOWN

SPOUT

(Society to Preserve Our Unbelievable Town)

As he walked up the dead-straight backbone of the town, he saw, on brand-new signs announcing each cross street, the same grinning, spouting whale. Why whales? He vaguely recalled being taught in school that Columbia had been a whaling port, with whales caught in the Hudson River. But wait a second. Whales live in sea water. The Hudson is fresh water. Whales in a freshwater river?

In the haze of this last leg of his journey up Washington, one sight stopped him.

Just above Third Street, across from the neglected Painted Lady Lounge, was the General Worth Hotel. Once grand, it was now falling down. It was three stories tall, nine windows wide, made of brick. Now all the windows were boarded up or broken, graffiti and bullet holes were prominent, and the classic portico held up by four Doric columns was sagging badly to the right. An old sign read GENERAL WO   HOT   . Orville had a vision of his mother, wearing a dazzling cobalt-blue satin gown, as President of the Hospital Auxiliary at the annual Spring Fling benefit, flanked by her beloved candy stripers as she made her grand entrance down the majestic staircase to the ballroom of the Worth.

In front of the hotel was a three-person picket line, each person carrying a sign that said "Worth Saving." They were circling a yellow plastic pail for donations. One of the picketers was an old, white-haired woman walking with a cane. Another was a boy with dazzlingly bright red hair, straight red hair that whirled like water as he hopped and twirled. The third was a woman about his own age with slightly darker straight red hair. She wore a work shirt and jeans and a purple scarf and she was limping.

16

As a doctor, Orville could not help but read bodies, as farmers read land and weather, or sailors weather and seas. Dimly, through his exhaustion, he took it all in at a glance—the muscular upper torso, the built-up shoe, the asymmetric pelvic tilt—all of which told a story of a chronic deformity, maybe a childhood injury or illness. Despite the heat he shivered. Why, he wondered, as he had wondered more and more lately, *do I have such trouble now with the deformed?*

Through the gauzy dusk the three circled silently.

He walked on. In the town of his childhood, the walk all the way from lower Washington up to Fourth and then a long stretch up Harry Howard past the Fireman's Home had been a great distance. Now, in the toy town of his less expansive vision, it was not far at all. Soon he was on the outskirts, in a development of ranch houses, and at the door of his sister Penny's ranch.

Wet, bruised, and bleeding, smelling like creosote and bitten all over by ferocious insects, several weeks late for his mother's funeral and dressed like a pizza, on August 14, 1983, Dr. Orville Rose arrived home in Columbia.

3

"Mom did *what?*" Orville shouted.

"Calm down," said his sister, Amelia "Penny" Sarah Rose Plotkin.

"Unbelievable! Barbarian! Selma the Visigoth! I'm outta here! I'm catching the next train back to Italy."

"You'll be rich. You're broke, you're drowning in debt—"

"I'd rather be dead." Orville struggled to free himself from the soft sofa. "Good-bye and good luck."

"Very rich," said Milt, Penny's husband. "In a year and thirteen days."

The three of them had settled deeply into the furniture of Penny and Milt's sunken living room, a sanctuary on a southwestern theme done all in "biscuit" and "Navajo White," a beige kiva. Plastic vinyl runners protected the white carpet in the high-traffic zones. Penny, he realized, had become almost as much of a neat freak as their mother. At the end of his marriage to Lily, Orville had lived in such a house in New Jersey, complete with—the phrase had become a derisive mantra for him—"clean guest towels for clean guests."

Orville, Penny, and Milt talked about the sad event of Selma's death, comforting themselves that the end was merciful: a massive heart attack while cleaning the kitchen floor in her house on Courthouse Square. It brought back their father, Sol's, death a decade ago, he too felled by a heart attack, again mercifully, after a massive swing in a tight match on the sixteenth hole of the Catskill Country Club, a tricky par three over a brook and up a tough hill to an undulating green. Brother and sister agreed that in the time since his death, their father had mellowed, and both children now had mostly happy memories of him. Sol, the "Toy Store King," seemed more present in death than he had ever been in life.

"How rich?" Orville now asked, having climbed up out of the arroyo of the living room to the vinyl runner on the ridge leading toward the door.

"Adding all assets," Milt said, "almost a cool mil."

"Okay, I'll stay." They stared at him. "A joke. Where the hell did she get that kind of money?"

"It helps to be the only toy store in town for forty years," Penny said. "Dad sold a lot of toy airplanes."

"And the Jolly Jews made a killing," Milt said, happily. The Jolly Jews had been Sol's investment and poker club. "Y'know how they always say that if you'd of only put ten grand into conservative stocks and waited forty years you'd make a bundle? They did, and they did. And the last coupla years, with Reagan, you'd have to be a chimpanzee to not get rich. It's like a miracle around here, how the New Yorkers have discovered Columbia. They'll snap at anything! Especially the artsy-fartsy crowd, setting up antique stores in the danger zones down below Fourth. They come up here to get away from the gunfire and drugs in New York City; we sell 'em a piece of crappy storefront where they can live upstairs and what do they find? Gunfire and drugs!" Milt laughed so hard he seemed to cramp up. "We get a lot of gays. Pretty soon the three meccas for the gays will be 'Frisco, Fire Island, and Columbia."

Orville stared at his brother-in-law. The tall body had gotten pudgy now, and the pink Ralph Lauren shirt stretched the polo player over significant male breasts. Milt had always played tennis, and the crisp white shorts were now cutting into legs more flabby than Orville recalled. Milt had been discovered by Selma through the synagogue sisterhood Hadassah. Penny, a senior at Columbia High, was in love with Polonia Scomparza, a nice boy but goyim. Milt saved the day. He came from Albany, an hour upriver, and was hell-bent on becoming a certified public accountant like his dad. At first, Milt had always seemed braced for pain, yet chatty. Now, around Penny, he seemed pain free but as silent as Sol had been around Selma.

In the past few years Milt had been less an accountant and more, in his words, "a man in development." He was making money, and money was making him. Bald, with a half-smile resting on his moon-face that widened to a laugh, making his eyes happy slits and his big head roll this way and that in wonderment at life's riches, Milt now seemed happy. Finally, Orville thought, the wolf of failure has been driven from his door. Here before me is a success. Dealing all his life with a sense of his own failure, Orville now looked at Milt with an electric fascination, asking himself, How the fuck has he done it? What the hell has happened to the concept of America as a meritocracy?

The terms of Selma's will had a certain elegance. Half went to Penny. The other half, and the family house and car, went to Orville.

There was a catch.

Orville got the money, the house, and the car only if he lived in the house continuously for one year and thirteen days, starting on the day he arrived home. "Why the extra thirteen days?" he asked Penny and Milt. No one knew. The house was a nineteenth-century Victorian sitting on Courthouse Square in the town center. The car was an elephantine '81 Chrysler New Yorker—"The biggest Chrysler makes," Milt said. "Your trunk space is amazing."

Staring down at his sister and brother-in-law from the vinyl runner, Orville said, "Live *here? Live* here?"

"We do."

"I'd die in a month. It's blackmail. How could she do this to me?"

"I believe, Orville Abraham," Penny said, "she did it out of love."

"Did you know about this?"

"No. It was news to me too."

"And if I leave?"

"You get nothing."

"Who gets my almost-mil?"

Penny looked to Milt. Milt looked to Penny.

"*All* of it? The whole other almost-mil? You get my mil?"

"Nowadays," Milt said, "a mil doesn't go all that far."

"Let me be clear," Penny said. "We'd rather have you here than have your money. Right Milt?"

"Oh, sure," Milt said. "Sure, sure. You're family. Sure."

"And if I go, what happens to the house?"

"It sits there empty for a year and thirteen days," Penny said. "It can't be sold or rented. Then Milt and I get it and we can sell it."

"And the car, too," Milt said. "The New Yorker."

"The house just sits there empty for a year?"

"Hayley keeps cleaning it and Buzzy keeps fixing it."

"No dice. I'll stay out the week, to see you guys and Amy."

"No you won't," Penny said.

"What do you mean I won't?"

"Amy's away at drama camp. Her first overnight camp and it's *killing* me!" Penny took out a hankie, started to cry. "I will not let you see her unless you're staying."

"She's my niece! She's my special—"

"She's my daughter, and I will not subject her to your comings and goings at this time of our grief. You know how close she was to Mom. I mean, she's taking it well—sometimes I think she's the most mature one in the whole family—but when we couldn't even find you, she got that look in her eye and said, 'It's like Orvy's dead, too.' She's doing okay at camp, but it just about killed me between not having Mom anymore and your not answering my telegram and calls and sending her off. . . ." Penny blew her nose, an astounding *hroonnnk!* She looked up at Orville and said, "I figured you'd say no to this. But this time, for once, I'm being smart. I'm cutting my losses."

"Wait. After we spoke last night—you didn't even tell Amy that you'd found me?"

"If you had a child, you would understand."

Orville felt as if he'd been punched in the gut. He rocked back on his heels, seeing in his sister the same genius for hurt their mother had. Penny was staring at him, chin up in self-righteousness. Orville's gaze fixed on her neck, on the prominent wrinkles encircling it; the swan's neck that when she was a young woman had been her pride and joy, to be shown off with a collection of necklaces that outstripped even Selma's; a neck that, always uncovered down past Tuesday, helped deflect attention from her slightly too long, too narrow face, her thin lips, her brown eyes set slightly too close to the nose. Her neck was now partly hidden by a high-ruffled black Victorian blouse. The skin never lies. Her connective tissue was going. He read in this woman of forty-four the skin of a sixty-year-old. She's too thin now, eaten with anxiety, and as nervous as a small bird. His eyes traveled back across her body and medical history to her overcheery girlhood in this overdepressing backwater, where culture was a yearly piano recital at the junior high by someone from out of town who was an unknown about to become a has-been, and where the nearest nice Jewish boy was an hour upriver in Albany.

And so Orville shifted, hearing in her voice, however vicious, the voice of his mostly helpful big sister, and his rage eased and he smiled.

Penny, too, awakened by her anger, suddenly saw her little brother more fully, these two years on. She thought he looked younger, more handsome, healthier, slimmer, with a dynamite tan. She noted that he was no longer wearing glasses.

"Contacts?" she asked, smiling. He nodded. "You look great, Orvy. Mom would've been proud—I mean, of your looks."

"Partly proud. Let us not forget The Incident of the Other Necktie."

Penny laughed. One Chanukah several years ago, Selma had given Orville two neckties. He went upstairs and came back down wearing one. She took a look, sighed, and said, "You didn't like the *other* necktie?"

"Partly proud maybe," Penny said. "So listen, kid, why not stay?"

"What the hell would I do for a year? Watch TV? Play golf?"

"Golf," Milt said sagely, "is good."

This comment led up a narrowing wash to dead silence. Orville noticed that Penny was grinning, and he knew it wasn't because of what Milt had said.

"What?" he asked. "C'mon, c'mon."

"Oh, nothing. I just remembered something. Bill asked after you."

And then Orville got it. Bill Starbuck, the aging town doctor, had been the one who'd led him into medicine.

"Oh, no," Orville said, backing away, his hands warding her off as if she were a ghost or were pointing a gun—or were a ghost with a gun. "You wouldn't, you didn't!"

"You'd be great, Orvy."

"Nice try, kid." He shouldered his backpack. "If you won't let me see Amy, I'm outta here now."

"I won't, but you can't leave now. There's no train 'til morning."

"I'll sleep on a park bench." He opened the door.

"You're welcome to bed down in our home, stranger," said Milt.

"Wait!" Penny said. Orville waited, his back still turned. "Here." She came up, slipped two keys into the palm of his hand. "The keys to the house and the car. I'll run you down."

Orville stared at her, then Milt. "Milt, I've got a question for you."

"Fire away."

"Why whales?"

"Huh?"

"Why all the whales, on the banner and the street signs and all?"

"Oh, because whales are the logo for our revival, for SPOUT."

"Yeah, I know. But why whales?" No response. "Why Columbia and whales?"

"Oh. Well, Columbia was built on whales. They used to catch 'em in the river."

"But whales live in the sea. *Sea* water. The Hudson's a river. *Fresh* water?"

"Oh. . . . Dunno. But I'll tell you one thing I do know, as a developer. They work. Those whales work. Those whales are putting us on the damn map."

◊ ◊ ◊

Sometime after midnight Orville found himself wandering around the cleaned-out, cleaned-up, urethaned old house of his childhood. It had grown small, an *Alice in Wonderland* house of tiny rooms, stairs, windows, and toilets. On the kitchen table he found a letter, addressed to him in his mother's hand and postmarked "Columbia, August 13."

It had been mailed yesterday, two weeks after her death.

To calm himself, he sought out his sanctuary, the flat tin roof. There, amid his friends the trees—the larch, the maple, the copper beech—under what as a child he'd secretly held to be sure signs of that something else, the stars, he clicked on a flashlight and opened the envelope. He set aside a thick old document and opened her letter. Handwritten, it was undated.

Dear son,

2 A.M. We old people don't sleep well. Strange to get a letter from a dead person, but such is life. You've been out gallivanting around Europe, but even though the apron strings are cut, I'm holding on for your good. The terms of my will will have upset you, but such is life. I did it so you'd come back to your roots, find someone, grow up and settle down. It's a two-by-two world—*unfortunately.* Penny grew up and settled down nicely, but oh no not you, not Mr. Bigshot Ornery oh no. Bet you're still not socialized, still don't know how to have fun. You can say no and go away again but you lose a lot of equity if you do. I'm offering you a way to live you never would otherwise. When your father dragged me here from the city in '46 I was appalled. The only two things Columbia values are money and mediocrity. But here you are *known.* You're just like me: shy and superstitious, but always leaning *into* life.

He stopped reading, astonished. She imagined that he was like her?

So here's your big chance, honey-bunny *Luftmensch!* And you can be with that other high-flier, sister Amelia, and that cute Amy. Over the course of the year and 13 days you'll be hearing from me from time to time by a secret method.

Love your mother

P.S. The enclosed document is your birth certificate, your real one. You were not born on July 24, 1944, but on August 6. The night of August 5 I had a bad dream about a big black dog and a Nazi. I got your dad to bribe the Air Force Registrar at Fort Bragg in North Carolina (the home of Wilbur and Orville's first flight!) and we had your birth certificate changed by a flyboy who was a forger named Arizona Lanquardo. And a year later on your real birthday wouldn't you know it but they dropped the Atom Bomb? You won't forgive me but your father and I and the Registrar and Arizona are the only ones who know and now we're all dead. That's why Sol and I might have acted just that little bit strange both on July 24 and on August 6 both. Is Leo better than Cancer? Do you believe in horoscopes and the astrology craze? Is it our stars or ourselves? The good news is that you're younger than you think—13 days younger in fact. Until I write again I remain, doll, with love, *Me!*

Orville stared at the treetops, at the stars, mouth open in disbelief. Suddenly he had a palpable sense that she was there, behind him, hovering like a hummingbird in the dark thick air just off the roof. He turned quickly, as in that child's game of red light where you try to creep up behind someone and tag them. For the briefest instant he could have sworn he caught a glimpse of her, flapping her arms in that cobalt-blue satin ball gown, flying away over the green copper dome of the courthouse toward St. Mary's, a vision straight out of Chagall, or Marquez.

Terrific, he thought, you're seeing your dead mother flying around the treetops. And she's planning to write again? Who's got the letters and who's mailing them? Penny?

Rising, seeing again as if it was only yesterday—and it was only yesterday!—the red rowboat and the walk around the island with his beloved Celestina, he faced the dome of the courthouse and said, "No way, Mom. I'm gone."

4

W. STARBUCK, M.D.
Office Hours
9–10, 1–3, ~~7–8~~ P.M.
Wed., 9–10

Orville stared at the sign in the window of Bill Starbuck's office in the small brick house at Fifth and Washington. It was the same sign that had been there ever since Orville could recall reading it, except that the 7–8 night slot had been crossed out. Bill had cut back.

It was the next afternoon. Penny was still dead set against him seeing Amy. Upping the ante, Orville had told her he'd made a reservation to fly to Italy the day after tomorrow. Maybe, he thought, knowing how important he and Amy were to each other, Penny would soften and change her mind.

Every time he came back to Columbia, Orville visited Bill. Now he opened the door, turned right into the waiting room, and was met with the familiar scent of sweat, tobacco, cheap perfume, ether, and pain. The small room was packed, the furniture insufficient, so that those who could stood against the walls. Children wailed, a demented man chattered about the FBI, old people creaked and sighed and groaned, and a slender man in a stunning Canali suit who, Orville figured, could only have been a New Yorker, stood reading *The New Yorker*.

Bill had never had a receptionist or nurse. You arrived, sat, stared at the stained-glass door marked IN, and, despite your worry and pain, tried to focus on keeping track of your turn. Orville stood near the door, trying to avoid making diagnoses on the others, staring at the YES SMOKING sign.

The IN door opened. There was Bill, ready for the next patient. Orville's image of him, as always, was of a benevolent Humpty Dumpty.

"Orvy?" Bill broke into a shy smile. "Well, well, well."

"Hi, Bill. I can wait my turn."

"Folks, you all remember *Doctor* Orville Rose? I'm sure you wouldn't mind if he came in for a few minutes?"

In the instant of that first glance, both doctors did the dance of diagnosis on each other, scanning the body for new decay or disease.

24

Orville was startled to find signs of Bill being a lot further down the road than two years before. A short, oval-shaped man whose crisp white shirt and clasped tie billowed over his plump tummy, his rumpled dark slacks slumped over his only fashion statement, pointy Italian shoes. On his bald head and round face, which sat on his collared neck like an egg in a cup, were dark senile keratoses and other plants in the skin-garden of aging. A recently burned-off basal cell carcinoma glowed on his sharp nose. The lenses of his glasses had thickened several diopters—question, cataracts?—magnifying his eyes so that they seemed to be peering up out of deep water, big and roaming, the eyes, Orville was surprised to think, of what else but a whale. Bill's girlish lips were now tinged with blue, a trace of cyanosis, a sign of the lessened ejection fraction of Bill's heart. The only exercise this body had known was poker. And once, Orville recalled, at Penny's wedding at the Elks Club, this body had swirled his wife, Babette, around the floor with surprising lightness, gliding, smiling, an Arthur Murray athlete. The two hearing aids were new. Orville felt in Bill's handshake the old firmness and yet a new fragility, the bones afloat in the puffy skin.

Ushering Orville in, Bill's hand was on his shoulder. As always. Bill was a toucher, a great toucher. You might forget what he told you was wrong with you or what he was going to do about it, but you remembered that touch. Hours later the place he'd touched still felt special. Warm in winter, cool in summer.

"Good t'see you, son," Bill said, settling in behind the big cluttered desk and another YES SMOKING sign. His words came out in a calm, deliberate way, with significant torsion of his lips, as if each word was being molded as delicately as an egg and required care to survive. His greeting blew the scent of fresh scallions at Orville. Bill's other addiction, besides nicotine, was fresh scallions. When in season, his rural patients kept him supplied. Bill "the Scallion" Starbuck. Bill shook a Camel free and lit up, blowing out two dragons of smoke in that relieved way that always reminded Orville of Bill delivering Amy by an emergency C-section.

Ten years ago, the summer that Sol died, Selma was holed up in her bedroom, weeping and growling, over and over, "How could he do this to me?" Penny, too, was in rough shape. Orville, an internist in New Jersey, heard that Penny was in labor and came back. To Orville, the labor seemed to be going along easily, more quickly than you'd expect for a nulliparous woman.

But all of a sudden Bill said to Orville, "Somethin's wrong. I'm goin' in." Milt, terrified, lost his spine and went catatonic, unable to talk or move.

25

When Amy was delivered, Milt was in the men's room vomiting. Bill, clad all in surgical green, handed the baby to Orville. "Gotta go back in," Bill said. "Total hysterectomy."

That moment, that first real moment in Amy's life, was with Orville. In his arms, she *looked* at him. Her face all wrinkled and red like a little old lady in no apparent distress, the baby kept right on looking into his eyes. Quietly, merely, looked. And he looked back. His heart twisted on its spindle like a ripe fruit on a tree of ribs, and he fell in love. He would never forget the feel of that eye contact. It was the beginning of their special bond. "I was imprinted on you, Uncle O.," Amy would say, as she grew up with the story, "like a duckling on a duck."

She was the only family member he loved absolutely. After Bill had finished the hysterectomy, he came out bloodied as a butcher and motioned Orville to walk him out into the hospital parking lot. There, Bill snapped out a Camel and lit up, blowing those two spirals of dragon fire out through his nostrils, relieved.

"Paper-thin," Bill had said, holding up two fingers close together. "The wall of that uterus was paper-thin. Never saw a thinner, more porous uterus. On the edge of rupturin'. Don't know how that baby ever made it to term in that paper bag of a womb. Reckon it's a miracle."

"How'd you know to go in?

"Didn't. I got lucky. That's the damn thing about doctorin'—you're always making 100 percent of the decision on 50 percent of the data."

From then on Orville and Bill called Amy "the Miracle." Every time Bill lit up and sighed with relief reminded Orville of it, and her.

Now, sitting in the patient's chair, Orville looked around the oak-paneled room, once the living room of the small house. From the time he was in high school, Orville had hung around with Bill, spending a lot of time in this office with him, learning what a small-town doctor did. Now it seemed so familiar, so well-worn, so much his real—the word came to him untarnished—home.

Over the fireplace was the fourteen-point buck, tilted a little, and on the wall was the photo of the man in the cowboy hat and scowl, his handlebar moustache drooping down, his arms crossed over his chest, and a revolver clasped in one hand, pointing up past his ear. *Josiah Macy, Columbian Doctor, 1834–1861.*

"Died in a gunfight," Bill always said with a measure of pride, "shot by a husband catchin' him in bed with his wife on a house call, heh heh."

In the corner was the massive old safe like you see in the saloon in a Western, and behind the curtain of the examining room Orville glimpsed the metal stirrups of the examining table. All of this—the fourteen-point buck, the lascivious gunslinger, the saloon safe, the stirrups—made it seem that you were getting doctored in a frontier town of the Wild West. Behind Bill, reaching to the high, stamped-tin ceiling, was the glassed-in medicine cabinet that seemed to hold everything, from musty old text-books to bottles of medicine to boxes with red crosses now gone pink from the sunlight to chrome instruments that may have been put down five minutes ago, or five years.

"Sorry about your mother, Orvy," Bill was saying, shaping his words slowly. "Massive MI. Went quick. I know you didn't have the . . . the perfect relationship with her, and that can make it all harder now. I'm sorry. Real sorry, son."

Sensing Bill's caring, Orville felt sadness rise in his throat, gritty, tin-gling his lip, his nostrils, presaging real tears. As he fought them down, he sensed how his whole life had been caringly held by this kind, maybe wise old man. He remembered himself as a sick child, body burning with fe-ver, thrashing around unable to breathe, and hallucinating in the middle of the interminable night in his parents' bed wondering if the terror of breathlessness would ever end, and dimly sensing the arrival of Dr. Bill in a cloud of scallions and tobacco and feeling the cooling stethoscope like a friendly flat hand on a riled burning chest and then turned face-down, butt-up, holding someone's—Sol's?—hand for the shot, the strange bite of the needle not hurting as much as you feared but just when you thought it was over the searing rush that seemed to last and last, like your butt was a hot skillet, and you tried to fight away the hand doing it to you and then it was over and the pain was being massaged to a dull ache by Bill and it was soporific and you eased down into the featherdown of sleep. And as a teenager embarked on a course of rank failure—his grades mediocre, too short and chubby and slow to make sports teams and too pimply and shy to get a girl—when he refused to talk with Selma or Sol or Penny about anything close to his heart, he was sent to Bill for advice.

Bill never gave any advice. He sat and smoked and told stories of the fourteen-point buck and the gunslinging doctor and the stirrups and what was in the safe. The summer after a desolate sophomore year when Orville was bored half out of his mind and depressed out of the other half, Bill began to take him around with him, let him help out in the office, go on house calls out in the county, learn about medicine. What a time that had been. Deliveries, deaths, and everything in between. The shy boy opened up to the kindly man.

Orville had been enthralled by the realness of doctoring, the intense contact with people at the crucial times of their lives that often helped them heal. Coming out of a family where nothing much ever seemed to take place between the sighing and the silence, it was incredible for the boy to see that things actually happened in life, actually got done.

Now, staring across the desk at the old doctor, Orville realized that for Bill, too, given his suffering with his handicapped only child who had died young, their friendship had been not only an opening, but a rejuvenation. Bill got in the habit of calling Orville when there was a particularly interesting house call or emergency. Some of it was rough for a boy—the accidents, the sights on the pathology slab of severed legs or hands or breasts or eviscerated viscera. The morgue itself was off-limits.

Have I ever felt more at peace, Orville wondered, than in the dawn light alongside Bill in his black Caddy on the drive home from delivering twins somewhere out in a godforsaken shack in the middle of nowhere? This man had grown him up. After that first summer with Bill, Orville began his junior year at Columbia High wanting to understand biology and science and math—and people. Even though he didn't make the basketball team, he managed the team—kind of doctored the team, really. And with the status (even if second-rate) of being the manager of the Fish Hawk hoopsters, he got the girls. But his grades only got him into his safety school, Syracuse, where, away from Bill, he plunged into pot and lethargy and watched the '60s protests from the sidelines. He managed to graduate but was rejected by every American medical school. It was Bill, through an old doctor friend in Ireland, who got him admitted to medical school at the working-class, Catholic, University College Dublin. There he bloomed. He did well in down-to-earth medicine and met and fell in love with Lily Wolf, an English major from NYU on an exchange program at the snooty, Anglican, Trinity College. They married, he interned back in New Jersey, set up a general practice, tripped over the hamster egg and watched the marriage detonate, and ran like hell around the world.

All in an instant.

From behind his desk Bill was smiling at him serenely, on a nicotine high.

"I'm leaving the day after tomorrow," Orville said. "Going back to Italy."

"Italy? Jeez!"

Orville told him about Celestina Polo. Bill smiled in delight. "I know there's this rumor going around, about my staying, joining up with you in your practice, and I'd love to, Bill, but it isn't true."

"You'd be crazy to stay here. I always told Babette the same thing—'I'm leavin' the day after tomorrow.' Now I'm finishin' up fifty-four years. Heh heh. Came here in '29. Bad year. Babette wants me to retire down to Boca Raton, but what the hell's a fella like me gonna do in Boca Raton? Golf? Surf? Shop? Son, get out while y'can." He stubbed out his butt. "Stuff that walks in here? Today I saw a girl—one of the Rope Alley half-wits? She's been tryin' to get pregnant, and last week on ultrasound we see somethin' in her uterus. So today she comes in and says to me, 'I told Spike I had somethin' in my uterus and he goes, Great, must be my Yankees cap. Been lookin' for that sucker for weeks!'" They laughed together.

Bill opened a drawer, took out a scallion, and bit into it. "Y'look good, Orvy. Contacts, eh? Thin, too. Been runnin'?" Orville nodded. "Toldja that right knee'd heal without surgery. Bodies almost always'll heal, if you get out of the way and give 'em time."

"Tincture of time. You taught me that. I've saved a lot of lives doing as much nothing as possible."

"Seen Amy yet?"

"Penny won't let me. Not unless I take this deal of my mom's."

"Yeah, I heard about her will—everybody in town did, I reckon. You'd be crazy, even with the cash. But you should see Amy. Our little miracle's become quite the thespian. Got the lead in a Shakespearean play at camp 'n' all. Too bad Penny won't let you see her before you leave." As if with reluctance, and difficulty, Bill rose. His hand on Orville's shoulder, he ushered him to the stained-glass door marked OUT.

"Sorry about that rumor, Bill—"

"Yeah, well, lotta rumors. Only person who really knows what's goin' on around here is me. People tell the truth in here. Fella like me gets to lift up the lid, peek in under the edge, see past the bullshit and—" Bill coughed hard and had trouble catching his breath. Orville recognized the wheeze and gurgle of congestive heart failure.

"Got my nitros right here." He took out a pillbox, fumbled, and spilled all the pills onto the floor. Bill stared down at them as if they were lost in the deep. He tried to bend down but couldn't.

Orville squatted and searched them out, one by one, on the worn linoleum. He was hit hard by the sight of those pointy-toed Italian shoes now tattered and scuffed and, where one trouser cuff had ridden up, the alarming way one puffy ankle was ballooning way out over the elastic top of a black sock. Heart failure big-time. Corralling the nitros, Orville wondered what would have happened if he hadn't been there. He handed Bill the pills and asked if he had a doctor of his own. Bill smiled sheepishly.

"A doctor who treats himself," Orville said, "has a fool for a patient."

"Gotta be a fool . . . ," he wheezed, "t'stay here . . . long's I did. I'm leavin' . . . th'day after tomor—" He was too breathless to go on. His hand on Orville's shoulder went from being supportive to needing support. The nails dug in.

"Open your mouth," Orville said. Bill did. Whoa those scallions! "Tongue up, scallion breath!" He popped a nitro under Bill's tongue. They waited.

Bill began breathing easier, and then smiled. "Good luck t'you, son. Say hi to Italy for me—never been, myself."

His hand on Orville's shoulder lightened and the OUT door was opening and there was that ushering out and then the door shut with a well-worn *click,* and Orville found himself in the dark hallway, unsure whether to go back or leave.

He waited, half-fearing he'd hear the body drop. But then he heard the IN door click open for the next patient. How can I leave him turning in this circle, old and sick and alone?

Out on the street, smacked by the remorseless dead weight of the wet summer heat, he realized that he might just have seen this old man for the last time.

5

Later that afternoon Penny and Orville sat together on a bench in the Courthouse Square, facing Selma's old turreted Victorian. In front of the large Greek revival courthouse, a Columbian in dark green work clothes and a baseball cap graced with a grinning spouting whale, was diddling an American flag to come down.

Orville was sipping George Dickel on ice. The bourbon and the jetlag made him woozy. He had tried to call Celestina Polo, to tell her what the situation was at home and that his flight would arrive in Milan the morning after the day after tomorrow. Getting no answer at her apartment in Rome, he remembered that she had said, on parting, that she would be on retreat in some Ayurvedic Buddhist center in Biella, west of Lake Orta.

She had written the name and number down, but he had lost it. Try as he might, he couldn't recall it. He missed her desperately. At the airport he'd told her that he had quit his job in Holland and was going to move to Rome to work as a doctor and make a future there with her. She cried and hugged him insanely hard. They'd stayed that close, heart to heart, until he boarded the plane. He could feel her with him even now.

He stared at the Columbian yanking at the flag, which was now stuck halfway down the pole. Orville sent out a thought toward the man: *Yank it harder!* The man yanked it harder. *Harder!* The man yanked it harder. The rope broke. The flag fluttered down. The man ran to catch it, but it caught him instead, shrouding him. He thrashed and then surfaced, crying out "Shit!"—which echoed off the granite facade of the courthouse and off Selma's house and then the post office—"Shit! . . . Shit shit . . ." and scurried after itself down Fourth across Washington to hit the limestone face of the Library, "shit."

"What would be so bad about staying and helping Bill?" Penny asked.

"It would be lethal."

"But Columbia's changed, Orvy. The New Yorkers are coming. We've got cultural events up the wazoo. Street fairs, even. It'd be over before you knew it."

"Pen, look." He showed her the watch Celestina had given him, with the NOWs instead of the numbers. "My whole life in this town—in this country, even—was spent looking ahead, looking for what's next. I don't want anything to be over before I know it—ever again. 'Cause that's what's lethal. For two years I've been free. The last three months, for the first time since the disaster with Lily, I've been in love, and I'm damn well not going to screw that—"

"Love? With who?"

"An Italian woman, Celestina Polo."

"Nice name. Tell me all about it."

He told her a lot about it, the romance, their plans, Celestina's work.

"Don't you just *love* all this New Age stuff?" she said. "We've got shiatsu out in the mall on Route 9 now, can you imagine?" His heart sank. "I can't wait to meet her. If you stay, she can come." Orville rolled his eyes. "Okay, then we'll go over there. Milt and I did Tuscany three years go. It's so gorgeous you could die. And the pasta!"

"What do you know about Mom's letter?"

"What letter, hon'?" He told her. "What? She wrote you a letter, and someone mailed it now?"

"Penny, it's very important that you don't hold this back from me—for the sake of you and me in the future. Is it you? Did she give you this letter to mail?"

"I swear to God, *Baruch atooh* and all that, that I know nothing about this, that it wasn't me, that the first I heard about it was right now. I promise."

"On Amy's soul?"

"On Amy's soul."

Orville knew that Penny, like Selma and even him, was superstitious, especially around Judaism, things like souls. Selma was always touching wood or throwing salt over her shoulder or, if she had to go back into the house after forgetting something, sitting and counting to ten before she left again. At times it seemed almost Kabbala. So he knew that Penny was telling the truth. She knew nothing about the letter.

"Thanks."

"Welcome, but I can't believe this! She wrote you a letter?"

"A number of letters. She said I'd be hearing from her from time to time during the year and thirteen days."

"So she wrote a bunch and somebody's got them and will be mailing them?"

"Anonymously. The first one had a Columbia postmark. Any idea who?"

"Could be a friend, maybe Minky Schenckberg. I can ask."

"No. Swear to me that you won't. I can't stand anyone else knowing." Orville was adamant. "Swear?"

"I swear." Penny thought for a moment. "What did she say?"

"Nothing much. Kind of chatty. Critical. The usual."

"Critical of me, too?"

"No. Even after her death, dear sister, you are a saint. Critical only of me."

"Yeah, well, I had a different relationship with her," Penny said. "Maybe because I didn't resist her as much—at least not face-to-face—and I never really left her, never went as far away. All the way to Syracuse? And then Dublin? I only went to Albany with Milt—until she convinced him to come back here."

"You know, when I'd come home from Syracuse to visit, she'd keep a record in her diary, by the phone in the kitchen—'Time Orvy Arrived, Time Orvy Departed'—and at the end of the visit she'd announce the total hours and minutes I'd been home. And when I was there, if I got up from her burned brisket to go out with my friends, she acted like I'd plunged a knife into her heart. She'd wait up until I came home. The drives back to Syracuse were murder. I felt like the worst son on earth. The guilt. Once, when I'd left her weeping her heart out, I couldn't stand it. I got as far as Catskill before I turned around. But when I walked back in she was on the phone with Minky, laughing, telling her what a great visit she'd had with me. She stared at me, puzzled, and asked why I'd come back."

Penny nodded. "I know. I always saw the difference between the 'Public Selma'—pillar of the community, proud mother of two great kids—and the 'Private Selma'—all *tsuris* and blame. But she was never as vicious to me. We reached an accord."

"Lucky you. When she put me on the train to go to Dublin for medicine, her last words to me were, '*I* want that degree!'" Penny laughed.

He then told her about the last time he'd seen Selma, two years ago as he was leaving for Europe for good. They'd sat in the living room—now empty of Sol's toy king laugh and signature tag at the end of his rare statements, "and so forth." That afternoon, Orville had opened up to Selma, telling her that his marriage to Lily was over.

"Lily never really loved you, honey-bunny," Selma had said. "I always knew that."

Orville's head had imploded. Sand rushed in. His belly went all watery. That was Selma: if you opened yourself up a crack, she would disembowel you. Guts on his shoe tops, he shut up. The grandfather clock ticked . . . tocked.

"Total selfishness," she had announced. "The thing about you, Orville, is your total selfishness."

"Thanks for sharing, Mom," he had said, getting up to go.

"Why didn't you invite me to New Jersey for your thirtieth birthday? You had a big celebration, I hear, and you didn't invite *me?* Your mother?"

"I didn't want a party," he said, asking himself, Is there no statute of limitations on imagined slights? "But Lily went ahead anyway."

"But it was your birthday. A milestone. Thirty is a definite milestone."

"It was *my* birthday, Mom!"

"Maybe," she said indignantly, "but *I* did it."

He got up to go.

She sighed, the sound of some large object collapsing into something deep. "Any words of wisdom for me?"

All he could think of was Sol's favorite expression, which was, in fact, a kind of wisdom. "It never rains on a golf course?"

At that Selma wept, out of her one good eye. When Selma was in her forties, she'd been diagnosed with a benign brain tumor, an acoustic neuroma. In taking it out, the neurosurgeon had cut a facial nerve. One side of her face went dead, disfiguring her. "It kills me," she'd said, that last day with him, "to cry out of only one eye."

Gutted, Orville wanted desperately to go to her, put his arm around her, hug her as any good son—any normal son—might to comfort his mother in her pain. He could not. Everything in him tried to get his feet to move toward her, but stiff-faced, he moved away. He left.

"I failed her," he said now to Penny. "I was never enough for her."

"Tell me about it. Back here, seeing her every day took its toll. I drove to Albany twice a week for years for therapy. The way Mom was, it's amazing we're not both on Stelazine."

"*You're* not on Stelazine?"

"You *are?*"

"Just joking."

"Oh you sto-op!" She punched his arm playfully. Then she, too, sighed, scarily like Selma. "Leaving's so easy, and staying's so hard."

"I've done enough hard things for one lifetime—"

"Tell it to Amy."

"Let me see her and I will. You're acting just like Mom."

"Don't start, don't you dare! This isn't about her anymore. It's about me and you and your family. Our family. Our very little family here in our godforsaken shitty little—as you put it—lethal town."

"I thought you said it had changed."

"Well, it's still *kind* of lethal, but c'mon, kid. Stop angst-ing around. Try it."

"Dream on."

"I don't, that well," Penny said sadly. "You were always our dreamer."

"If I stay, she wins."

"You've got it ass-backwards."

"If I stay, she loses?"

"If you run, she wins. You confirm her idea that you're a bad son, so she wins. And so do Milt and I, financially."

He stared at her. "You'd rather have the money, wouldn't you?"

"Milt would. I would not, no."

"Yeah, I believe that." He got up to go. "Celestina has your phone number. If she calls, please don't tell her anything about any of this. Just get her number and tell her to call me at Selma's."

"Okay."

34

"Thanks." He walked across the street and into the house.

Between the jetlag and the bourbon he was asleep on the couch by seven that evening. Sometime around two in the morning, he sat bolt upright, sure that someone was there. Not seeing anyone, he tiptoed through each bare, clean room. Nothing.

He found himself in the seven-sided turret overlooking the square, his childhood bedroom. The room was empty, the floor freshly urethaned. Looking around, Orville was overwhelmed by a sense of barrenness, a sense of all that had happened in this room that had been lonely and sad and crazy. He backed up against a wall as if for protection, but felt dizzy, as though he were balancing on tilting planes of a recurrent childhood nightmare. He closed his eyes and slid down the wall to the floor, grabbing his knees and pulling them up to his chest. He thought of all the hours, all the years he'd spent alone in this room in this town.

What a waste. What a damn waste.

A desperate sadness filled his chest and rose in his throat. His heart beat fast and his mind went shallow, like a lake at night or a field in winter. The shallowness ran to the horizon. Blinking, he looked again around the empty room, recalled the lonely effort to understand without being understood. He felt the losses, the loss of the possibility of being brave and daring rather than shy, of being a believer instead of a cynic, of being loving rather than being—at those key moments of closest approach to anyone—awash in dread.

"Barren," he whispered, and in the empty urethaned heptagon a faint echo overlapped his whispering "barren" again.

"Who's barren, honey-bunny?"

He jumped, looked around. She was hovering outside at the level of the second story turret window, one hand resting on the golden ball on top of the flagpole. Once again wearing the cobalt-blue gown with hair and makeup in the style of the early '50s: black eyebrow pencil, blue mascara, red rouge, and lipstick the scarlet of those pesky little bleeders you get in scalp lacerations. And her face was beautiful! Unmutilated. It was Selma before the operation. She hovered, an expectant look on her face, waiting for an answer.

He blinked, shook himself, looked away, then looked back. Still there. He walked closer to the window. She let go of her hold on the flagpole and floated up and down slightly, as if on ripples of the breeze. Had he gone crazy? He knew from his doctoring that the bereaved often have visions of the dead in the weeks and months following the death—not only visions but conversations, as if they were really present. "Presences," they sometimes called them. Should I talk to her? Why not? Maybe, dead, she'll be nicer?

"*This* is barren," he said, gesturing around the room, and in as conversational a tone as he could muster. "All of this. My life here."

"Now wait a sec, Mr. Big Shot. *We* weren't barren. Sol and I raised two kids, one very successful, and you, well, moderately successful. One grandchild. We waited for a grandchild from you, but oh no, not you, you just wouldn't give us one. Not even *one!* The barren one is *you*."

"Go away," he said.

"I am away."

"Leave me alone."

"That's not how it works."

"How does it work?"

"You leave *me* alone! I gave my life to you and your sister and now you run away again? Just like your whole life. Run away from love. Run, run, run. Runaway. And then you sit here in your old room mooning around about yourself? Total selfishness. I mean, did I sweeten the pie or what? Sol's hard-earned dollars, the very lovely home, the customized New Yorker with only 34,000 and some miles on it? *Oy gevalt!*"

"What do you mean I have to leave you alone?"

"Dare you to stay, honey-bunny. *Ciao!*"

Doing a barrel roll like one of Sol's radio-controlled fighters, Selma flew stomach down in a nosedive toward the square, pulling out at the last second and then rising, rising, that hefty nose cutting the air like a rocket, banking around the green copper dome of the courthouse and away. Gone.

Orville ran downstairs and out into the town.

It was a hot, hazy summer night. The particular NOW on his watch was where the three might have been. He walked along Washington Street, the spine of the town, the spine of a humpbacked whale whose ribs were the eight ruler-straight cross-streets numbered First through Eighth, each curling down into the South Swamp through which he'd walked into town, and down into the North Swamp stretching toward Albany. Why the meticulous grid? Bizarre, in this town where breakage rules.

He found himself facing the General Worth Hotel. In the dead quiet on the deserted street, he stared at the condemned hotel's sagging front portico, the whole right side flaccid—like his mother's half-paralyzed face. It was almost as if it, too, were talking to him, talking awkwardly, slurring its words the way she, with the half-dead lip and tongue, often slurred hers:

36

"Save me! I'm half-dead. They wanna blow me up and finish me off. You're a doctor, save me! I'm 'Worth Saving,' aren't I?"

Orville blinked in astonishment. Now a building is talking to me? He listened more closely. Nothing.

He ran home. Drank some more bourbon, lit a Parodi, and turned on the TV.

Nuns were dancing, interrupted by The Man With the Vegematic.

The phone rang. His heart raced.

"Hello?"

"*Caro?*"

"Thank God!"

"I was so worried when you didn't call."

"I lost the number, forgot the name of the place."

"Tell me *tutto*—everything!"

"I love you!" Orville said, choking up.

"And I love you, too!"

"I love you so!"

"And I you. I was so afraid, not hearing anything, maybe you fell out of our love."

"Never! I've got my flight back."

"And now I am glowing all over my body with your words, your spirit. In my very toes, *mio dito del piedes!* When do you arrive and where?" He told her. "*Bene.* I will meet you in Milano. Now, tell me *tutto, pronto.*"

He told her about Selma's will, although, taking heed of her warning never to talk to her about money, merely said that there was possibility of some money if he stayed. "But the reason she demanded that I—"

"How much money?" Celestina asked.

"But you said never to—"

"*Si, si,* but this is *fatto,* the fact. It is okay to tell me."

"Just under a million dollars. And the house and the Chrysler."

Silence on the line.

"Hello?" Orville said. "Celestina? Hello? *Hello?*"

"I am here, *caro.* Tell me everything else."

He told her some things but couldn't tell her about his desperate sense of barrenness, about the chilling letter and the flights of Selma Rose, or of the Worth Hotel seeming to talk to him. Feeling again the desolation, he hid it. He chatted cheerily about Amy and Penny and Milt and Bill.

"I'm so happy to be coming back to you," he said. "Less than two days! I'm counting the hours."

"Me, too. But what is wrong?" There was alarm in her voice.

"Nothing."

"No, no, tell me. I am picking up *oscurita.* Dark."

"It's okay."

"I sense it like iron. Tell me at once."

How does she do it? he wondered, pick up these things? Still, he couldn't tell her.

"I love you," she said, "and you love me. Tell me."

"I, uh, well, I've seen my dead mother flying around outside the house. Twice."

"*Avemaria!* Go on."

He told her, and even told her about his creepy feeling that the Worth almost seemed to be talking to him. He didn't mention Selma's lying about his real birthday, unwilling to spoil the magic of their joint celebrations the past July.

"*Caro,* listen to me. You must stay there."

"*What?* I can't stay here!"

"You must stay. Do not come back here."

"I've got my ticket—"

"Cancel it. I will not see you. Do not attempt to see me."

"Because I've gone crazy?" he joked. Half-joked.

"Because, *caro,* this is a gift. Her gift to you."

"Come *on!* This place is a shit hole! I'll die here!"

"And come to life! In the compost pile the seed comes to life. In the shit the flower blooms. Do not forget—*Jesus* flew."

"Jesus *flew?*"

"*Si, l'Ascensione,*" she said. " Jesus flew for us all. On a Thursday, Holy Thursday. Your suffering among the Columbians will bring the healing *essenza* of sorrow."

"No chance of that."

"If your mother is not flying around, I agree. With her flying around, with the very buildings of your home town talking to you, your chances are good."

"I'll come to Europe. She can fly around Europe. She and Sol always loved their trips to Europe."

"I doubt she has the fuel for this. I will bet she flies only there."

"I can't stay here. I'm coming back."

"I will not see you."

"I'll bang down your door."

"You cannot bang down my heart."

"It's the money, isn't it?"

"Do not talk to me about money! Never!"

"But you were the one who—"

"If you come, I will not see you. But if you stay, I will come."

"For how long?"

"How the hell do I know? Jesus!"

"Promise?"

"*Si, si,* promise. You will be the rich American doctor, I will be the sensation of the shit hole, teaching them to breathe. Do they have there bufalo mozzarella?"

"Bring some. When will you come?"

"I check my book." Orville could hear the flutter of pages being turned. "*Allora.* Starting next week, I am teaching in Rome for six weeks. A yoga and meditation retreat on the *Piazza Navone.* Students from seven countries. Then I come."

"For sure?"

"*Si, si, certo.* Send me the ticket."

"Seven weeks?" His heart fell. "It seems like forever."

"Forever is now. And as long as you do not come here, I am loving you with all my heart and breasts and nipples and toes."

With kisses into receivers and promises to stay in the most intimate touch, they hung up.

◊ ◊ ◊

Later that morning Orville walked over to Bill Starbuck's ranch house and rang the bell. Babette led him into their breakfast nook, where Bill was reading *The Columbia Crier* and smoking a cigarette.

"Bill," Orville said, "I've decided to stay and help you out."

"You're crazy!"

"Bill!" cried Babette. "We can go back to Boca!"

"No, no," Orville said. "I'm not taking over. I'm helping out. Part-time. Some days, some nights, some weekends. We do it together."

"Wait a second," Bill said, his fingers drumming what sounded like a foxtrot on the yellow formica, clearly upset at this news. "You doin' this under duress?"

"Yup. A lot of duress. You bet."

"So it ain't your choice?"

"Nope. Like you said, I'm crazy."

"Well, that makes sense." He smiled. "One thing I've learned is, is that whenever you think you're choosin' things based on the facts, ten years later you look back and see you didn't know shit from Shinola about what was really going on in the world and in your life to push you to think *you* were choosin' things one way or another." He took a deep drag on the Camel and blew it back out contentedly. "Stay, leave, what the hell difference does it make anyway? You get that nice Chrysler, though, and a helluva lotta cash."

"And the house."

"Y'know, Orvy, they say that house has ghosts."

"Ghosts would be an improvement."

Bill laughed. "Maybe we'll have a little fun. Like we used to?"

"Maybe," Orville said glumly, "and maybe not."

"Hear that, Babs? Same old card. A joker." He chuckled. "Okay, partner, you've got yourself a deal."

The two shook hands. Orville started walking away.

"Dr. Rose?"

"Dr. Starbuck?"

"Son," he said, choked up. "For me, this is a dream come true."

6

Seven weeks later, Orville was in the emergency room tending to a Columbian garbageman who had fallen into the business end of his truck and had seen the bottom half of his body compacted to the thinness of a door. The man was going to die and, horribly, knew it. His screams and curses filled the small circle of cubicles. No one wanted to go near him. The only way Orville could deal with it was to shift into "Distanced Doctor" mode and go into the room periodically to push morphine.

It was the morning of October 12, a day of singular importance to Columbians—Columbus Day. The parade, filled with pomp and trepidation, was to start soon. Orville had promised Amy that he would take her. He was trying to finish up fast and make a smooth handoff of patients to Bill so he could run up to Penny's ranch to pick up his niece.

He was coming out of the garbageman's room for what he hoped was the last time when he got an urgent call at the nursing station.

"*Caro!*"

"Celestina?"

"*Si, si,* Celestina."

"*Cara!*" Screams interrupted. "I'm in the emergency. You have to shout."

"What?"

"Shout!" he shouted.

In the six weeks that she had been on retreat, they had spoken often. Their love was still intense. More intense, even, for their physical absence and their passionate phone calls.

"The retreat was *fantastico* and I have one favor to ask, *caro.*"

"What is that?"

"I need two more weeks."

"*What?*" His heart did a flip-flop and started to sink. "Why?"

As best he could hear, she was saying that the retreat had gone so well that the participants were revved up to try and set up an all-European *sangha,* or Buddhist community. Something about a Swiss banker from Zug who owned half an elephant in Nepal and had wandered into the *Piazza Navone* retreat by mistake (the banker not the elephant), stayed, had his eyes opened, and, now in a kind of dazed philanthropic state, was talking about helping finance the ongoing endeavor, and would Orville mind terribly if she delayed her arrival in Columbia for two weeks?

"Give me a firm date," he shouted.

She said something he couldn't hear.

"What? I can't hear you."

"What?"

"Keep shouting!" he yelled over the dying man's screams. "You've got to shout!"

"*Ottobre* 30," she shouted. Just two more weeks."

"Okay. October 30."

"October 30, *si, si.* I love you!"

"I love you, too!" he shouted back, but suddenly was embarrassed because everything had gone silent. The garbageman had died.

"And have you seen your mother flying around?" she screamed.

Orville spoke normally, "You don't have to shout anymore."

"Okay."

"No, I haven't."

"And no buildings are talking to you?"

"The hotel never actually *talked* to me. It was just a—I don't know, but nothing since, no."

"This is the bad sign," she said, sounding worried. "Something's fishy."

"After my mother's third letter the other day, if I never hear from her again it'll be too soon. I still don't know who's mailing her letters."

"Poor Orvio," she said, "to have to deal with these *pazzi* Columbians."

They said how much they missed each other and how they longed for the feel of their toes intertwined. With shared avowals of their love and the sheer impossibility of waiting two more weeks with such yearning, they hung up.

Orville pronounced the garbageman dead and changed out of his green surgical scrubs. He was hustling out the door to get down to the office and Bill when an ambulance rushed up screaming, and out of the back came a small body with tubes going in and blood coming out.

"Eleven-year-old girl," said the emergency tech. "Shot by a nine-year-old boy."

Orville turned around and followed the stretcher in. A little older than Amy. A sweet girl, shot in the chest, looking like she was about to die. Her color was turning from healthy pink to cyanotic blue—soon it would be deathly white. Everything in Orville clicked in to save her. He did the usual things, but nothing was working. It was puzzling. Her heart didn't seem to have been hit by the bullet, nor had the aorta or vena cava, but her heart was straining, as if drowning, beating but not pumping out much blood. The girl was going under.

Her parents were there on the other side of the curtain, waiting.

What the hell's going on? He felt a flicker of panic—of missing something that might save her, of failing. The nurses went silent, avoiding his eyes, waiting for him to come up with something else to try. One nurse, a friend of the parents, was sitting with them. The mother prayed. The father paced. Orville realized that the thread of the whole thing—the girl, the parents, the nurses—was unraveling fast.

He stood over the little girl, watching and waiting. He'd been in situations like this often before, in various hellholes all over the world, with someone who was dying, often from a bullet. If he were lucky, now, something else might happen.

Time slowed.

And then, as if a hand were on his shoulder, Orville felt himself pulled back—it was, he realized, a kind of Celestina moment—pulled back in order to truly *see*, seeing the girl, seeing the chest, seeing the heart, seeing— yes! *Not* the heart. The sac *around* the heart. The bullet must have nicked the pericardium. Blood was leaking into the pericardial sac and, trapped there between the heart and the sac, was compressing the heart—like a swimmer held under. Cardiac tamponade.

Quickly he jerry-rigged a large-bore needle to a lead of the EKG machine and pushed it between the ribs gently until the current of the heart showed him to be in contact with the pericardium, and then he popped it through the sac and with a whoosh, like the rush of air out of the mozarella Pappa's windpipe, bright red blood and tiny raisins of clots blew out of the open end of the needle and the heart, like a swimmer surfacing, expanded fully and contracted fully, and he watched as the girl turned from white to blue to pink. He waited, monitoring her for a while until he was sure. She would live.

He went out to face her parents. In their eyes was the question.

"She's going to be okay," he said.

They collapsed into each other's arms.

"You can go in and see her."   .

"Thank God, thank God!" they cried and rushed to her.

He arranged for the medi-vac helicopter to fly the girl up to Albany Medical to have a cardiac surgeon remove the bullet. Walking out of the hospital, he realized how lucky she'd been—there wasn't even much of a risk of infection, since bullets, going in hot, are sterile. It wasn't until he sat behind the wheel of the Chrysler that he started to shake.

Hey, wait a second, he thought. *Why* did a nine-year-old boy shoot her?

Getting no answer, he floated the car down to Bill's office and walked through the full waiting room and in the IN door. Bill, cigarette in hand, had already taken over his shift and was listening to a woman named Tracy Liebowski. Orville had known her in high school, she a junior to his senior. Cute, and in the band—flute. Bill and Tracy were discussing Tracy's five-year-old boy, Wally, who had become unmanageable. She was confused and unsure how to handle him.

"Wally has behavior problems. He bites other kids, he won't read, he flies into rages, and he *never* sleeps through the night." She sounded fed up, bitter. "Worst is the pooping. He won't poop in the potty or the toilet. He poops in his bed at night, and it wakes him up and he wakes us up. He poops all over the house—under the dining room table, behind the Lay-Z-Boy, yesterday in my husband's motorcycle helmet." She turned to Orville. "Which he didn't notice 'til he put it on."

Despite himself, Orville smiled.

"I'm exhausted," she said to Bill. "Jeffrey is threatening divorce. Wally's killin' us. Like he's from another planet or somethin'. He's in the waitin' room."

"Bring him on in," Bill said.

Orville braced himself for the encounter with the little alien.

In walked an angel, a beautiful boy all silken blond hair and cowlick and clear blue eyes and freckled nose. Orville wondered what Bill would do.

"Hi there, little tyke," Bill started, handing the boy a lollipop. "How 'bout we talk about your poopin'?"

The boy said nothing. Bill started talking. The boy seemed to listen. Bill kept talking. Soon, to Orville and Tracy's surprise, the boy started to talk, too.

"Wally," Bill explained, "it's about having a job. Your mom's job is at Columbia Cold Storage, right?" Wally nodded. "And your dad's job is at Scomparza Demolition and Upholstery, right?" Another nod. "Well, son, *your* job is to poop in the potty. And I'm gonna give you your very own poop-juice, to help you." He handed him a bottle. "Take a drink every night—*every* night, got it?" Wally nodded. "And take a drink of this every morning." Bill handed him a cute little bottle with a label that read "Elixir of Starbusol." "And whenever you poop in the potty, you get a star!" He handed him a packet of stars. Little Wally had trouble holding all these gifts. "Okay?" He nodded. "You do your job, and I'll see you again next week and you can show me your stars."

Wally jumped up, eager to start, and scampered out the OUT.

In the doorway, Orville said to Tracy, "He's beautiful."

"Yeah," she said, her eyes brightening for the first time. With a sudden sureness she went on, "There's a reason for that."

Startled, again Orville felt the feathery touch of whatever Celestina was talking about, say the spirit—why not? He smiled at Tracy, seeing once again the cheery high school girl, playing her flute. Placing a Starbuckian hand on her shoulder, he ushered her OUT.

Handing off the practice to Bill, Orville told him about the patients he had an ongoing concern about, ending with the girl shot by the boy.

"Good work," Bill said. "Jeez, that's a tough diagnosis to make, especially when you're on the spot like that. Damn good work, Orvy."

"Why all the guns, Bill?"

"What's that?"

"Why all the guns? Last week that migrant worker got shot right in the hospital parking lot, today this girl. It's like the Wild West around here, Bill."

"Yep, it is. Only here they're not as good an aim, heh heh. Hell, did you see that the First Lady announced on TV the other day that she's even packin' a gun now. They say that soon there'll be a gun for every American—250 million guns."

"But a *nine*-year-old with a gun?"

"Wasn't his, of course. Probably his dad's. But that age is unusual. That ain't a trend, nope, nope."

"Not yet," Orville said.

◊ ◊ ◊

Between contempt and compassion doctors run their course. Years ago in New Jersey, the trauma of Orville's failing marriage to Lily Wolf had affected his work with his patients, tilting the balance toward contempt. He had been trained to keep his practice walled off from his marriage, but the wall began to crumble. His heightened contempt at work—and his self-loathing—had spilled back into his marriage. He would come home a sulking, snarling bear. After a while everything about Lily seemed mean-spirited, tight, and too neat and clean. As did suburban New Jersey. Infertility brought him to his knees. His desperation seeped into his doctoring. To protect his patients from his contempt, the doctor had run.

But shy men carry a secret daring. At sixteen, afraid of heights, Orville had taken a job 158 feet over the Hudson River on the Rip Van Winkle Bridge. At thirty-six, afraid of leaving his wife and suburban medicine, he'd run straight toward the worst medical situations imaginable. Whether in atonement for failing Lily or in nihilistic rage to destroy himself, or in some Hemingwayesque macho-shit testing of himself, or maybe even just wanting—after all those clean guest towels for clean guests—to feel the poverty of dirt, he'd run full blast toward pain and suffering. Black bag in hand, *Médecins Sans Frontières* as his umbrella, he worked in hellholes like Haiti, Madagascar, Rwanda, Somalia, Lebanon, and East Timor. He'd ended up in sight of Bikini Atoll, in the post–H-bomb test islands in the Pacific, where frogs lacked testicles and lizards had bird wings and birds laid eggs with shells thin as glass and humans had too few fingers or too many or cleft palates or spina bifida, and sat around wondering why a lot of their kids were strabismic or leukemic or dead.

He figured he'd done his part. Nothing much had improved.

And Columbia? he asked himself now, as he eased his dead mother's floating Chrysler over to Penny's ranch house to pick up Amy for the parade. Well, ever since he'd started with Bill, Columbia had surprised him.

Columbia, in its own way, was about as bad as any of the other places he'd seen. His Sakhalin Island.

Alcohol and violence. Not only gunplay and knife play but ax play and chainsaw play. Murder as grisly as in Angola. Malnutrition as bad as in the Third World. Car crashes as creative as on the Autobahns or the sorry roads of India—whole families of Columbians turned to a mush of metal and blood and bone and brain by a drunken kid in a five-ton truck. Ninety-year-olds driving sixteen miles an hour meeting sixteen-year-olds driving ninety. A cornucopia of drugs to make the East Bronx, and the shamans of Peru, proud. Despite an epidemic of smoking, an epidemic of obesity—"Be *glad* they smoke," Bill had said, "think how heavy they'd be if they din't."

Sexual violence and perversions, including, in the rural zones out in the county where the hills were made of lush green grasses all alfalfas and timothys and the woods of towering oaks and maples and chestnuts and pines and the streams ran splashing like kids and spilled diamonds over waterfalls to collect in pools of silvery blue and lakes of chill deep purple with names like Bash Bish Falls and Roeliff Jansen Kill and there, always there like good grandparents anchoring it all, were the Catskills and the Hudson, there out in those wondrous rural zones where he captained the Chrysler on house calls to the impoverished farms and trailer parks, he saw daisy chains of brutality, sodomy, rape, pedophilia, and the raw neglect of children so that when they were discovered they were ten-year-olds with the bodies and minds of fives. And in the office, as study after study of doctors had shown, 80 percent of the patients revolving in that IN-OUT circle of hell had no identifiable physical disease. 80 percent of the time in our offices, Orville mused, we doctors are treating phantoms.

Why was Bill's practice so bad? The wealthier, and often healthier, Columbians and New Yorkers had stopped coming to Bill. He was old, half-blind and half-deaf, and his office was outdated and scruffy. He no longer took any insurance payments; he was unwilling to fill out the crossword-puzzles of forms. He accepted cash, check, or barter, and he always carried a big wad of bills neatly ordered in ascending denominations, like a gas station attendant. He wasn't up on the latest medical technology. He had no receptionist, so you had to wait your turn—the death knell for yuppies. He smoked, and often smelled like an onion.

Another strike against Bill was his increasing reliance on his own special medicine, Starbusol. For decades, he had made the stuff himself. It came in bottles, smelled of pine, and tasted like a cross between cherry cough medicine and Coca-Cola. In extreme cases, it could be injected. No

one, not even Orville, knew what was in it. Bill swore by it. He often with-
held it as treatment until the crucial moment, when he claimed it would
have maximal effect.

"But it's a placebo, Bill, right?" Orville had asked him the other day.

Bill said nothing.

"It's just the placebo effect?"

"Whatsamatter with havin' an effect? And it's never made anybody
worse. Most treatments make people worse. Even antibiotics, in the long
run, are makin' humanity worse. You just wait, son. There'll come a day
when nothin'll be workin' for you, and you might just be ready for some
Starbusol."

"For my patients or myself?

"Yep. Heh, heh."

And so the better-off people, including Milt and Penny, had stopped
coming to Bill. Instead, they drove nearly an hour out to the wealthy enclave of Spook Rock, where a very tall and handsome young doctor named
Edward R. Shapiro, who seemed straight out of a TV sitcom about a very
tall and handsome young doctor in a wealthy enclave, would serve up a
kind of Disney medicine seen on TV as well as fresh coffee, caf or decaf. It
didn't take long for Orville to realize, from Shapiro's lethal mistakes, that
he was as bad a doctor as Bill and Orville had ever seen, a kind of poster
boy for both mental illness and medical malpractice. The worst. As was
often the case in medicine, the worst charged the most.

The rest came to Bill and, now, Orville. They were mostly poor, native
Columbians, often people of color. The walking wounded and the walking
worried. For Orville, every day in the hospital and in the endless circle of
IN-OUT-IN of the office and every night he was on call, was dispiriting.

Again, he was doing his part. Again, nothing much was improving.

◊ ◊ ◊

Orville docked the Chrysler at the end of Penny and Milt's flagstone walk
and honked the horn. To him, it sounded ugly and too loud and he was
always sorry he'd honked it, afterward. As usual, he was late.

Amy shot out of the door and raced down the walk toward him, a big
smile on her face. As always when he saw her, Orville lit up.

At Penny's "Welcome Home Orvy" party, they had screeched each
other's names and she had rushed into his arms. They had hugged each
other so long and hard that the noise of the party went away, and all they
heard was their hearts beating in their temples. Drawing back but holding

47

on, they had looked into each other's eyes with a shared curiosity. Orville saw again those wide-open eyes, just as at her miraculous birth, and Amy saw the dear outrageous uncle who had always been her safe haven. For a moment, then, as they held each other's gaze, his blue to her brown, they felt safe, two birds caught in an empty pocket of the wind. Protected from Penny's frantic and perfect party. Home.

Penny had assigned Orville Sunday afternoons and Wednesday evenings with Amy. Sunday afternoons were Ascot Riding Lessons out at the Spook Rock Hunt Club followed by Greenie's Budapest Drama Lessons in the Opera House down past Fourth followed by dinner with Penny and Milt at Chinese Restaurant, run by two guys from New York who owned Unique Antique next door. Wednesday evenings were Math For Girls Lessons followed by an hour of free time. Amy's other afternoons were also wall-to-wall lessons.

"Why all the lessons?" Orville had asked Penny. "Don't kids just go out and play anymore?"

"Too dangerous. A child was kidnapped last year, right on the street in front of her house."

Orville thought back to Ethiopia. A war zone. Everybody's hungry. Kids play.

"All the mothers do it now, the lessons. I spend my life in the car—thank God for the tape deck. Lessons are the only way to break their addiction to TV." She had smiled at him, seeing in him a seasoned doctor with a hard-won measuredness. "It'll be great for her to be with you, Orvy. She's crazy about you. Ever since she spent that week with you last year in Paris, she's thrown you up to us—'Uncle O. wouldn't say that, and if he were here he wouldn't let *you* say that either.' It's all manipulation but still. What she needs from you, kid, is advice. It'll be great for you, too. Good fun."

It had been great, mostly. Probably because he never gave her advice. In fact, it was often the other way around. Amy had a self-assurance that was astonishing to him and a voice that could sing the birds out of the trees. Even standing in the horseshit Sunday after Sunday watching Amy ride animals that he regarded as mere paraplegia in horsehide, the burnt-out almost-forty-year-old felt like a young father, a dad at last. From time to time in the oblique October light, the shadow of "She's not yours" would canter out from his feet toward her on her horse. But it was just a shadow, not the feeling, which threw none.

"Hi, Unc!" Amy said now, slipping into the seat and throwing her arms around his neck, hugging him hard.

"Hi, Ame!" In a glance he took her in—Yankees cap with her auburn hair poking out the back in a pony tail, sweatshirt with a whale logo and Leviathan Players (her drama group), and her long slim legs in jeans and Reeboks—and felt a rush of love.

She drew away. They stared into each other's eyes for a second—as they always did, a gut check. He watched her brow knit in concern.

"What's wrong?" she asked.

"Nothing. I'm fine."

"Hey, don't be phony with me. It'll come back and bite you!"

"Okay," he said, laughing. "Just being a doc, that's all."

"So tell Doctor Amy. Where doth thou hurt?"

He laughed. "C'mon. No more medicine talk for today. Let's get to that parade."

She reflexively snapped on her seatbelt—a generational difference. She looked over at him frowning. "C'mon, Uncle O. Buckle up."

He buckled up and started the mammoth Chrysler on its way downtown to Selma's house on the Courthouse Square, where the speeches would take place.

They arrived just as the Columbus Day parade was grinding to a halt. The lone float was a Chevy gussied up as a ship, representing the Nina, the Pinta, and the Santa Maria. It carried the mayor's cousin-in-law, Warsaw Gologpzyk, dressed as Christopher Columbus. The Fish Hawk Marching Band was playing a tentative rendition of "Columbia, the Gem of the Ocean." Blinky the Clown, the town drunk, performed tricks that were failing to amuse even the youngest Columbian. Mayor Americo Scomparza stood on the steps of the courthouse preparing to speak.

Orville and Amy could sense a rising tension in the crowd. The native Columbians nervously moved away from any overhanging streetlamps, limbs, and phone lines. The gaggle of New Yorkers, glasses of white wine in hand, chatted to each other noisily, happily.

Americo's string of platitudes was passing for a speech. Near the end he launched into his "Columbus Day Appeal" for money for "our terrific bankrupt little town" and unveiled the sail-covered "mast" of the Chevy, a large thermometer with a series of ascending colored lightbulbs. This was designed to track the progress of fund-raising toward the goal—what else but $14,920—marked by a gold whale at the top. The thermometer would sit on the square until January 1, 1984.

"And so," Americo said proudly, "it gives me great pleasure to light the lights to start the appeal."

He threw the switch. The lights went on, just as they were supposed to. Columbians cheered. But then there was a flash and a soft *poof,* followed by an extended *pfizzzzzzll.* The lights went out.

The slumming New Yorkers, seeing the breakage as a quaint quirk in this amusing folk festival, giggled and applauded and raised their glasses and called out "Yes! Yes!" The native Columbians, including Amy and Orville, moved back quickly, seeing the start of another episode in the Columbian Curse of Breakage and fearing the worst.

The mayor, thinking that the microphone had also broken, muttered "Shit. Nuthin' ever works right in this fuckin' place," which boomed out over the square.

The New Yorkers' sniggers were cut off suddenly by an explosion from the Chevy. Someone cried out, "The gas tank!" In an instant the float was engulfed in flames. Columbus abandoned Chevy, his robe on fire. He dropped to the ground and rolled. Telling Amy to stay put, Orville rushed to him.

The fire department, which was part of the parade, sprayed everything with foam. Soon the Discovery of America celebration looked less like a heroic appeal for funds and more like an ad for a new-and-improved laundry detergent.

Orville was covered head to toe with foam and had to scrape it off to see the burned man. Reaching for his black bag, he realized that Amy was beside him, also covered in foam. She had already opened the bag and was handing him his stethoscope. With the fire now out, he felt okay to have her there beside him, and smiled at her. He took the stethoscope and called out "Bandages and tape!" She handed them to him. Sometimes on their Sundays and Wednesdays he'd been called away for emergencies, and Amy had come with him, hanging around as he doctored, asking questions, curious about it all. She'd seemed fearless, cool in the theater of trauma, and had learned quickly how to assist him. He soon stabilized the singed Columbian.

The ship was totaled, the Appeal-o-Meter in ruins, and the mayor pissed off.

"It's the Democrats!" he hissed in Orville's ear. "An election year and they're making life miserable!"

Warsaw was not much burned. More dazed and embarrassed than hurt, smelling like a gas barbecue gone bad, he insisted on walking with Orville and Amy to Bill's office for further treatment. As they walked along, Amy took Orville's hand. He looked down at her. How tall she had gotten, he thought, lanky like Penny. Her brown eyes were wide-open, ablaze with the excitement of helping. Her ponytail poking through the back opening of her baseball cap flicked as she bounced along, like a foal's tail. There was, he thought, a dose of Milt in her baby-fat jaw, but mostly there was Penny and the slender Sol. And maybe, just maybe, in her leaning into life a little right now, a touch of her crazy uncle.

7

Ever since Orville had arrived home there had been a drought, the worst in living memory. Rain, real rain, had been rare. Not only had it been dry, but hot. Now, at the end of October, apples were withering on trees, cows were melting, chickens were going crazy, rabid skunks and raccoons and an odd red fox were attacking even in backyards, cherries were flaccid, peaches were leathery, and grapes were more raisinlike than otherwise. Farmers, often silent, were sullenly so, and farmers' wives were appearing in Bill and Orville's waiting room with the florid trappings of nineteenth-century hysteria and melancholia.

Orville had been fat as a child and by now had pretty much licked it. He had been shocked by how fat Americans had become, the epidemic of overweight. His obese patients found the relentless heat intolerable. Their ailments inflamed, and excoriated. Cigarette sales soared. Whole families would walk into the office puffing away like old-time steam engines, a three-hundred-and-something-pound dad with a fake satin jacket reading "Earl," a wife tipping the scales well over two-forty reading "Marge," and two teenage fleshballoons reading "Junior" and "Peg," all revved up on nicotine. Much like, Orville mused as he treated their phantom complaints, what he and Lily had seen at Disney World during the cousin's wedding in "Wedding Pavilion"—whole tribes of American families dressed like bowling teams, looking like they'd eaten the balls. Nicotine revved them up, but couldn't bring rain.

Orville and Bill were wilting as well. Orville was a man who loved rain, every kind of rain. Holland had been heaven. He loved living below sea level, pummeled daily by precipitation, taking long walks through the tall, straight evergreens outside of Zeist, where the drizzle served up a pine scent so solid you could almost chew it. Parched skies were hard for him. Bill, corralled by Babette, worked fewer hours, seldom taking night call. His care seemed a few degrees off. Orville was constantly repairing his mistakes.

But Celestina was coming. The day after tomorrow. On Monday the 30th Orville would pilot the Chrysler down to JFK to meet her. Her return ticket was open-ended. In their last phone call, the day before yesterday, she had said she might stay the whole year. What an image, he thought. Celestina among the Columbians? Buckle up!

But first he had a party to get through.

"You don't go out!" Penny had decided, and Penny decided was Penny not to be denied. He waited for the blow to fall. She had coaxed him to a dinner party that night at the home of Henry Schooner, who lived in another grand old Victorian, restored perfectly and painted gaily in peach with burgundy trim, and resting exactly 134 strides across the Courthouse Square from Selma's house. The only strange part about his going to Schooner's dinner party was that Henry had been the sadistic bully who had made a good part of Orville's childhood a living hell.

The dinner finished, the guests sat at the table chatting. It was an intimate affair, Penny and Milt, Henry and Nelda Jo, and Orville and the woman Penny had arranged as his "date," his childhood girlfriend Faith Schenckberg O'Herlihy, with whom, playing doctor in his basement as the furnace roared and the woodpile stank of rats, he'd had his first public erection. Faith, a religious Jew, wore a low-cut dress and push-em-up bra that brought to Orville's mind the Hebraic phrase "a sunburnt offering." During dinner Orville had the recurring feeling that his mother was hovering nearby. From time to time, furtively, he would glance up out a window, scanning the sky, but no.

The aged port and top-shelf brandy circulated the mahogany table on rimmed silver trays, and Henry offered real Havana cigars along with a heavy silver cigar cutter. To Orville, the surprising thing was how sophisticated the evening was. He had grown up in a family one generation shy of immigrants who'd had no real tether to the rituals of the Old World and whose take on the New World was ad-driven toward "looks," the "look" of a car or of an outfit of or a person was the currency. A man was summed up by the size of his neck, a woman by how ugly or lovely she was, as if getting away from the thin necks and ugliness of the *shtetls* of the Old World was more important than finding out the complex truth of the person. For Orville to dine elegantly so close to home was bizarre. And to have this come from *Schooner?* From the kid who, in the soaring vulgarity of the town, had been the most vulgar of all? *Mousse saumon* and *coq au vin* with a *trou* of palate-refreshing raspberry sorbet in between—from sadistic, pornographic, anti-Semitic Schooner, the only kid he knew who was ever expelled from Columbia High.

Orville stared across the table at Schooner, seeing in his bulky body and square face and the neatly combed Andy Warhol–white hair and weird dark eyes—seeing in all this adulthood the same tough kid of twelve with the same block of a body and the same eyes that had filled him with terror. He could not help but see, in the smiling man, the vile boy.

Reflexively Orville found himself fingering a raised nubbin of scar tissue on the back of his neck. When he was twelve, sitting in the front row of a sock hop in the Mount Carmel Church basement watching the girls jitterbug with each other, Orville had felt a sudden searing pain on the back of his neck. Jumping to his feet, turning around, he was face-to-face with a leering Schooner holding the cigarette butt he'd just put out on Orville's neck. Schooner was daring him to do something about it. Bigger, tougher, stronger—first kid on the block with pubic hair, first on the block to sell dirty postcards from Mexico—Henry, seemingly at whim, would chase Orville and beat him up and tell him that if he told his mother or father he would beat him worse the next time. Orville, terrified, had never told. Schooner started extorting money from him for protection.

He remembered Schooner sitting next to him in seventh grade and, during a Studebaker math drill, tapping him on the arm; when Orville looked over he saw Henry's dick laid out on his desktop next to a ruler, and not to solve a math problem either. Another day, Schooner and another thug at Boy Scouts in the Lutheran Church basement dragged Orville into the men's room "to see what a Jew dick looks like." They pulled down his pants, did their mocking inspection, and, with a threat, let him go.

The worst, in a way, were the basketball games at the Boy's Club on South Third. Orville loved basketball. Schooner played, too, on an opposing team, played like a bull in a china shop, throwing elbows, cracking knees. Orville knew that if Schooner's team lost, Henry would be waiting for him, and so toward the end of games, Orville tried to lose. If it looked like a win, he'd get ready as the clock ticked down, and the final whistle was like a starting pistol at a race and Orville would run like hell through the locker room down the stairs and up Prison Alley toward the Courthouse Square, Schooner chasing. If he was caught, he was extorted and/or beaten.

Downstreet below Fourth was Henry's home turf. He was poor and lived with his father, who worked nights as a security guard at Iron Mountain out near Tivoli. Their tiny house was close by the North Swamp among the poor Italian and Hungarian and Ukrainian immigrants, just a street away from the black section of town, near the Colored Citizens Club. Henry came from the bad part of town, without toys; Orville from the good, with a storeful.

Before Orville had come back last August, the last time he had seen Henry Schooner was more than twenty years ago. Orville had been manager of the league champion Fish Hawk basketball team. The starting five—Whiz the black star, Konopski the tall farmer who played a solid center, Scomparza the kid who could rough 'em up under the boards, Basch the dentist's son who could drill shots from long range, and Tommy Kline of Kline's Whale Oil And Gas who was the sizzling, savvy playmaker—had made it clear to Schooner that if he messed with Orville he was dead meat. The Fish Hawks were hot. Tickets were in demand. Henry Schooner stole a roll of tickets for the big game against Troy and was scalping them. He got caught and was expelled.

The last time he had seen Schooner was when the starting five and Orville, from the steps of the gym, watched Henry trudge away, his refrigerator body moving as if on wheels, his white-blond head unbowed. Just before he walked into the woods on the path that was a shortcut around Kleek's Pond to the rough, impoverished zones of Downstreet, he turned and raised a middle finger at the team, mouthed a "Fuck you!" and disappeared into the woods.

"A toast," Henry was saying, rising from the table, raising his glass of port. "To Doctor Orville Rose, a welcome home, and to the memory of a fine lady of Columbia, a woman I often looked at as a kid wishing, since I had no mom to speak of, she could've been my mom. I'm talking about your mom, yours and our dear Penny's, Selma Rose."

"To Orville and Selma Rose!" shouted all.

"A wonderful couple!" shouted Milt.

All eyes turned to Orville for a response. Given a whole childhood of Schooner's threatening him with "If you tell anyone, especially your mother, I'll kill you!" and given the smarminess of the toast that made Orville feel like throwing up the mousse, the coq, the sorbet in between and the two wines, it was only with the greatest discipline that he was able to rise, swallow his revulsion at Schooner's current duplicity, and speak.

"Thank you, Henry. Being back here again after so many years has been, well, sort of great, and I greatly appreciate your kind, great, really, words about my—our—mother. It's been the greatest evening, a really great dinner. Penny and I greatly appreciate it."

It sufficed. The conversation rolled on. He sat there quietly drinking until Penny, in a lull, visibly perturbed that Orville was silent, said, "Penny for your thoughts."

"Oh," Orville said, startled, for he had been in a reverie about Celestina Polo and the twenty tiny chapels set among the cypresses and gravestones on the pilgrimage site on top of the Sacre Monte. "I . . . uh, I was just wondering, why whales?"

"Oh, Christ!" Milt said, in mock horror. "Him and his whales!"

"What about the whales, dahlin'?" asked Nelda Jo. She was a dazzling, elegant blond from Tulsa, with a nose just a touch too flat. She taught aerobics at Schooner's Spa out on Route 9 near the mall and seemed to have a body made all of pectorals and gluteals, a body that reminded Orville of the female athletes in Zeist and of the women leading the exercise shows on TV. She was wearing a silky, casually draped beige dress with a V-neck that both showed a necklace of significant diamonds and two un-bra'd nipples, which seemed, to the slightly drunk Orville, as big as muscat grapes.

Just my luck, he thought. She goes to Dr. Edward R. the Sociopath Shapiro.

"I mean," Nelda Jo went on, "are we talkin' Moby-damn-Dick?"

"I was wondering, with whales being the logo of Columbia, why *whales?*"

"Oh, I get it," Nelda Jo said. "You're wondering *why* whales?"

"Columbya wassa whalin' port," Faith said, slurring her words. "Caught 'em in the river." Faith had recently come out of a nasty divorce but had not come out too sober.

"But whales live in sea water, right?" Orville asked. "The river is fresh water, right?" Everybody said right. "So?" No one knew. The conversation veered back toward the known. Soon Orville got beeped out. Schooner accompanied him to the door.

"I am sensing that you are not comfortable here tonight," Henry said. "Ever since you've come back, you've been avoiding me, and I just want you to know two things. Number one, I understand why. Number two, I'm sorry."

"It's okay," Orville said, "I really—"

"No, it is not okay, not okay at all. I have to earn your respect."

The beeper went off. "Gotta go."

"It's early. Hope you finish up quick, maybe you can come back?"

"I'll try."

"I believe it." Henry was shaking Orville's hand in the way experienced politicians do: one hand in the voter's, the other clasping the elbow in the most friendly way. This reminded Orville of Bill showing him how the old docs also did this to palpate the olecranon fossa of the elbow in unsuspecting patients, searching for nodules of syphilis.

"One more thing," Henry went on, "before you disappear for your noble rounds?"

"Yeah?"

"People change."

"Some don't."

"As Shakespeare said, 'The past is past.'"

"What he said, Henry," Orville said, seeing in those eyes the sadist, "is, 'the past is prologue.'"

"And 'the play's the thing!' I don't want anymore confrontations between the both of us."

Orville noted the lapse of grammar, the old Schooner slipping out. And then he was surprised to see that Henry was noting his noting something.

"It'll take time, Orvy, to win your respect. I'm game if you are." Orville said nothing. "We're on the same team now."

"What team is that?"

"Columbia. America. The world. We're global now." Schooner smiled. "You know, in the last couple of years I got close to your mom, real close. Great lady."

Orville had a sickening thought: he's mailing the letters.

"I'd go over to the house from time to time, look in on her, have a cup of tea, chat. It's okay if you don't come back tonight. It already means a lot that you came at all."

◊ ◊ ◊

The funny thing, Orville thought in the emergency room, trying to deal with the carnage of a Saturday night in Columbia, is that Schooner seemed to have meant it.

Doctoring tipsily is like tightrope walking without a net. As Orville popped a peppermint Lifesaver and revived a teenage girl overdosed on her mom's Valium and Barbados rum, he tried to wrestle his mind into balance.

He moved on to a hysterical Mrs. Len Date, wife of the Columbia town lawyer. Len had come home drunk. Mrs. Len had confronted him in the driveway, berating him until she noticed, in the bed of his pickup truck, the severed head of a woman. The rest of the woman was soon found by troopers in a sharp curve of a road way out past Omi. Orville sedated Mrs. Len and went next to tend to a three-year-old boy with a popcorn kernel stuck in his ear.

The kid was screaming. Orvy tried to be nice. He let the anxious young mother hold the scared boy as he tried to pick the kernel out with a probe. No go. Then he tried to suck it out with a sucker, also with no luck. He tried this and that, the kid increasingly frantic and wailing, the mother trying to hold him steady. At that moment Orville felt the whole world of care turn, the way it does when things go wrong and the Emergency Gods are angry. He got frustrated, irritated, and called for a nurse to strap the screaming, flailing kid down to a papoose board so he could get a better take on the ear. The mother objected. Other patients were piling up. The emergency room was taking on a surreal feel, with word of another car crash on the way in. Disasters were waiting and more were brewing out there and the Great Doctor Rose couldn't get the damn popcorn kernel out of the kid's ear, and everybody was getting nasty, including him.

"Hi there, little tyke, heh heh."

It was Bill, shuffling in toward the bedside, putting a hand on the mother's shoulder and a hand on Orville's, and breathing scallion into the air.

"What're you doing here?" Orville asked, but then realizing that the head nurse must have called him.

"Me? Oh, I got this popcorn kernel stuck in my ear . . . Heh heh. Hi, Gloria," Bill said to the mother and then, waving a red teddy bear at the boy, said, "Hi there, Benji boy. Got a red teddy for you here." The boy stopped screaming and reached for it. "Y'know, Gloria, one of the hardest things in doctorin' is getting a popcorn kernel out of a kid's ear. It can get very frustratin', right Dr. Rose?"

Orville bristled, feeling a hit of criticism. But then, feeling the warmth of Bill's hand on his shoulder, as if now the hand itself were telling him— "Take it easy, it's just a damn popcorn kernal"—he relaxed, and said, "Very."

"Want me to take a shot at it?" Bill offered.

"Be my guest."

Bending over the ear, he took out of his pocket a homemade chrome and rubber thing and, still playing with the kid and the red teddy, worked the ear and with a whispering plucking sound like a string of a harp, out came the popcorn kernel. Orville was amazed, and was about to ask how the hell he'd done it when he got called away to attend to the car crash. Refreshed by Bill's caring and skill, he took care with the victims, none of whom was badly hurt. He spoke to the families, glad to bring them good news. The Emergency Gods had come through.

After one in the morning, he walked out of the hospital and guided the Chrysler with its liquid power steering back down to Courthouse Square. Across the way, the party was still going strong. The porch light cast an amber glow, the house was alight. Peals of laughter scurried through the tiny holes in the screen door out into the warm fall night.

Should I go back? Orville wondered, as he pulled into his mother's drive? No.

Not feeling sleepy, he got a beer and came back out and sat on the porch. In the hot, still night, a kind of Indian summer's Indian summer, a last batch of confused crickets sang out as if there were no tomorrow—which might well be, for them. Staring across the way at the party, Orville was unwilling to join in again, yet unable to get his mind off Henry Schooner.

Henry was a mirror image of Gatsby—his past known, his present mysterious. Orville knew that Schooner had walked into the woods and joined the Navy, had risen like a rocket, done tours in Vietnam, gotten his high school degree, had gone on to college and business school, and, in his own words, "had played a significant role in clandestine activities, national intelligence and security." Just after Orville left America two years ago, Schooner returned home to Columbia with a dynamite wife of some wealth with a dancer's body that wouldn't quit, and two young boys, Henry Jr. and Max, both thick-bodied and blond, two compact refrigerators of the same brand.

He bought one of the most expensive houses in town, on the most elegant square, and with a team of Filipinos renovated it to period elegance in record time with no breakages. Two Filipinos stayed on, husband and wife, and did all the childcare and household chores. At dinner parties they cooked fine meals in many cuisines of the world and, in stiff-starched white, served them. In addition to Schooner's Spa, Henry had formed a company with Milt—Schooner and Plotkin, Developers—which was making a fortune. Word was out among New Yorkers that these were the people to see, not only for property but for financing and all the little extras that Schooner, well-connected on every level, could provide. Schooner and Plotkin were heavy into SPOUT. Henry was now a pillar of the community, on the boards of a hospital and bank, a member of the Chamber of Commerce and Episcopal Church, and an alderman.

"My alderman? Orville said aloud now to himself. "That jerk is my alderman?"

"What's wrong with that, Mr. Bigshot Doctor? He's goyim, but nice."

Selma was floating low over the front walk, just off the edge of the porch, dressed in a yellow golf skirt, red blouse, and pink hat with a purple tuft on the top. She carried a golf club, maybe a wedge.

"You?"

"Yes, and you did a nice job up there at the hospital, though let's face it, with that mother and her son you could have been a lot nicer. Try a little tenderness, will you? I know it's hard for someone like you, but try."

"Did you give your letters to Henry to mail? Is he the one?"

"Letters? *Moi?*" She smiled coquettishly, a full smile—her facial nerve hadn't yet been cut, or had healed after death. "Adios, bubbula! Fore!" She flew up, up, and away.

Orville sat on the porch staring at the dark sky into which she'd vanished. Warm laughter from Schooner's snapped him back to his senses. Suddenly he felt lonely, left out.

He walked across the square back to the party, and found them all in the oak-paneled den. Burnished, tasteful, costly antiques furnished the room. Henry was standing in front of the mantelpiece. Something had changed. Instead of everyone talking with everyone, everyone was listening to Schooner. All attention was being paid to him. More than attention. The others were rapt, awed. Even Faith, who was swaying, but listening. What was going on?

World affairs was going on. Someone would ask about the recent terrorist bombing of the Marine barracks in Beirut that had killed 250 soldiers. Schooner had done a tour of duty in Beirut, and answered, "Our nation is the greatest force for good in history. The bad guys can't stand it. Thus, this tragedy of the peacekeepers—our brave fighting men." Two days after the bombing, the president announced that American armed forces had invaded Grenada. Many Americans thought that the rapidly aging patriarch must have misspoken. Surely he meant that they invaded Lebanon. An easy mixup, Lebanon, Grenada. Three syllables, sound a lot the same, no one really knew where either of them were. But no, Grenada it was, wherever it was. And Schooner knew exactly where Grenada was, from his tour of duty in the region: "a small island in the Caribbean with a dangerous pro-Castro Communist faction building an airstrip."

Schooner's answers were calm, expert, humble, brief, sure, and telegenic. Clearly he had been touched by the magic of TV. He had, in fact, been on TV several times, commenting on the crisis. He was now a TV personality. Parlaying his recent links to national security and intelligence, Schooner had become an authority and a star.

All five of us, Orville realized, are deferring to him.

He seemed bigger, taller, in command. Orville could almost see tiny flecks of glitter, the glitter of fame bestowed in the studio by the TV camera, as sometimes you see bright glitter on a woman's cheek the morning after a party. With a sense of horror Orville understood that the next time Schooner was on TV there would be a redoubling of this process, more magic TV dust would rub off, leaving more left to rub off here at home in person. Schooner would be even more a person to be listened to than before.

And if someone in the group disagreed, well, Henry would take this in and gently but surely turn it to his cause.

This went on until Nelda Jo said, "They want old Henry to run for Congress this year, but I said only if he buys me a Ferrari and a week in Venice, Italy, and the boys one 37-inch TV each for their rooms."

"Do you take VISA?" Henry asked.

Everyone roared.

"Why Congress?" Milt asked. "Why not the whole enchilada?"

"Damnright," Faith slurred, "runfer the goddamn Wide House."

Henry considered this. "Maybe, someday. My job now is to help our sweet little hometown. Let's face it my friends, we in Columbia have problems. The mayor, the other day, said to us Aldermen that Columbians are CAVE people, you know C-A-V-E?"

The dinner guests asked what did these letters stand for?

"Citizens Against Virtually Everything!" Laughter. "We all got our work cut out for us. And nobody knows that better than our good doctor. He sees the worst of us, and he's tryin' like hell, with that great old guy Bill Starbuck, to make us better."

The party broke up. Orville was impressed at how well the Schooners ended their party, disengaging slowly with just the right words, as if they never wanted their guests to leave. Henry suggested to Milt and Penny that they bring their kids and guns out to the Federation of Polish Sportsmen's Club for a turkey shoot and barbecue again soon.

"You've got guns? Orville asked Penny, startled.

"You got to, the way things are. We're trying to get Amy interested, but she's in between the Schooner boys and won't play with either." A knowing glance. "Yet."

"Milt, too?" Orville said, stunned.

"Just a deer rifle, for hunting season," Milt said. "And a 9-millimeter pistol."

"Jews with guns," Orville said indignantly. "What's wrong with this picture?"

"Tell it to an Israeli!" Milt cried out drunkenly. "Talk about tough mothers. Two eyes for an eye! Teeth for a tooth! Never again!"

Faith tugged hard at Orville's arm, making him lose his balance and sending him into a floor-to-ceiling heavy antique breakfront, which wobbled ominously as if it, too, were loaded and about to crash to the floor.

"Whoa! Dangerous!" Orville said. "An accident waiting to happen. You oughta get that trued up, Henry."

"Thanks, doc!" Henry said delightedly. "My man will see to it tomorra."

Wobbly himself from the booze, Orville dimly felt Faith pressed tightly to him out on the porch, everybody saying good night to the excellent Schooners.

"Henry," Orville said mockingly, "you're a great American."

"Thanks, old friend," Henry said, taking it as a compliment. "Can't tell you how much it means to me and my family that you're back home, and that you came to our home tonight. It's a start, a good start, and I look forward to keepin' this friendship goin'."

"Come back 'n' see us, doctor," Nelda Jo said, hugging Orville hard, so that he felt those grapes pressing through her thin fabric and his thin shirt, muscats set in breasts firm as mangoes. "Or I'll be all over you like white on rice!"

"Works for me," Orville heard himself reply.

"Be good, you two!" Schooner called out.

"Be bad!" Nelda Jo called out after them. "Go for it! Feel the burn!"

As he walked across the square holding up Faith, Orville looked back at Henry and Nelda Jo, side by side, arms around each other under that golden globe of a porch light, waving them on to good luck in sex.

Orville was horny and drunk, Faith drunk and willing. But no. Celestina was way too much with him. He put Faith in Penny's old bed, he in his own. His last thoughts, as boozy sleep slid down over him like a big eyelid over the day: I'm a young man with a bright future hidden somewhere in my past. It's hard to be a doctor for a town that you despise. And why in the world does Henry Schooner care about earning my respect?

Honey-bunny,

Hiya! How are you? I imagine I'm fine. Heaven can't be worse than life, can it? I can't imagine I'm in Hell.

By now you've settled in, so you and I can get comfy and talk. Your sister always talked to me, except when she was going through her adolescent phase with that Scomparza boy—Catholic, but nice. But you never did. Here's a question: Why, in all the photos Sol took of the family, you're never smiling? He always said things to make us smile, the usual "Say cheese" or one of his dumb jokes. Never worked on you, oh no. Were you depressed? Just thought I'd ask.

By now I bet you've got a girl. My guess and hope is that the lucky one is Rebecca Shapiro, sister of the nice young doctor. Not the most attractive girl, but smart. It takes a special kind of girl to become a CPA don't you agree? Her brother the doctor told me she's a tiger in bed, so you might look into her. Tigress. But I tigress. I hope you find a nice Jewish girl—except that Faith Schenckberg! Do not—repeat—do not mess with her. Jewish, but a tramp. For once, listen to me. Like with dessert: do not indulge.

Orville put down the letter in disgust, his head throbbing. It was eleven Sunday morning, the day after the Schooner party. He felt like shit. His tongue felt like an army had marched across it during the night, and his head like it was now marching through his brain, up over the gyri, down into the sulci, using spare fissures for latrines.

Facing Faith in the morning had been tough. In the glare of daylight the tracks of her plastic surgery—nose job, chin tuck—were all too apparent to his doctor's eye. They'd sat across the table at a breakfast of strong coffee, aspirin, untouched halved grapefruits, and cigarettes.

Faith had wanted to chat, Orville did not. He'd tried to be polite but felt that if he didn't get her out in twenty minutes he would plunge a serrated grapefruit spoon into her heart, or maybe into his own. Secretly he'd had himself beeped for "an emergency," and with a promise to see Faith again soon, he'd ushered her out.

He picked up the letter and read on:

Love is a many-splendored thing, but then there are the Sols of the world. I never told you this, but as soon as Penny was born I decided I'd had enough of Sol. But I couldn't go through with it. Was I a coward? Well, it was wartime and for all his faults the man had a certain earning power. But I'll never forgive him for dragging me to Columbia.

I bet you're practicing with Bill. I mean, what else would you do, sell toys? Bill's Christian, but nice. Nice man, terrible doctor. I went to him with that pain in my groin and he gave me that Ointment of Starbusol, so I went around even to social functions smelling like a pine tree and it turned out to be a hernia! And all my years of dizziness and tinnitus in one ear that he misdiagnosed as inner ear until I went to Sinai and they found the brain tumor. So that's another reason I brought you home: Good health care for Columbians. But I'm writing for another reason: suicide.

Do you know it runs in the family, on my side? (Sol's side is full of pathetic, *meshuggeneh* optimists.) You know Aunt Bernice who supposedly "fell" in the kitchen? Nope. Head in the oven. You remember in the Old Country my father's father Abraham, at the height of his success selling hides to the Russian Army for the Japanese War, supposedly died in combat? Wrong again. Slit his own throat. Do you know how blue I used to get, not hearing from you, not even a postcard or a call? Knowing you were angry at me? I got suicidal, too, you bet. Old people think a lot about death. Getting old is not for sissies. Especially disfigured and handicapped, from all those nerves being cut. "Do you have hobbies?" someone asked me the other day. "No, I have doctors." Sol tried hard, taking me on trips, but he never took me on my dream trip—doing Russia, that boat trip down the Vodka. So, suicide. You never understood me, never. I was brave, and well-informed. You don't really know about life until you're dead, and now I am (well, not now, but now) and now I do. So read every word as if it were carved in stone, like Genesis was, and treat me right—which, for you, would be a *first!*

Love Mom

Orville threw the letter aside. He poured himself a Dickel on ice and cracked a Budweiser—neither seemed enough, on its own—and glanced out the kitchen window to make sure she wasn't flying around.

Well, she was and she wasn't. There she was, more hovering than flying. Outfitted for travel—brown worsted jacket and skirt, pumps, navy blue pillbox hat. She looked tired, bedraggled. He stared at her.

"Of course I'm tired, doll, I just flew in from the coast."

"The Gulf Coast? The condo in Naples?"

"The West Coast, Hollywood. It's not easy, flying all the way cross-country on a broomstick! Haha!" She floated away over the copper dome of the courthouse.

Dead, she's funny? Relieved that Bill was taking call, he picked up the phone and dialed Celestina in Rome to make final arrangements for her arrival the next day.

It rang for a long time.

"*Ja? Ja? Sprechen?*" A man's voice—groggy, as if just awakened. It was five in the afternoon in Rome.

"Celestina? Celestina Polo? Is Celestina there?"

"Vait."

Ohhh shit, Orville thought, waiting. And waiting.

A rustling, maybe sheets. "*Pronto?*" Celestina.

"It's me." His heart was pounding.

"This is not the very good time to talk."

"Okay." He tried to stay calm. "I just wanted to make sure everything's okay."

"Bad news."

"What?"

"Hold, *per favore.*" A phone moving, a door closing. He felt his heart fall into his gut, as when, with her in Orta, he'd gotten the telegram of his mother's death.

An extension picked up. Celestina said, "I cannot come tomorrow."

"What do you mean? You've got to come! You have no choice but to come!"

"I'm going to Nepal."

"Nepal?" He was screaming. "With a *German?*"

"Swiss."

"You can't. I won't stand for it. I'll come."

"It is not what you think. The banker owns half an elephant. In a hidden valley filled with yogis and monks. It is the chance of a lifetime, a spiritual journey. Rafting. Venture capital for the all-Euro *sangha!* Not for me, for the *dharma.* It is life, *caro,* life—either you grab it or you miss it."

"Wait. Hold it." He breathed. "I'm breathing."

"Good. I feel your sensual breath through the very phone."

"What about us?"

"I love you still with all my heart."

"Well, then come! Come here! Don't go to Nepal!"

"I will be back. I will come to you. I promise."

"You've been promising for three months!"

"But it seems like only yesterday that we were in Orta, no?"

"No. It seems like a year! I can't believe you're doing this to me. For a German?"

"A Swiss. In the war, they were neutral."

"In *that* war, they were neutral."

"I feel your hurt, but I—"

"Hey, it's simple, baby. I love you. Come."

She was crying, sobbing. "Dearest one, my heart is breaking."

"Then come. Come now."

She hesitated. "Tomorrow I leave for Nepal. When I come back, perhaps—"

"No. If you don't come tomorrow, it's over. Either you grab it or you miss it."

"Then I shall miss it now. But it is merely now. *Carissimo, arrivederci!* Always remember, it is—"

"No, I didn't mean—"

"—a *gift*." She sobbed.

"But I can't live—"

Click.

Orville stood there dazed, the phone buzzing in his ear. Then, frantic, feeling he had forced her to choose when she was holding open the choice, he frantically redialed. The phone rang and rang. He redialed again. It rang and rang. He hung up.

Suicide? He had barbiturates, a needle, good veins. A strange thought came to his mind: I'd kill myself, but I don't want to make my mother happy.

He began pacing around the dead house. Pacing, pacing.

Everything's falling apart. Gotta get out of this house. Run.

Going out the front door, black bag in hand, he saw a sight that blasted him again. The Family Schooner Raking Leaves. Two blond boys were being chased around the front yard by the athletic blond mom, all three diving into the big pile of leaves and scattering a rainbow up into the autumn air, while the white-haired dad stood by, smiling, in one hand a rake, the other cradling a pipe out of which an enticing, even healthy, wire of smoke arose as if hooking into a higher good, even a common good. Schooner saw Orville and waved gaily, gesturing to his neighbor to come join the Sunday fun.

A molten pulse of envy hit Orville in his solar plexus, sparking the filigree of tiny nerves to fire, knocking the breath out of him. He staggered, trying to hide it from Schooner. He hoisted his black bag as an explanation.

Schooner gave him a thumbs-up and then a clenched fist "Go for it!" The pipe stem pointed to the heavens.

Heart in shreds, feeling transparent and with no idea of who he was now or what he was doing except that he was mortally wounded and alone with the pain, Orville reflexively raised his own fist and smiled.

He closed the coffinlike door of the Chrysler on himself and was filled with self-loathing. He smashed the steering wheel as hard as he could, feeling a welcome pain in his fists and screamed at himself, "Asshole! You asshole! You jerk!"

◊ ◊ ◊

Driving aimlessly around what now seemed remarkably desolate and ugly countryside, sometimes enraged and screaming and banging the steering wheel and sometimes feeling as sad and lonely as all the men he'd doctored as they'd died with no one else there—in the end, from the whole world, no one else there!—he tried to keep afloat. He found himself way out on 9H, driving fast past Lindenwald, the home of President Martin Van Buren whoever he was, and then whizzing past a small pond bordered with two peculiar tiny old houses—one brick, one white clapboard. For some reason he stopped, turned around, and went back.

In the parking lot was an old, beaten-up Ford station wagon with fake wooden paneling, a Country Squire. On its bumper was the message WORTH SAVING. The sign on the brick house read LUYKAS VAN ALEN HOMESTEAD 1737. On the white clapboard one, ICHABOD CRANE SCHOOLHOUSE 19TH C. An old woman with her gray hair in a badly done bun beckoned him to the homestead.

On his suicidal afternoon off, Orville was not ready for old women in badly done buns. He skulked into the schoolhouse.

A single small room. Rows of kid-sized one-piece wooden desks and chairs, facing, to his left, a blackboard above which hung a nineteenth-century American flag, George Washington and Abraham Lincoln, and A Dog and A Cat. Across the room were two tall windows, half-open. The room, like all the distemperate schoolrooms of his past that had been either too hot or too cold, was too hot. Through the century-old glass the red-leafed maples and white birches wobbled.

Orville put a fingertip into a groove carved in a desktop, tracing a Cupid's heart and arrow linking one JS & SB. Feeling a rush of sorrow for these long-dead children and whatever was now dying inside himself, he raised his eyes to the windows to get away to get out, and lifted his hands to his chin, his fingers on his cheeks as if they could keep things in place, aligned, alive.

His hands dropped to his sides, hanging down helplessly. His nose clogged up and his throat ached dryly, presaging real tears, and for the first time since his divorce from his first love—from innocence itself, re-ally—he lost the fight and stood there with tears easing down his cheeks. He felt he had lost his place in the world—no Celestina, no Lily, no real friends, even—nothing to run away to anymore, but nothing to stay for either. No place in the world and a lot of time left.

All at once he sensed he was not alone. He turned. In the corner to his right, a woman sat at a desk.

Their eyes caught and held. Hers, in the low light from those two west-facing windows, glinted a fresh light green. Her hair was bright red, pulled back into a girlish ponytail, and her skin was that redhead's cream, sparsely freckled. Revealed by her sleeveless scoop-necked dress, the muscles of her shoulders and neck seemed prominent for her slender-ness. She'd made up her eyes with care, liner and shadow, which seemed strange, to make your eyes up for a lonely volunteer Sunday afternoon where she might encounter only a few blue-haired ladies or some lumber-ing dodoes looking for some free activity for their kids. Her plump scarlet lips were pursed, and her head was tilted, in curiosity. It seemed terribly still in the room, as if time had stopped, leaving something else.

He wiped his cheeks. Embarrassed at her seeing him so opened up, he walked over to her and stood in front of her schoolmarmish desk. "Brings back a lot of memories," he said with a deliberate casualness.

"I know. For me, too. It's a faithful restoration. Any questions?"

Just why are you so stunningly beautiful? is what went through his mind. And why is your voice like music? And why no wedding ring? Shyly, he said only, "No."

"Well, if you do, just ask." She smiled brightly and went back to her book, a thick, oversized volume with tiny print.

Unwilling to break off, Orville searched for something—anything—to engage her in conversation. He noticed, hanging above the desk where she sat, one of those old prints of a whale being harpooned by a whaler. Four dollars. Amy might like it.

"Excuse me?" She looked up. "Could I have one of those?"

"Sure. There should be one right here." She leaned over from her chair to search in a cardboard box on the floor. Orville couldn't help glancing down her scoop-necked dress, seeing in all that healthy musculature healthy breasts, bulging up out of a white bra like waves breasting the ocean, all alabaster. He looked away. She riffled through the tubes of prints and sat back up, face flushed. "You picked our most popular print. We may be sold out. If you have time, I can look in the cloakroom."

"I've got time, yes."

He watched her gather herself and place both arms solidly on the desk and kind of hoist herself up and start to walk away from him across the room and—Oh, God, she's walking with a limp? His heart went out to her, seeming to strain against his ribs with each step, rooting for her to make it. What he had thought was her dress was actually a blouse. To cover her leg—was it childhood polio?, she looked the right age for it—she would always wear pants. What pain, to see this! Something about seeing this exquisitely lovely woman his age who had seemed to be in the prime of life and health, with practiced difficulty lurching hard on one foreshortened and probably withered leg, rolling on it at the hip as if about to fall before catching herself on the good leg, planting herself solidly once again, and limping on, threading a path through the desks. He was shocked, and touched. More touched for her making that journey away from him without looking back, without asking for help, without hiding a thing, knowing she was being seen. As he, too, had just made a journey to sorrow so frankly before her, but with the safety net of thinking he was alone. More—she walked with dignity. He found himself tearing up again.

Pretending to inspect the other maps and posters and gag items such as a Day-Glo Orange whale hat with flippers for earflaps, he heard her limp back—*Ka-plott . . . Ka-plott . . .*—and heard her call out happily, "We're in luck!"

He turned, smiled at her smile. She handed him the tightly rolled whale, went back behind the desk and braced herself on her arms again and lowered herself into her seat. Orville's reaction to her was so powerful that he had to fight it down into nonchalance. He handed her five dollars. She handed him one back. Now what?

"Why whales?" he asked, prolonging the time with her.

"What?"

"Why whales?"

"'Why whales' *what?*" she asked, coaxing him as if he were a slow learner.

He felt like an eleven-year-old boy flirting with an eleven-year-old girl, his yearning making him so nervous that he sounded like a moron. "Why, in Columbia, the whale-thing? The logo, the street signs, SPOUT? I grew up here. I've been away twenty years, and I keep asking Columbians 'Why whales?' and all they say is 'Caught 'em in the river.' I was taught that, too, in school here. So I say, 'But whales live in seawater, right? And the Hudson is freshwater, right?' And the Columbians go, 'Duhh ...'" She chuckled. "And then they think it over some more, and they go, 'Duhhh ...'"

She laughed, runs of Mozart. Their eyes met. She laughed harder, now doubled over. It was contagious. He laughed with her. Finally, she surfaced, blushing, the blush spilling down her throat, her chest, and that lovely cleavage.

"You really want to know?"

"*You* know?"

"I know."

"My life is saved." She seemed startled by this. "Just joking," he said. "Tell me."

As if to collect herself, she closed her eyes and took a deep breath in and then slowly let it out. "It's the American Revolution, okay?"

"I remember."

"Good. It's good to remember American Revolutions. During it, the Nantucket whaling fleet is at the mercy of the British Navy, which destroys it. After the war, the rich Nantucket merchants decide that they don't want to go through that again. They form a group to search out a deepwater port, safe from attack. They're Quakers, peace-loving, spiritual folk. Very thrifty. Very wealthy. They send a delegation from Nantucket on a journey to this part of the world, in a three-masted whaling ship, to find a new home. They poodle around Long Island, almost buy a farm on the East River in Manhattan, and stop at Kingston—then called Esopus. One day, in 1784, they sail around a bend in the river to where Columbia is now. Is this boring?"

"Fascinating."

"I talk too much history, my friends say. It's my job. I'm the town historian. My name's Miranda Braak."

"Orvy Rose. I'm a doctor, working with Bill Starbuck. Temporarily."

"Oh," she said, as if surprised. "Yes, dear old Bill. I'd heard he'd gotten some help. And it's you."

"Yeah. But I had no idea Columbia had a town historian."

"I pushed for it. Columbia's bicentennial is next year. I convinced the Columbians there might be tourist money in it. The job doesn't pay much, but at least it's a job. I supplement it by volunteering—figure *that* one out." They laughed again. "So, there's no 'Columbia' here, then, just two stores and a ferry. Actually, we'd better back up a bit. Henry Hudson lands his ship the *Half Moon* here—*maybe* here—in 1609." She glanced at her watch. "I've got to go soon. I'll give you the *Reader's Digest* version, condensed?"

Orville nodded.

"Okay. So. The wealthy, upper-class Dutch settle here in the mid-1600s. Wanting wetland and farmland and not river frontage, they build their village miles inland, to the northeast, at Spook Rock. 'Spook' comes from an old Indian legend, I think Iroquois. The river landing is owned by two feuding Dutch families, lower class, with some Mohican blood. There are two wharves, two stores, two of everything—and not enough trade—both families keep getting even poorer. A group of Mohicans, ostracized from their tribe because they're drunks, do the heavy lifting, for booze. The Dutch storekeepers own the North and South Bays and the cliff we call Parade Hill. The place is called Claverack Landing, after the clay cliffs, or *klavers*. You can still see them rising above the North Swamp. *Rack* is reach."

She glanced at him, as if to check if he were still interested. Leaning back against a child's desk, he said, "I'm with you. Go on."

"One day a huge, three-masted whaling ship comes upriver and docks. Out of it come white men in the homespun gray suits and tall hats of the Quakers. They speak no Dutch. The Dutch speak no English. Nobody knows what the Mohicans speak. The Quakers, led by Seth Jenkins, like what they see: two deepwater ports north and south, protected by the high escarpment overlooking the river, the bays, and the mountains. So they offer—"

"*Escarpment?*" he asked, delighting in the word.

She smiled. "Escarpment, yes." A glance. "So . . . they buy it and settle it at once, bringing a few houses off the boat that day. Thirty Proprietors from Nantucket form the governance of the town. They start fresh, build their utopia."

"Utopia? This?" She laughed at his astonishment, a little riff of Lizst. "Wait a second," he went on. "They brought houses off of the boat?"

"They dismantled some houses in Nantucket and reassembled them here. Check out the Curtiss House, at Washington and First. It has a Widow's Walk, 128 miles from the ocean. So they lay out their utopia, first on big sheets of paper, then on the land. The streets are perfectly ruled, and—"

"Which is," he said, beaming, "why the grid!"

"Which is why the grid, exactly. Five long straight streets, eight cross streets, dead-true square corners. Alleys between the long streets for sanitation and freight. And in a grand flourish of Quaker imagination, the cross streets are named First, Second, Third—"

"Hurry, the tension's unbearable!" he said with a smile.

She laughed. "Fourth through Eighth! Anyway, they rebuild their whaling port here. Start Quaker meetings, Quaker culture, the Society of Friends." She seemed to consider this and then embrace it. "Wonderful phrase, don't you think?"

"Yes. Do you think it's possible?"

"Historically not, for any length of time."

"Why haven't I seen any pictures of these Quakers?"

"They didn't—still don't—believe in images. The whaling industry—sperm oil, permaceti for perfumes, whalebone corset stays—attracts all kinds of other shipping-related business, like rope making and—"

"As in Rope Alley?"

"Yes. They stretch the strands of hemp for a hundred yards up Rope Alley, to braid rope, yes. They're at a perfect crossroads: farm goods from the east, timber from the Catskills to the west, able to send goods upriver and down between Albany and New Amsterdam. The utopia gets a name—Columbia—and becomes a boomtown. Within five years, 4,000 people live here. It's the third biggest port on the East Coast. And the life blood of the port is . . . are—"

"Whales! Those cute whales!"

"Yes! Ships are sent out all over the world—to the South Atlantic all the way to Tierra del Fuego, to the South Pacific, to Japan. You could walk all the way across the South Bay on the decks of ships anchored there side by side waiting to unload."

"It's not a bay, though. It's a swamp."

"They killed the bay with the railroad decades later. But here's the good part, the irony. There's *always* an irony." She squinched her eyes up conspiratorily. "The town, this 'good' town of strict, moral, orderly, religious folk, attracts those classically 'bad' elements that boomtowns do: gamblers, thieves, con men, whores. The Quakers attract the whores!" She smiled, then sighed. "But we have to stop. My son's soccer game's almost over. Can't be late, you know."

"No," Orville said, startled, then saddened. "Actually I don't."

"Oh. I see." Miranda seemed to pick up on his sadness, the red thread in the weave. "Sorry, but I do have to go."

"But it's a cliffhanger."

She chuckled, gathered up her things, and hoisted herself up. They walked together quietly to the door. "I'd love to hear more," he said, holding the door open for her.

"Well, you're in luck, because we're only up to 1803. I live in the old Staats House, on the river north of town. I'm in the book."

"I'm always in the office or the hospital. Occasionally in my mother's house, on Courthouse Square."

Together they noticed that rain, its arrival unnoticed, was now beating down hard on the tin roof of the schoolhouse. Lightning. One thousand one, one thousand two, one thous—*boom!* A crack of thunder, a roll, *Ka-rrr-rrb-bbooom!* And then the echo off the mountains, and the echo of the echo.

"Rip Van Winkle and his men are bowling in the Catskills," Orville shouted over the din.

"Is that what it is?" she shouted back.

"I was taught that in school."

"Well, at least you learned one thing that was true."

"Need a hand?"

"Thanks. I'm fine." She opened her umbrella. "Want to get in under?"

"Nope. I love rain!" Miranda looked at him quizzically and then laughed.

Orville strolled nonchalantly toward the Chrysler, thinking Handel's *Water Music.* Rain was popping off the bald patch on the top of his head, sluicing over his eyes, funneling down either cheek, washing away the scratchy salt residue, soaking his trim beard, his white shirt, his khaki pants. The soaking reminded him of Holland and Celestina Polo.

He felt a surge of grief, a pinching in his tear ducts. It passed. His heart felt wet too, all senses wet too, so that he caught the scent of wintergreen and thought Starbusol but it was coming from a small grove of finally-drenched and relieved blue spruce and he felt happy, happy as a dog's nose in spring, which was of course strange because winter was coming. His eyes climbed a spruce trunk up to a bough near the top where a big bird perched, huddling against the downpour. He and the bird stared at each other through the curtain of rain and alleged evolution. The bird gathered itself and sprang up and out into the wet air and started to fly in a circle, its cry a high-pitched *scree, scree,* so that the man knew it was a red-tailed hawk.

The hawk in the rain circled tiltingly above the man as if on the rim of a plate spinning on a stick. They were tethered together by their shared sight.

In the man's eyes? A blurred shape in flight, a dreamhawk.

In the hawk's eyes? Too big to eat too earthbound to fear.

Man and bird, doctor and hawk, general practitioner and red-tailed, Orville Abraham Rose and Unnamed, did the dance of shared and differing creaturedness for a moment and then the bird flew off into speckhood, leaving a few red tailfeathers of hope clutched in the man's and the woman's memories and imaginations, maybe, as these things go in these moments, forever.

Orville looked back. Miranda, under her umbrella, was nearing her car. He noticed again the bumper sticker: WORTH SAVING. That's it! She was the limping woman in the picket line in front of the General Worth Hotel his first evening home.

"Worth Saving?" he called out to her through the clattering rain.

"What?"

"Worth Saving?"

"Yes! 'Worth Saving,' most definitely, yes!"

Part Two

◇ ◇ ◇

No one is responsible for their face
until they're forty.

—*Abraham Lincoln (apocryphal)*

9

The next Sunday afternoon, Miranda Braak was driving into Columbia toward the Worth Hotel to meet Mrs. Tarr and Orville and his niece, Amy. Orville had called the morning after their schoolhouse meeting, saying he'd like to see her again and how about the next Sunday afternoon.

"We could talk more history," he said. "Starting at 1803."

"Why talk when we can do?" she answered. "I mean, if you'd like, we could visit a historical site. I promised Mrs. Tarr—she's my coconspirator from the DAR—that I'd do an hour's picketing with her at the Worth. We could start there."

"Deal."

Miranda still felt high from the afternoon in the schoolhouse. Like a kid anticipating a great tomorrow, she'd had a restless night and had awakened early, even before her son, Cray. All week long she'd been trying to match the reality of the man with what his mother had told her.

Selma had said that in the summer of 1961, when Orville was sixteen, she had come home from brain surgery at Albany Medical Center. She left home a beautiful woman. Two months later she came back with one side of her face slack, an eye sewn shut, and her shaven head in a turban. Back then, the normal way to handle such a thing was not to tell your children what the surgery was and not to allow them to visit. Weak and depressed and wanting to die, the only thing that kept her alive, Selma said to Miranda, was her children, "wanting to see them grow up and settle down."

When she came home that June, Sol tried his hardest to help, but hey, it was golf season. Her daughter, Penny, at loose ends after graduating from New Paltz State Teachers College and dating Milt Plotkin up in Albany, was skittish about caring for her. Milt was about to take off on a Beth El Synagogue Summer Program to a *kibbutz* and had invited Penny to join in the Dead Sea fun. Selma encouraged Penny to go, to pursue being pursued by Milt—as Selma had put it, "sacrificing my happiness for my only daughter's only chance at her own."

Which left Orville. That summer he had fallen in love for the first time, with a Columbian girl named Laurice. "Nice, but Lithuanian," Selma had said. He finally seemed to be coming out of his shyness, Selma thought, having friends on the basketball team, and hanging around with Bill Starbuck. He was blossoming at last, his days and nights full of adventure.

"But you know what?" Selma had said. "Despite the pull of his very exciting life, Orville was there for me. Day after day, week after week, my son sat with me out on the back porch, helping me learn to use my face again, my brain again. I told him, over and over, don't stay with me today. Go out and play with your friends, go swim at Taconic, go to Catskill and golf with Sol, hang out with Bill, go out even with Laurice—but don't don't don't sacrifice your summer for me. You're free to go, honey-bunny. Fly!" With a grand humility, Selma looked Miranda in the eye and said, "And you know what? That boy would have none of it. He stayed. Stayed and took care of his mother. My son took care of me."

When Miranda realized who it was standing before her in tears that afternoon in the schoolhouse, her heart floated up to her throat and in an instant it all made sense. His tears were from the recent death of his beloved mother. Loving her so much, how could he have gotten over it in just three months? Especially after missing the funeral. She saw, then, that the whole thrust of his life, the conjunction of his caring for his mother with his finding a kindly old doctor to hang around with, had been determined by that summer of helping, that summer in which a shy boy had learned compassion and had grown into what Miranda had come to feel was a rarity in her world: a truly caring man. And now a caring doctor besides? She knew from her own long history with doctors how rare that was.

Yet there was no way that Miranda would have volunteered to Orville that she had heard about him from Selma, or even that she had known his mother. Miranda had a love affair with secrets. From the time she was a girl, keeping secrets was at the core of her being. It began in earnest on the day when she was almost seven, as she was walking from the living room into the lanai of her parents' house in Boca Grande, Florida, and she fell down. She got up, surprised, but when she tried to walk, again she fell down. Poliomyelitis had entered her life, and it would never leave. Like a tree growing around a spike, the girl grew around the crippled part, taller and stronger, and more muscular for the paralysis.

But she grew differently. In the face of the other children's small cruelties about her limp and her steel brace, she grew a will of iron. She learned to keep her rage secret, ironclad. After the war, her father, a postal clerk, and her mother, a junior high schoolteacher, had migrated from Minnesota to the Gulf Coast. Their cool northern reticence melded into a southern courtesy; in her family, anger was transformed to politeness, hurt to feigned interest. She learned to keep her steel brace secret under her pant legs, her leg secret under dashboards and desks and tables and counters. Only occasionally did it come to frank attention, such as when someone could not get past her in the aisle of a darkened theater and she had to say out loud the humiliating, "I'm sorry, I'm disabled. You'll have to go around." The iron spike inside even prevented her from getting a car sticker for handicapped parking.

Miranda came to think that, in a world she saw as often unkind, secrecy worked. To be open, to tell the truth, meant being vulnerable. And to be vulnerable was to be powerless. It was out of the question. Secrecy for her became a virtual daring.

Her husband, Cray's father, was an actual daredevil. He was a young engineer on a series of oil-drilling platforms in the Gulf. They had met when he was vacationing for a week at the Gasparilla Inn in Boca Grande, where she was waitressing, earning money for history graduate school in Tallahassee—she had always loved history, first going with her parents to the sites, then the study. He overwhelmed her with his passion for action, and for her. He was always pushing the edge, from fast cars to fast boats to fast planes to, finally, in those planes used for stunts in the movies, aerobatics.

Soon after Cray turned two, her husband dared too much. At an air show in Clearwater, which she refused to attend, in front of hundreds of people in a viewing stand, he took off and did a daring flip too close to the ground and crashed. Both of Miranda's parents were dead by then, so she was left with no one but her two-year-old son and a spinster aunt in Grand Forks, North Dakota. So three years ago she and Cray had moved up to a piece of property left her by an uncle, a house on the banks of the Hudson River north of Columbia. She had spent parts of her summers there as a girl and loved it. Cray and she were poor, but okay.

Miranda grew around the tragedy of her husband's sudden death, but again grew differently. Except when Cray or someone else asked, she never talked about it. It went up into her attic of secrets. Over the four years since his death she came to realize that, in a sense, secrets are lies told to the world, and each has a price. But for her the price was acceptable. Her virtual daring was now overlaid with a certain fear. She had opened herself up to the world and had fallen down, opened herself up to loving a man and had lost him.

So when Orville called that Monday morning and asked to see her again, she was thrilled and scared. She feared being thrilled. Hadn't he said, about working with Bill Starbuck, that he was only there "temporarily"?

Much as she had opened up to him at that first moment, she could not afford a temporary man. Her fear was not only for her being left. The life in her life was her son.

Then there was Selma. The two women met about a year before Selma's death, in the Columbia Area Library. Miranda was working in the archives, researching her thesis. Selma was volunteering at the main desk. Seeing Selma's facial disfigurement, Miranda's heart opened to her. They talked. It turned out that Selma was involved in many civic projects in Columbia and out in Kinderhook County. She said Miranda would be perfect to join the committee planning the faithful restoration of the Library. Miranda agreed.

After one of the meetings, Selma invited Miranda back to her house for tea. Driving up Washington in the Chrysler, Selma took a detour at Second Street, before going back across Fourth to the Courthouse Square. Miranda asked why.

"I'm superstitious," Selma said. "I never drive by the Worth Hotel. It's the one project I won't get involved in."

"Why not?

"It reminds me of when I was still beautiful. When we first came here in '46, there was only one place where all the gala events were held—the Worth. It was a grand hotel then. I volunteered in anything that would have me, and when I was in charge—president of the Hospital Auxiliary, the library, even the Junior League (first Jew, imagine!)—I had all my affairs there. It and I were beautiful. After, I never went back."

That afternoon and into the evening, the two women had a heart-to-heart. Their handicaps drew them together. Not only the sagging face and withered leg but the mutual understanding of a life-tree trying to grow around that spike pounded in. The younger woman had many more years to grow around her insult. She would not talk about it, but she listened to the older woman with understanding.

Selma, having lived through conflicts with her own daughter and the increasingly long flights of her only son, and having felt the stirrings of new love for her only granddaughter, reassured Miranda about the ability of the life force to compel endurance in the face of losing a loved one. Miranda saw Selma as so blunt that she dared reveal a core of truth. Selma saw Miranda as so shy that she could be trusted. Both were daughters and mothers. Both had lost men. Lost men were in the air.

Selma told Miranda about Orville's kindness after her operation and about the terms of her will—his getting the money and house and car if he lived there continuously for a year and thirteen days. Why thirteen days? Selma smiled mischievously but didn't say.

Hearing this, at first Miranda was startled. It seemed controlling, and weird. But as she listened further to Selma, listened to how two years ago her son had gone "gallivanting around the world" and how "every day I think of him and it's like the worst heartburn on earth," it resonated with how she herself was starting to feel about her own son, Cray, now six. He had started moving away from her. She saw in Selma's pain where her lesser pain was pointing. She identified with her as a mother of a son. She admired Selma's spunk; the lady was *gutsy*.

Miranda could see how badly Selma wanted to give her son a chance to come home to his family and how, as weird as they seemed, the terms of her will might just work. After all, those times when Cray didn't want to be with her or didn't want her around was like death, was it not?

When Orville walked in, Miranda was sitting behind the desk staring at an oversized facsimile volume of Ellis's 1848 *History of Kinderhook County*. Usually she read it with such fascination that she lost sight of time, finding herself awake at 3 A.M. when she thought it was only about eleven or, like a few weeks ago, almost forgetting to pick up Cray from his play date at his friend Steffie's house, over in Ghent. But that afternoon she couldn't make the words make sense. She kept reading the same passage over and over. She was worried about her son. In particular, she was worried about how for the last four years he hadn't had a father, or any other man, consistently in his life. She felt she was failing him. Lately she felt him spiraling out.

Earlier that afternoon Cray had his sixth birthday party, which she held at her house. Nine boys and Steffie. Cray and his friend Maxie Schooner, who had recently broken his wrist and was in a cast, had been playing baseball cards when Cray traded one to Maxie and then decided he wanted it back. Maxie didn't want to give it back. They argued. Theo Geiger, of the junkyard Geigers, and Cray's best friend, tried to intervene, but suddenly Cray hit Maxie as hard as he could on the cast. Miranda was stunned. He'd never done anything like that before. Maxie was more surprised than hurt. Cray was the one who started to cry. Shaken, she made it through the end of the party, the cake and the favors.

When Maxie's mom, Nelda Jo, learned about it, she was angry. "I've been meaning to tell you this, Miranda," she said at the door before she took him home, "you need to do something about your son—he's impulsive. That boy needs a man around to straighten him out."

Miranda had always felt fairly good about how she'd raised Cray since his father's death, but she always had doubts. Suddenly all she had were doubts. Her whole mothering world seemed to be collapsing around her. What mother wants her son to be cruel?

After the party, Cray and some of the other boys were supposed to go to their soccer game in Stuyvesant Landing.

"Do you still want to go, Cray?" she had asked.

"Yeah, but I don't want you to come."

Swallowing her pain, she said, "fine," dropped him and his friends off, and, fearing the thought of being alone, called Mrs. Tarr and arranged to volunteer with her that afternoon at the Ichabod Crane Schoolhouse.

Being in historical sites always made her feel safer, even safe. She had been sitting in the one-room schoolhouse feeling a little more safe, but her heart felt raw—raw about her failure as a mother and about celebrating a son's day of birth that echoed down the hollow where his dead father lay, raw about the losses and failures in her life—and then Orville walked in. He thought he was alone. It was one of those times, she thought, when you see a person absolutely the way they are. When he noticed her, his tears touched her deeply. His eyes were so open. A few minutes later, when she realized who he was, her heart went out to him—he was a son crying for his mother.

By the time she'd driven back out to the soccer field, there was no one there. The rain must have started sooner up in Stuyvesant. She stared at the soggy field, at a single soaked orange jersey left behind. Mike Fredrickson, Zeke's dad, must have driven Cray home. Nice going, lady, she thought. Yet another shred of evidence of your being a Bad Single Mom. She got out, put up her umbrella, walked carefully out onto the battered grass, picked up the orphaned jersey, and sloshed back to the car.

She drove home through the downpour to find Mike's pickup in the driveway. He and Zeke were sitting in the cab. She waved a thanks, and they took off. A light was on in Cray's room upstairs.

Miranda went in and called up the steep, narrow old stairs. "Cray?"

Nothing. Then, "Yeah?"

As gaily as possible, she called up, "I'm home, dear."

"'Kay, Mom." A little space of time. She barely breathed. "Look on the table."

"'Kay." On the kitchen table was a letter, sealed, addressed to "My Mom." She opened it. On a piece of porous lavender construction paper, in block capital letters done in black Magic Marker that had run fuzzy at the edges, was "Plez See My Hart."

◇ ◇ ◇ .

Now, a week later, as she pulled up in front of the Worth Hotel, she still felt the glow from that affirmation, from his just plain resilience—and hers, too. *Our* resilience, she thought. I've jiggled the red thread stretched between me and my son. He'd felt it and jiggled his end in return.

Mrs. Tarr of the DAR, her white hair in what, with each passing month of their picketing, seemed to Miranda an evermore eternal bun, was already wearing her sandwich board that declared either her or the hotel WORTH SAVING. The pail for donations was carefully positioned on the pavement, blaring plastic yellow into the crisp, sunny, and windy November day. Even though Miranda was fifteen minutes late, Orville and Amy were not there.

Miranda had never met Amy or spent any real time with Penny or Milt. After that heart-to-heart talk, Selma and Miranda had served together on committees and projects and occasionally had tea together, but they never again reached the same level of intimacy. It was as if they'd said enough, or maybe too much. Miranda lived several miles outside Columbia, and her circle of friends was up in Kinderhook, so she and Selma didn't see each other socially. And so their brief deep connection remained their secret.

This made Selma's sudden death hard for Miranda. At the surprisingly large funeral, standing on the fringe, she felt like an outsider. She searched the family members for Orville and was amazed that, given his closeness to his mother, he hadn't come. Eavesdropping as the mourners walked from the cemetery, Miranda heard that Orville was away somewhere in Europe, unreachable. Driving home alone from Selma's funeral, she was surprised at how sad she felt.

The day after Selma's funeral, Selma's maid, Hayley, showed up at Miranda's door. A short, plump, cocoa-skinned woman wearing thick-lensed glasses, a neat plaid dress, and a stylish red straw hat. She stood there with a large cardboard box in her arms from Scomparza Moving and Funeral. Hayley explained that she was on a secret mission from Selma. Sometime before her death, Selma had shown Hayley the sealed Scomparza box with a note "For Hayley" taped to it. If Selma died, Hayley was to take the box at once to Miranda, address enclosed. Selma made Hayley promise not to tell anyone, ever, that she had done so. Hayley had been the one to find

Selma dead in the kitchen. Keeping her wits about her, Hayley had put the box in the trunk of her car and then had gone back into the house to call Bill Starbuck.

"Now that she's passed," Hayley said to Miranda that August afternoon, getting up to go, "my mission done. Don't know what all's in it, but it's meant only for you." At the door she hesitated. "Miz Rose was a little strange, but *very* strong."

"Very. Strong and zany, yes."

"Amen."

Miranda opened the box. On top was a letter to her from Selma.

Dear Miranda,

Hi there! I'm dead now. I hope you are well. I hope I am well, too. Is "well" relevant in the Afterlife? Our rabbi knew nothing—couldn't even tell me if there's a Heaven or not. Nice man, but fat.

In a separate sealed shoebox is $5,000 in twenties—my secret bequest to you. Things with Sol were always tense, and just in case we decided to divorce I kept my own cash. Count it. I trust Hayley, but you know, you never know, with money.

In the big box are wrapped-up framed photographs, and a series of letters, from me to my son Orville. They are addressed to him at my house on the Courthouse Square. Each is sealed and stamped double (just in case the U.S. Postal Service raises the rates—nice group, but Irish). On each letter is a yellow Post-It note with a number—they are numbered in order—and with the number of weeks after Orvy arrives back in town at which time each letter is to be mailed. The first says, "To Be Mailed the Day before He Arrives." The second, "To Be Mailed Three Weeks after He Arrives," and so forth. They are to be mailed every two or three weeks for the year and thirteen days. At the end of that time, the remaining contents of the nice box are to be mailed to Orville. You must never reveal that you are the one mailing the letters!

Miranda was shocked. Bizarre! Why me? We'd had a heart-to-heart, a few other talks, served together on the Library committee, but that was it. Why *me?* Strange.

I know this may seem strange to you, dear, but it is the most important wish I leave you with. Even though we didn't spend much time together, I know I can trust you. That night we talked was so special! We both deserve a pat on the back—if I still *have* a back. If you are touched right now the way I am touched by writing this, dear, please mail these letters and never tell anyone.

This is my dying wish.

You are a mother. You have a son. We talked about our sons. Mine stayed and cared for me, and to pay him back I let him go, let him fly from the nest. But he flew too far and couldn't get back. My will, and these letters—love letters, really, with all the things I never got to tell him—are to help him see what he flew away from, and maybe help him find his way back.

Now I'll ask you one more thing. Walk outside. Look up in the sky and imagine me and put your hand on a rock or a Bible or cute little Cray's red hair and say, "I promise." I might not hear you—do the dead still have ears?—but I'll know. Or, God forbid, I'll know you didn't. Do it now. Feel good about it. Spend!

Love Your Selma

P.S. Do not open and read the letters. Love letters between a mother and a son are sacred and sound a little mushy and mawky to outsiders. Think of a similar correspondence between that beautiful Cray and you.

Miranda put down the letter. Unbelievable! She unsealed the shoebox (Mouse Schmerz Shoes). As she counted down through the bills she noticed they went from crisper newer ones to raggedy older ones—some seemed once-crumpled, hidden in a pocket or a change purse maybe. Five thousand exactly. It would go a long way for Cray and her. She thought it over. It was masterful, in a way. The whole thing had a certain logic of the heart. And how could she refuse Selma's dying wish?

She closed the Scomparza box and hauled it up to the attic, hiding it behind the big steamer trunk with the relics of her girlhood in Boca Grande and the mementos of her marriage. Then, feeling foolish, she went out to the river and sat on a boulder and put her hand on it and looked up at the hazy August sky and thought back to her girlish notion of Heaven—the feathered wings and golden halos and white choir robes—and said: "Okay, Selma, I promise."

Two weeks later, while she was doing research at the library, one of the volunteer librarians happened to mention that Selma's son, Orville, was due back the next day. That afternoon Miranda drove into Columbia and mailed the first letter.

"Sorry I'm late," Orville said now, as he and Amy stepped out of the Chrysler in front of the Worth Hotel. "Bill's on call and he's already swamped—I had to stay and help out." Miranda wore a white fisherman's sweater and knit cap, which set off her bright-red hair. To him, she looked stunning. "But here we are."

"I'm glad," she said. His worn leather jacket was open over a white shirt and a wild purple tie that fluttered in the strong breeze, giving him a jaunty, carefree look.

Silence, that paralytic silence known only to shy people.

Mrs. Tarr took over, introducing everyone to everyone. And then she started circling, Miranda following. Next, awkwardly, Orville. Then, happily, Amy.

"Didn't they have fashion shows here?" Orville asked.

"Righto!" said Mrs. Tarr. "The door's locked, but you can see in."

She ushered them beneath the sagging mouth of the portico to a window beside the front door. Leading down into the foyer were the remains of a grand curve of staircase. Orville dimly recalled seeing Selma come down that staircase in the cobalt-blue satin ball gown that she now was flying around in. The mahogany banister was mostly intact, but many of the black walnut steps were missing, probably stolen and sold for drugs. The foyer was littered with beer cans and Styrofoam thises-and-thats and a mangy sleeping bag and the charred remains of a campfire. Druggies and squatters and rats were the only guests.

"The fashion shows were benefits," said Mrs. Tarr, "put on by the Junior League or the Hospital Auxiliary. Your mother organized several. I miss her very much."

"Grandma Selma?" Amy asked, surprised.

"That's right, dear. Before you were born. I can still see how lovely she looked, coming down that staircase and then announcing the other girls one by one."

Amy considered this. "I wish I had seen her . . . I mean, lovely?"

"Oh she was divine!" said Mrs. Tarr, smiling. "It's chilly. Let's walk." She led the others in a tight ellipse as the wind picked up.

"Why Worth?" Orville asked Miranda.

"'Why Worth *what?*'" she asked back, a twinkle in her eye.

"Uncle O.?" Amy shouted, over the wind. "Why are we picketing?"

"Because, Amy," Miranda said, smiling at her, "your father wants to knock it down and put up a supermarket."

Amy's mouth made a little o. "My father?"

"Plotkin and Schooner are trying to knock it down."

Amy considered this. She stared at the decrepit hotel. "He wants to knock down this . . . this beautiful historical hotel where my Grandma Selma was a fashion model? What a *reeker!*" The others laughed. Miranda looked at Orville and winked. "Milt'd knock down his own mother for money! How can we stop him?"

"This is how," Miranda said.

"Let's go!"

They started circling again. But the wind had picked up, colder and stronger, a premature Canadian blast funneled by the Catskills and Berkshires into the Hudson Valley and then, at Columbia, breaking over the humpback of the town and turning into a whirlwind circling from North Swamp to South, blowing down the bright dying leaves of the Columbian fall and tormenting the unprepared people. The sandwich boards acted like sails, the big gusts catching and lifting them. Mrs. Tarr and Miranda clutched at the wooden edges as if holding onto the masts of a ship. Orville helped push them upwind and then, on the downwind leg, helped hold them steady.

"I'm freezing!" Amy cried. "I'm really, really cold!"

"Me, too!" Miranda shouted over the gusts. "Let's stop."

"Come to the DAR," said Mrs. Tarr. "We'll have hot chocolate."

The solid brick DAR was right next door, and soon they were cozily settled in the private library, cupping their mugs for warmth. Miranda and Orville smiled at each other once or twice, shyly.

Orville was surprised to find, still there after all these years, two immense whale jawbones set on end, spanning the lending desk like a bony arch. He recalled standing under them as a boy, the desk looming over him and those scary, pointy-teethed whales soaring up to the ceiling as he asked the woman if he could sign out one more book than normal—just *one* more, please?—and when his request was denied hearing Selma, looming even larger behind him, arguing with her, screaming in the dead silent library so that he wanted to crawl into one of the cracks in the floor. And suddenly his mind filled with the night when the Worth seemed to talk to him and—worse still—he pictured Celestina Polo in Nepal with the Swiss banker and the half-an-elephant, rafting and meditating and making love, and he began to feel really bad. Waves of longing and grief washed over him. The only things he knew that might just take away the pain were alcohol and what Celestina herself had taught him, to breathe. The first was unavailable, and the second brought her back even more intensely, making it worse. Desperate, afraid of casting a pall over all this warm and cozy and happy with them, he asked, with feigned interest, "So. Why Worth?"

"Why *what?*" Mrs. Tarr asked, cupping her ear. "Whatwhatwhat?" She was a patient of his, and Orville knew just how hard of hearing she was.

"Why Worth?" he repeated more loudly, looking to Miranda for help.

"Why Worth *what?*" Miranda teased, again.

"Who was he and what did he do to deserve a hotel?"

Shyly, Miranda smiled. They were back into their conversation at the schoolhouse. Feeling even more attracted to him now, Miranda found it easy to move with him that way, even a relief. "William Jenkins Worth is born in 1794 on Coffin Street, a son of two original Nantucket Quakers. In 1812, at eighteen, he's working as a clerk at Gadicke's Feed and Grain, up on Eighth, measuring out barley and oats and doing a lot of heavy lifting. He's bored stiff. General Winfield Scott, with seven hundred soldiers in snappy uniforms and the latest guns all aglitter and lots of big healthy horses and fifes and drums, camps overnight right on Courthouse Square on his way north to fight the War of 1812."

Amy and Orville asked, more or less together, "Which war was that?"

"Americans fighting the British and the Indians. Worth joins up, runs away from home. With General Apocalypse Smyth and General Scott, he's a hero at the Battle of Niagara, leads a massacre of the Indians at Chippewa, and becomes the Fourth Commandant of West Point. Restless, he runs off to massacre more Indians, this time in Florida in the Seminole War—Lake Worth, Florida, is named after him. All through the 1840s he's leading massacres, this time of Mexicans in the Mexican War."

"Yech!" Amy said. "Killing Native Americans? What a jerk."

"But jerks tend to rule, Amy dear," said Mrs. Tarr.

"No joke! In school, the boys go down the halls in groups so you can't get by, shouting 'Boys rule! Boys rule!' But we go, 'Boys drool! Boys drool!'"

"Jolly good for you!" said Mrs. Tarr. "I wish we girls had such guts in my day, yes."

"When I was little," Amy went on, "we chanted back at them, 'Girls go to college, to get more knowledge; boys go to Jupiter, to get more stupider.'"

"Which is," Miranda went on, laughing, "probably true of General Worth. He's stupid, but he looks great. He's said to be the most handsome man in the American army. Sitting on a horse he looks gorgeous, and he's a terrific dancer. The most popular dance of the day is 'The General Worth Quick-Step.' America falls in love with him. And here in his hometown, they name this, the best hotel in Kinderhook County, after him. Famous people stay here—politicians, itinerant opera singers, titans of industry. Because of his talent for massacre and his gorgeousness on horseback and his dancing, he's a natural to run for president. But he has a . . ." she smiled mischievously, "a *fatal flaw.* He was one of the most stupidly arrogant, self-centered men in history, and it brought him down. Talk about shooting yourself in the foot? He tries to hog the limelight of the Mexican War by personally receiving the surrender, upstaging the same General Winfield Scott who'd lifted him up out of being a nothing here in Columbia. When chastised by Scott, he writes bitter, self-serving letters to newspapers, ripping his benefactor to shreds. The powers-that-be retaliate, stationing him out in the middle of nowhere to fortify the new border with Mexico. To honor him they name the first fort in Texas after him."

"Fort Worth?" Amy asked. "I've been there with my parents. It's so uncool, like all yucky with golf courses. Milt plays there."

"It's a thrilling story," Orville said. "Columbia Boy Makes Good."

"Not so good," Miranda said. "He dies of cholera in San Antonio before he knows of the honor."

"A great American," Orville said cynically.

"In fact," Miranda said, "he almost is."

"Do they exist?"

"Try George Washington. Incredible man. After the Revolution he could have become a dictator, another Napoleon, but he gave the country back to the people. Steered us clear of becoming a banana republic."

"So now we've got a regular republic," he teased, "but with a banana in charge?"

Happily the group sipped hot chocolate and chatted bananas and Indians, whale jaws and Revolutions, while the howling wind rattled the huge old windows of the Federal-style house until Miranda had to leave to pick up Cray at soccer. And Amy and Orville would end their Sunday afternoon as usual at the Hudson Diner up at the Seventh Street Park with the lard-fried everythings of Orville's, and now Amy's, youth.

"And he's buried up there on Cemetery Hill?" Orville asked, as the group broke.

"Oh no!" Mrs. Tarr said, shocked. "That would be much too lowly for him. He's buried under an obelisk in Manhattan, Fifth and 25th, facing the Flatiron Building. All of his battles are carved on the obelisk. Chapulte-pec, Vera Cruz, Puebla, Lundy's Lane, Chippewa, Chorobusco—quite musical actually, are they not?"

All agreed that they were incredibly musical.

"And the historical irony, of course," Miranda said, "is that no one notices he's there. It's a traffic island now, railed in, and there's not much free sidewalk. Even if you did notice, it's such a busy spot, noisy and frantic with traffic, few people stop. If you looked casually you'd think it was a relic stolen from some tomb in Egypt. Nobody reads what's on it. Poor Worth."

As Mrs. Tarr flipped off the old light switches one by one, each with a sharp *clack,* Orville asked Miranda, "About the hotel, is there a chance you could win?"

"Almost certainly not. We've petitioned to have it put on the National Register of Historic Places, which delays things a little. To restore it would cost half a million. The people of Columbia want to tear it down. Most of our support comes from the people out in the county, but they don't have a vote. The feds have agreed to pay two-thirds of the demolition costs. We're waiting for the National Register to decide."

"It could be the centerpiece of the resurrection of downtown," said Mrs. Tarr. "The antiquers are with us, but they are few."

"So what are your chances?" Orville asked.

"Uncle O.!" Amy cried out. "You mean what are our chances, right? You're with us, right?"

"Totally. What are our chances."

"Just about zero," Miranda said. "Even if it's declared a historic site, if no one comes up with the money to restore it, the mayor can still knock it down. Plotkin and Schooner get to develop a brand-new history-making Price Slasher supermarket."

"Those reekers! We've got to stop them."

"So the bottom line is," Miranda went on, "that it's just about hopeless, wouldn't you say, Mrs. Tarr?"

"Quite hopeless actually, yes."

"Then why," Orville asked, "are we doing this?"

Miranda felt a sense of relief. She was suddenly on familiar ground. It was as if he were asking her "Why try to walk?" or "Why try to mother?" or "Why try to avoid falling in love or avoid falling out?"

Given the dim prospects, Orville was surprised when, as she answered him, her voice was light and musical, as in that flirtatious moment of possibility in the dreary schoolhouse the week before.

"Why, Dr. Rose," she said, touching his hand, looking him straight in the eye, "do we only do things for the results?"

10

"Babs said this mornin' that since you're doin' such a fine job with the practice, and since it's gettin' cold, maybe her and me'll take a little vacation down in Boca. Now, I don't know, I mean what the hell is an old feller like me gonna do down in Boca Raton? Funny name, ain't it, Boca Raton?

"Mouth of the Rat," Orville said, comforted by the waft of scallions.

"That so? Even with Babs so nuts about animals, I doubt she has much affection for a rat, heh heh. Her idea is we do Thanksgiving down there with the other snowbirds. But then we come back for Christmas. We'd be gone just a couple, three weeks?"

"Uh-huh," Orville said, leaning back in Bill's chair behind the old desk. Bill was sitting in the patient's chair and looked disoriented. "You want to change seats?"

"What's that? Nah. Feels kinda good bein' on this side. Say, doc, I've had this problem in my groin for about ten, fifteen years, and—heh heh." He blew out two plumes of smoke, coughed spasmodically, turned a little bluish, turned back to pinkish, and, pointing the Camel at Orville, went on. "I promised you you wouldn't have to carry the whole load, Orvy, so if you say no, then *I* can say no, and, hell, I'm happy."

"The practice has been kind of slow, Bill. Three weeks is okay by me."

"Shit. Kinda wish'd you hadn't of said that. I told Babs I can last two, maybe three weeks in Boca before my brain busts. We'd be back the first week in December?"

"Go for it, Bill."

"I was afraid you'd say that."

"When are you leaving?"

"Day after tomorrow. 'Course I been sayin' that for fifty-odd years, so we'll see."

But he in fact had left on that tomorrow, and that was two weeks ago now, and since then the practice had turned sour.

Orville soon realized that Bill hadn't told him about deer hunting season—drunken hunters trying to bring into focus the twists and turns of the woodsy hog-backed roads out in the county, crashing into trees, cremating cars and humans. Unhappy hunters back home blasting away at family and friends. To Orville, it often seemed like Columbians were bagging more Columbians than deer. One day it would be a hunter bagging a propane tank of a house, exploding a family of six into the air. Another day a hunter bagging a schoolbus, showering the kids with glass—only one eye was lost but still. Housewives hanging up wash on the line getting a barrelful of buckshot. Several Columbians blasting off parts of their own bodies—a toe, a foot, a finger, a hand, an arm, a leg, a head—yes, even a head—leaving gaping wounds behind.

Exhausted by all this, Orville worked like crazy to find creative solutions, ways to take these remnants of the severings and eviscerations and amputations and gapings and, out of them, as the New York antiquers were always putting it, *make art*—that is, make not necessarily humans but bodies. Exhaustion and the intense focus on his work lengthened the intervals at which the loss of Celestina Polo tormented him. But for the enlivening carnage and the Sunday afternoons with Miranda and Amy, he was living in a blackout, carrying his exhaustion on his back like a curse, simmering with resentment. He became outspoken in his critique of hunters and hunting, and this stirred up a lot of anger among the Columbians. More and more he found himself arguing with his patients. Not good, he would say to himself, trying to cool off after another sharp exchange in the office or the hospital, definitely not good. I mean, doctors are supposed to be neutral, right?

Even during those precious few hours on Sunday, his one afternoon a week off, his bitterness moved in. He was mostly okay visiting historical sites with Amy and Miranda and even the tough Mrs. Tarr, but often he would encounter his patients. They would want to talk about their problem or someone else's or about his attitude toward deer hunting. Try as he might to listen patiently and respond courteously, he felt that he was failing, seeing himself at best as stiff and standoffish and at worst as oafish, even harsh. Bitter, yes. He worried what Miranda was making of all this.

As if the overwhelming workload weren't enough, Orville had gotten mugged. Early one morning a few weeks ago on a house call down below Fourth, he had been walking back to the Chrysler when a steel arm went around his neck from behind and his lights went out. He awoke in the hospital with Packy Scomparza the cop staring anxiously at him. His bag had been emptied of syringes and drugs. No suspects. Diagnosis: concussion. Orville thought he might have a chance to rest a little, but they yanked him out of bed that very morning and wheelchaired him down to emergency to tend to a 300-pound young man whose giant red-and-white checkerboard hunting jacket made him look like a billboard for Purina Dog Chow in a space warp. The kid was a hunter who had tracked a deer into a swamp and sunk in. He had to be sucked out by the Schwermann Well Driller. His core body temperature was 87. Despite efforts to fricassie him back up to liveable, he died.

The good thing about the mugging was the arrival on his doorstep of a single red rose and a postcard of the Worth in its former glory with the message: "Feel better! Affectionately, Miranda."

Writing it, Miranda had hesitated how to sign it. Over the several Sundays that she had visited historical sites with Orville and Amy, she found herself liking him more and more. She kept looking for evidence in Orville of the kindness and compassion that Selma said he'd shown by staying with her. She thought that she had found it—not only in the way he acted toward his niece and her and Mrs. Tarr but in the way he was with the patients he often met. She watched him respond to their questions and complaints with frank care and concern, with patience and compassion, even as they took up precious time on his one afternoon off a week. He seemed a kind, generous, loving man who, like her, was always fighting a certain shyness. As she had seen this part of him, her affection had grown. She thought to sign the card "Love," but at the moment her pen point touched the cardboard, her fear came back. It was the fear of his saying "temporarily," of his being only temporarily there for her and for her son. The fear of again being left. And so the "L" became, with a little nudging and fudging, an "A."

Orville ran the fingers of his mind over the five syllables of that "Affectionately," a braille that brought back the music of her voice. "Affectionately"—it seemed like a lot. He kept the card in his pocket as he fought through the days and nights of butchery, replaying that music in his mind. It wasn't "Love," but in the face of his growing rage at what he had gotten himself into, doctoring Columbians alone, it was a comfort.

◊ ◊ ◊

Awaking the next Sunday morning after only two hours' sleep, Orville felt a bee sting of pain about Celestina, closely followed by a hit of rage at the latest letter from his mother, which had been awaiting him when he'd gotten home from the hospital at 3 A.M. But then he settled into a glow of, yes, affection for Miranda, for what he saw as her groundedness, her living out a kind of historical accuracy, her *authenticity.* So unlike Celestina,

93

with her fuzzy flights in the name of *karma* or *dharma* or whatever, with her secrets, her surprises, and her lies. Her betrayal—how meeting a rich banker had turned her "just two weeks more, *caro*" into forever.

The day dawned badly, an overnight mist sheening a first snow with ice. Driving and footing were treacherous. The night wind had been from the Universal Atlas Cement Plant, out past the storied hamlet of Katieville, so the town was covered with cement dust. Not only trees, houses, and cars but Columbians themselves, out shoveling or salting, were turned to dusty, ghostly shades. The cement dust mixed with the moisture in the air to coat the windshields of cars and trucks left out overnight with a thin sheet of cement. Water wouldn't touch it. The only way to remove it was to dissolve it with vinegar. This left the whole town smelling vaguely like a green salad gone bad.

As Orvy worked his windshield with vinegar, he watched the procession of dust-colored Columbians snaking their way across the icy, slippery Courthouse Square toward mass at St. Mary's. He pictured their pulmonary alveoli—imagine what this cement shit is doing to all of our lungs.

That Sunday's historical site was the Quaker Meeting House, down Coffin from the Square. For the first time in their several Sundays, Amy would not be with them. She had a rehearsal for the Christmas opening of *The Greenie Sellers Midsummer Night's Dream*. After that first day at the Worth, Amy had gotten fanatical about saving the hotel. Just last week the *Columbia Crier* published a front-page photo of Amy and Miranda and Mrs. Tarr picketing on the future site of Milt and Schooner's dream development.

Milt had gone ballistic, Penny all acid. Amy refused to talk to them. They asked Orvy to dinner to give some advice. While Penny and he sat at the table, Milt had taken Amy aside, down into the sunken living room. Orville and Penny watched Milt, on the verge of an explosion, patiently explaining the situation to his daughter. His hands traced logical fiscal scenarios of healthy urban development in the air of the all-beige *kiva*. Finally he sat back, inviting his daughter's response.

"You've got bad breath," Amy said, and stormed up, and out, to her room.

Milt blew. "No horses or drama-shit with that faggoty dwarf Sellers *forever!*"

"How can you date *her?*" Penny shouted at Orville, over Milt's raving.

"I'm not dating her, I'm just walking with her at—"

"Take it from Milt and me, she's a character!"

"What's wrong with that for Chrissakes?"

"Character stands in the way of progress!" Milt shouted. He seemed surprised at having said this and more calmly added, "and so forth."

"Just what this world needs, eh, Milt? Another Price Slasher?"

"Yes."

"Well, good luck, Milt. I hope you make a mint."

"As they say in Yiddish, Orvy: *From your lips to God's ear.*"

Now, outside the Quaker Meeting House, Orville offered his arm to Miranda as she got out of her car. The curb and walk were icy. For him, the feel of her leaning on him brought back the times that his mother, dizzy from her as-yet-undiagnosed brain tumor, would suddenly lurch into him, holding on for dear life. For a boy, a shock.

Miranda, leaning on so many arms in her lifetime, could read a lot in the Samaritan's touch. Now she picked up Orville's struggle, thinking of Selma telling her how her son had helped her to balance. But Miranda had a lot else on her mind. In the weeks since Cray's "Plez See My Hart" note, sometimes he had in fact allowed her to do that, but mostly not. He seemed to have gotten argumentative, a little lawyer. Her other friends who were mothers told her that it was typical for a six-year-old, this lawerly arguing his way out of even her smallest request. But she found it hellish. Her historian's mind labeled them "The Cray Wars: The Daily War of the Wakeup for School" or "The Great War of the Turning Off of the TV" or "The Eat Your Apple War" or "The Seasonal War of the Wearing of Your Winter Coat." She wondered if Cray sensed that something new was up with her on Sunday afternoons. Usually she had stayed at his soccer games to watch, but the last several Sundays she hadn't. Miranda had not told him why. Given her penchant for secrets, and her unwillingness to risk involving her son in this temporary little history with Orville, she felt it was better to hide it.

Separately and privately, Miranda and Orville shared an excitement about seeing each other again this Sunday. But when they actually did meet at the curb, shyness dusted them, graying them both. Alone together for the first time since the meeting in the schoolhouse, without Mrs. Tarr or Amy as their human vinegars, each saw the other with that pale cast of their own inner worry.

Bravely, they each tried hard to go against their natures. They said to themselves things like, "When you say hello, look into his eyes," or "Make a casual remark about how she looks or what she's wearing." But it was awkward. In just a few careful steps across the icy sidewalk small talk became big silence. Each of their minds filled with variants of "What the hell was I thinking of, saying yes to this?" or "Okay I'll just try to make it through this final Sunday politely and that's it." Wordlessly they went into the Meeting House.

The Meeting House was a tiny single room. Two windows next to the door were mirrored across the room by two looking out into Prison Alley. Old, worn, varnished benches formed a square around nothing. The benches were covered with dark blue cushions. A child's small plastic tricycle was parked in a corner. Few Quakers were left in Columbia. Five sat there around the square, as if around a boxing ring with the fights long banned. They were sitting in silence. Miranda and Orville joined them.

An elderly man spoke up about a young woman killed by a drunken driver two nights before out near Bells Pond. Orville had seen the mangled body, pronounced her dead. The man told the victim's story. She'd led an exemplary life of service, doing Quaker missions for peace in Central America in the Witness for Peace program, first protesting President Ronald Reagan's using the CIA in his first six months in office in 1981 to assassinate the elected presidents Omar Torrijos of Panama and Jaime Roldos of Ecuador, and ever since then to secretly run the contra war in Nicaragua. After Nixon and 'Nam, Orville thought it couldn't get worse. But now, in what was happening and the slick denial that it was happening, it was starting to.

A woman spoke of organizing a nonviolent local protest against the president's building five thousand new nuclear bombs and basing new "Peacekeeper" missiles in Europe.

More silence. They left early, leaving the others sitting there. Out on the street again, Miranda and Orville now felt not only shy but gloomy. So far the day was a dud. Together they faced but one question: Now what?

"How was that for you?" she asked in order to say *something*.

"Busy mind, going *flit flit flit flit help!* I've had better meditations."

"You meditate?"

"I did. Not much since I've been back. I did in Italy."

"What was her name?"

Orville was startled. "Celestina Polo."

Miranda heard in the way he said it his love for her. She thought, Okay, lady, you and he are nothing—be generous. "As my son would say, 'Awesome name.'"

"Used to be. It's over. Thanks to my mother and Columbia."

"How's that?"

He told her about the terms of the will and of Celestina's stalling and then dumping him for a Swiss banker. He didn't mention Selma's letters or her flying around or the Worth's seeming to plead with him.

And then a funny thing happened. Something about how she was looking at him, with such attentive curiosity, set him off. He told her about the hellish time he was having being back in town doctoring the Columbians. He talked about guns, about the endless drunken car crashes that left innocent Witnesses for Peace who'd never done anything wrong in their lives in smudges of blood and bone and guts and brain on the pavement, about the alcohol and drugs and muggings and violence as bad as anything he'd seen anywhere, hey maybe even as bad as on TV—and he talked about how everybody seemed to want to deny that it existed.

"I'm the guy at the bad end of it all!" he cried out, standing there on the icy street. "I'm the one they call to sew them up, cast their bones, pronounce them dead. I'm the one called in for a dose of reality and I'm sick of it! Do you know how much effort it takes just to sew up a wound, let alone try to repair a blown-off leg? How many years—hard, disciplined years—it takes to learn it? I put out enormous effort, superhuman effort on a daily basis, and they put out none! The Columbians eat crap and lie around like pigs and smoke so the nicotine makes them feel a little jazzed up while the carcinogenic tars mix with the PCBs from the river and the cement dust to destroy their lungs and livers, and then they say to themselves, 'Gosh, I think I'll go to the doctor!'"

He tried to stop himself but couldn't.

"The irony here is that the Columbians act in what they think is their own self-interest and wind up doing exactly what will hurt themselves the most! The true Columbian is always shooting himself in the foot. And who's my alderman? Who's gonna probably run for Congress? Henry Schooner—the neo-Nazi of my childhood. I've had it! Columbians, in total selfishness, do the worst things for themselves and I damn well don't want to be the guy that tries to patch 'em up anymore! Breakage! Self-centeredness! Looking Out for Number One! I mean, Jesus Christ, where's the kindness, the compassion for the other guy, Looking Out for Number Two? What about taking care of somebody *else*? Taking care of your neighbor, your town? Me and Bill try to care for bodies and maybe minds, but we're just treating symptoms, not anything that matters, not souls—we're just pissing in the ocean! It can't be just you and Mrs. Tarr, no matter how great a lady she is. God knows it can't be the children, the Amys of the world. I've had it. I've got nine months and change left trying to deal with this human breakage and then I am history! Every day I feel like giving up and running away again and the only good thing I've found here is *you*!"

YOU . . . You . . . youyouuuu echoed between the houses on Coffin.

Miranda felt a kind of *zing* go through her body, leaving her tingling all over, all senses heightened, deepened. For the first time since her husband's death, she knew that a man loved her. He was looking away, embarrassed, as if he felt he'd lost her—at the moment he'd found her! She couldn't speak.

Orville was sure he'd blown it. The silence killed him. He watched a pickup truck approach, on its front bumper a sticker saying DRIVER CARRIES NO CASH—HE IS MARRIED, and on its back bumper MY CHILD WAS INMATE-OF-THE-MONTH.

He turned back to Miranda, ready to say good-bye. To his surprise, she was smiling. She seemed to be trying not to laugh.

She *was* trying not to laugh. She said only, "Yes."

"Yes?"

"Yes!"

"Yes, *what?*"

"You *got* it. For as long as anyone can remember or kept written records, Columbians have been just as you describe. For two hundred years it's been the most mean-spirited, self-destructive little town that anyone else has seen either. It's been *known* for that! I've researched this for my thesis—'The Columbian Spirit'—and the more I learn, the more I feel like, at this moment, the way you look." She stared at him—standing there with his jaw dropped and eyes wide—and laughed, more freely now. "That look of—what? Incredulity? Disbelief?"

"No, no, no—belief!"

"Exactly! Sometimes I sit there reading the documents and I say, 'Oh my God, they didn't!' You see, it's hor—" she couldn't suppress her laughter. "It's *horrible!* C'mon." She crooked her arm for him to support. He took it.

She drove them up Washington and then north on Fourth to the Columbia Area Library, a two-story building made of chiseled limestone blocks all glazed golden in the noon light, with a central Federalist body and two symmetric wings. As they got out and walked toward the entrance, she told him that it had been built in 1818 as an almshouse in tardy and resentful compliance with a state law of 1778 that forced towns to take care of their poor, then in 1830 it became the first insane asylum in America, in the Quaker tradition of trying to be humane with the lunatics. Next, when the State Asylum in Utica opened in 1850, it was refurbished as the Columbia Female

Academy, where the great painter Henry Ary taught young ladies art, and then—as Orville must have known from his childhood—it became an orphanage.

"The Orphanage," he said, looking at it afresh. "I remember. Ominous, back then."

He helped her up the granite steps to the door guarded by two stone lions—miniatures, it seemed to him, of the two grand lions in front of the New York Public Library, the meeting point for him and his ex-wife, Lily, whenever they were in the City.

Miranda took out a key and unlocked the door and flicked on the lights. She led him upstairs to a tiny room labeled *Archives,* its tables covered with notes and typed manuscripts.

"This is where I work," she said. "Have a seat." He faced her across the table.

She told him that the early history of the Dutch and the Indians was full of folly. A ferry built at the exact spot on the east bank of the Hudson that guaranteed that its most direct route west across the river would be blocked by an island, Middleground Flats. A waterwheel at Kleek's Pond for grinding grain, fed by a stream that, in the dry months of the harvest, was too enfeebled to turn it. A bigger waterwheel at the same stream, which worked worse. Von Hogeboom's Giant Windmill, for grinding grain, built on the highest point of Cemetery Hill, caught the wind beautifully but was so high up that few wagon teams could reach it. But, she pointed out, such follies were not uncommon in such towns at such times. The New World, after all, was learning. The unique Columbian spirit was something else: a comic genius for self-destruction.

"We left off in 1803," Miranda said cheerfully. "The religious utopia of the Quakers is coexisting nervously with the sexual circus of the whores. Things don't go well. By 1837 the town is broke. Asked to increase their tax payments, Columbians refuse. Instead, the town sells off all the land encircling it to the hamlet of Spook Rock. This ensures that, forever after, the town will *always* be broke—its tax base is capped."

"Columbians strangled Columbia?"

"Good phrase—I'll use it. Soon Columbia becomes known as 'a finished city.' Ignatius Jones, a native son returning home in 1847, writes a memoir—*Whither Columbia?*" She opened a book and read. "An all-pervading air of listless indolence, and a Sabbath-like stillness, hung like a pall over what I remembered as busy, lively, bustling streets. Columbians are reluctant to risk one farthing for the common good." She closed the book and went on. "In 1859 oil is discovered by a wildcatter in Titusville, Pennsylvania—soon making whale oil worthless. The Quakers begin to leave. The remaining Columbians are offered money by the railroad to lay tracks across the two deepwater bays, which will destroy forever the possibility of Columbia being a port. They take the money. The bays turn into swamps, breeding pestilential insects. By the end of the Civil War the Quakers are gone, leaving the utopia in the hands of the whores and gamblers. In 1866 fires destroy much of Washington Street. Columbians are asked to finance a bond to buy a steam fire engine to replace a hand-operated pump. They vote 'No.' 1867 sees the town spending less than a third of what any other town its size in the state spends on itself. In 1876 there are schools enough for only half the children, which leads to truancy and crime, and when Columbians are asked to approve a bond issue for more schools and teachers, they vote 'No.' Columbia is the last town in the state to have a board of education or a public library. I mean, Andrew Carnegie was *giving* away money to every town in America to build libraries in the early 1900s. Even we, in tiny Boca Grande, Florida, population ninety-three, took the cash and built a library. Columbians were offered the money and voted 'No.' You know when this place became a library?"

"I never thought about it. Maybe when I was in high school?"

"In 1961! Last in the state. Dead last." She shook her head in puzzlement. "But the most amazing thing, I think, is the Columbian attitude toward light. I've really gotten into light."

"Tell me."

"Since 1797 there are gas streetlamps. But Columbians don't want to spend the money to keep them lit. They're only lit on nights when *The Farmer's Almanac* predicts there won't be much moonlight—sixteen nights a month, six hours a night. Never mind that even on the nights of moonlight there might be clouds or rain or snow. No light. By 1855 the town runs out of money again and shuts off the gas in the lamps. Columbians are outraged. Until they are asked for a special tax levy, at which point they say No. The streets stay dark. Gangs of young hooligans roam at night. Fires get harder to fight." She paused and winked. "But all is not lost. Finally, Columbians rally!"

"Thank God."

"They send out a call for more police and fire."

"As they should."

"The town council responds."

"We're saved!"

"They propose a small tax raise to pay for more police and fire."

"Who wouldn't pay for that?" Orville asked. "Why, no one wouldn't, no one wouldn't at all!"

"And what do the Columbians vote?" Miranda asked.

"Why, finally they break their streak and vote 'Yes'!"

She smiled and shook her head.

Together, they said, "They vote 'No'!"

They chuckled, and Miranda went on, "Columbia remains the most poorly lighted town on the Hudson—maybe in America, perhaps in the civilized world."

"And so when my fellow Columbians are given the choice between whether it's better to light just that one little candle or live in the dark?"

"They choose the dark. The only light is on Diamond Street, in the whorehouses. When the Quakers leave, Columbia becomes a boomtown in whores."

"From Whales to Whores: An American Story."

"But in 1953 Governor Dewey shuts Diamond Street down. Thirty years ago now, Columbia loses its last glitter. It goes dark. The same town that in 1790-something missed by one vote being named the capital of New York State is now dead." She looked at him curiously. "Were you born here?"

"No."

"When did you come here?"

"1946."

"Oh. I see." To him, her expression seemed like what you see at a funeral.

"Why?"

"Of all the bad periods of this town's self-destructive history, you might have chosen the very worst."

"Great," he said in mock appreciation. "You know, I remember Diamond Street. At night it *was* all lit up. We'd see fancy cars, license plates from Massachusetts, New Jersey—even Canada. Music floated out of the open windows. Women were all dressed up—men, too. Bill Starbuck was their doc. He told me about it. 'Two dollars for a house call,' he'd say, 'or I'd take it in kind. Never came outta there empty-handed.'"

"Yes, it was famous all over the world," she went on. "In the Jazz Age, Legs Diamond ran a speakeasy here and a big gambling operation. Look at this." She handed him a New York Central train ticket. "There was a conductor in Grand Central who, if he saw you were going to Columbia, would punch your ticket like this."

Orville looked. "A heart-shaped hole?"

"For a hundred years, the name 'Columbia' was synonymous with vice."

"That's it! That's why!" He was astonished. "Whenever anyone asked me where I was from, I *never* said Columbia. I always said, 'a little town south of Albany.' And I never knew why. Was I told not to tell? Had I been laughed at, the times I did?"

"I hate to tell you this, Dr. Rose," she said in mock seriousness, "but from the time they shut down Diamond Street—you were what, maybe ten?—you grew up in a town that was living in the dark."

"I love it!" He grinned from ear to ear. "I wasn't nuts—I mean, about being bored and beaten up and living with breakage and stinginess and meanness, feeling weird and dead—it wasn't me who was crazy!"

"No. It's always been a pretty mean and crazy town."

But then Orville understood what he was saying, and it suddenly seemed more serious, more like that sense of waste he'd felt when he'd seen his cleaned-out bedroom that first night back in town, when he leaned his back against the wall and slid down to sit splay-legged on the hardwood floor. He recalled the deadness, the expense of spirit, the just plain waste of life. Linked, always, to his mother. His mother alive, his mother dead. He sat there in silence for a few moments.

"You have to understand," he said, quietly "I mean . . . um . . . growing up here, you know, I always felt, deep down, that there was something really wrong with me."

Miranda thought of her own son, of his exquisite sensitivity to her and others, of how easily he could be hurt and how, lately now, he was resisting her reaching out to him whenever she tried to help him, even show her love for him. She felt a wave of sadness. She turned to Orville.

"A sensitive kid like you, here? How could you feel anything else?"

Understanding shared. They sat together in the tiny room cluttered with a historian's attempt to understand and a native's relief at being understood, sat in the stone-walled room that had been a cell for a pauper or ten and then for a lunatic or five and then for a young lady learning to paint and then for an abandoned baby or child and now for books telling it all. They sat with the frail winter sunlight hobbling around the jumbles of papers and then lying quite still on the old tabletop of Becraft Quarry limestone pocked with trilobites from a time when Columbia was a tropical lagoon like Orlando. Each sensed their shared sorrow, and without knowing it understood how close sorrow is to love.

"And it's still happening," Miranda said at last. "Milt and Henry are being so stupid! They're just the latest in a long line of idiots destroying the town and themselves for short money. The only thing that'll work here is to restore the town. Turn it into Antique Heaven, a mecca for interior decorators. Antique shops bring in rich people, spawn neat little places to buy a cappucino, to order pasta with sun-dried tomatoes and a glass of Chardonnay. Second homes for TV stars. Then, tourists gawking at the TV stars. Get it known for being known. Plotkin and Schooner think they're acting rationally of their own free will. They don't realize that they're being pushed along by hidden forces, historical forces, the old secret spirit of the town."

"Are we being pushed along, too? You and me?"

"Of course." She put her papers in order. "I've got to pick up Cray."

"When do I get to meet Cray?"

"Maybe next Sunday? After soccer?"

"Great."

"One more thing," she said, reaching for a drawer. She pulled. Nothing. Pulled harder. More nothing. Orville reached over and helped her. The knob broke off and the drawer jumped out spilling papers all over the floor. They looked at each other and laughed. She picked up a document, a color photo. "I wanted you to see this. It's the Town Seal of Columbia. Eighteenth century, in fact."

They looked, together, heads close. The seal was circular, like a porthole view of the ocean. Neptune, holding a trident, sat astride a spouting whale facing backwards. In the background a woman was doing something to a bird. Orville asked what that was.

"Officially, it's said to be a mermaid caressing a dove."

A scroll, scalloped like a fancy ribbon on a gift, made an arc over this peaceful aquatic scene. On it was inscribed the town motto: *et decus et pretium recti.* Orville asked what it meant.

"The Glory and Reward of Virtue."

Again they laughed and walked downstairs past the main borrowing desk and then out onto the front steps flanked by the cat-sized lions. They braced against the astonishing cold that now seemed more crisp and lively than ominous, so that they felt less chilled by the rawness than snug in the bundling up against it. As they walked to her car, Miranda's hand on Orville's arm felt newly familiar to both. She got in and rolled down the window, looking up at him.

"And do you know," she asked him, "who it is, in 1960, who finally leads the fight to create this library?"

"No, who?"

"A Columbian named Selma Rose."

"What?" he cried out, stunned, feeling a kind of slippage in his brain. "Selma Rose? Not *my* Selma Rose, no way. Must be *another* Selma Rose?"

"Nope. Your mom. A long hard fight, and against all the odds she won it."

Reeling, Orville tried to reconcile this clear evidence of Selma's altruism with all the evidence in his life with her and in her letters of her ruthless self-focus. He failed. He stood there in the cold, suddenly feeling like a few convolutions of his brain were being unrolled. He might have laughed but for the letter in his pocket. A cloud crossed his face. He wanted to let it keep passing across, and tried hard.

"Your mom, yes," she said again. She was looking at him expectantly.

"My mom." he said finally, failing to hide his bitterness. "I'll tell you about my mom. I got a letter from my mom last night."

"A letter?"

"You haven't lived 'til you've gotten a letter from your dead mother." He took off his gloves, fumbling in his pockets with freezing fingers. "She wrote a whole series to me, to be mailed after her death. They're postmarked 'Columbia'—someone around here has them and is mailing them, but I don't know who. Listen to this."

He started to scan it, searching for a piece that he could read without shame. The beginning, as usual, wasn't too bad. He read to her.

Hi honey-bunny!

He glanced at Miranda. She was smiling. He read on.

Were your ears burning? I was bragging about you. I never tell anyone anything bad about you—though as you know, there is *lots!*

"'Lots,'" he said to Miranda, barely hiding his contempt, "is underlined."

His harshness surprised her. To her it didn't seem that bad, it just seemed like Selma. A little weird, sure, but weird-funny. "Go on."

By now you've been here almost five months. Fun, eh? I imagine that right now—whether I'm in Heaven or that hot other place—I'll be feeling a sense of accomplishment. I figure you're helping Bill out, as a dear and glorious physician for our little town. My philosophy in life can be summed up in two short Sayings To Live By:

1) SO *WHAT?*

and

2) WHAT *NEXT?*

The first is good for the past. The second is even better for the future. God knows you can't do anything about the present. You were always stuck up in the mud of the present, which, if you think about it, and as opposed to dealing with the past and future, is *very strange.* One of the last letters you wrote me—and mind you there *were not many*—was all about your Buddhist Philosophy. I wrote back that it was wonderful. Now that I'm dead I can tell you the truth—"

Orville, realizing what followed, broke off reading. The sentence in fact ended with "—that it was just one more example of your *total selfishness!*"

He said to Miranda, even more bitterly, "It gets worse."

"It's a little weird, sure," she said, "zany even, but do you really feel it's that bad?"

"Bad? I'll give you bad! Try paragraph three!"

"Okay. Let's have paragraph three."

But Orville knew, from reading the letter late last night and feeling the knife twist in his gut, that what came next was too humiliating to read to anyone. He squatted down beside the car window and scanned it in silence.

There's something else I've always wanted to say. Your running away from me. The summer of '61 when I came home from my brain surgery and could barely see or hear or walk or talk, that long summer when I kept asking you, *begging* you, to stay with me. And what did you do? You ran. You never stayed. You didn't care and I'll never forgive you. And that's why my will, flyboy. My will is that this time you *stay.* To keep you from flying away, to make you for once in your life when you yourself don't really want to, to stay. Like I did. If you run now—

Miranda's voice brought him back. He found himself on a level with two light-green eyes framed by red hair. Eyes the color of tropical water close in to shore, full of concern.

He asked, "What'd you say?"

"It's okay," she said. "You can read it to me. I'd like to hear."

"No. It's too goddamn humiliating."

Again, Miranda was startled by the depth of his reaction to what she—knowing how much Selma loved her son—heard as basically a caring, loving letter. But, she thought, mourning a loved one is hard. All kinds of unexpected feelings and thoughts come up at the strangest times, surprising you. God knows I went through it all, too, when Joe died and when my parents died, the anger, the bitterness. He's having a hard time.

She took off her glove and reached out through the open car window and put her palm to his cheek. It felt icy.

Her touch on his cheek felt warm, even hot—less soothing than exciting. He asked, "Did you know her?"

"No."

11

All that night Miranda tossed and turned, wondering why she had said No. Should she call him back and tell him?

Two days before, she had gone up to her attic where the box marked Scomparza Moving and Funeral was hidden. She had taken out a sealed letter addressed to Orville, the next one on the pile. On it a yellow Post-It read, "To Be Mailed on the Third Week of the Third Month After He Arrives." She drove into town and dropped it in a mailbox, ensuring that the letter would be postmarked Columbia. As she had done five times before. All in total secrecy. Carefully. Wearing gloves. Making sure the mailbox flapper didn't stick, and flipped back, home.

In the three months before she met Orville, she had felt a certain satisfaction with being the agent of Selma's love, helping heal the rift between Selma and her son. She imagined the letters to be as Selma had described them, letters of a mother telling her absent son all the things she hadn't been able to when they were together. The letters were meant to help her son feel closer to her, help him work through his pain.

I wonder, Miranda asked herself in the middle of the night, if ever Cray goes off and I'm out of touch with him and I die, would there be someone I could ask to do that for me? It's a wonderful thing to do, isn't it?

All that night her secret ate at her. Why hadn't she said, "Yes, I met her. We were on committees together. But I didn't know her, really." Why couldn't she just have said the sensible thing? Why so flustered?

She knew, of course, that it was because of her secret, and that even to say Yes was dangerous—that's how secrets are. But more, she realized that it was her sense of the precariousness of love in general, and of this new love between them now.

Lying awake, she asked herself, "What was I going to say? 'That I'm just falling in love with you and oh, by the way, I'm the one who's been sending you your dead mother's letters in secret'?"

How can I tell him that, now? It's all too fragile now, too new. Besides, I promised Selma. Took her money—$5,000! I swore on a rock by the river. A promise is a promise, a secret a secret. He'll never find out. Let it go. Besides, I don't want her in here, getting between him and me.

But isn't it cruel to keep this kind of secret from someone you love?

Yes, it is. I'll tell him. Now.

She picked up the phone.

Put it down.

Picked it up again and dialed.

Put it down.

She picked it up again and dialed and let it ring until someone picked it up.

"Hello?"

It was him.

She hung up.

12

"Do you love Dr. Rose?"

This question came out of the blue of the backseat of the station wagon as Miranda was driving Cray to his last soccer game of the season.

Cray was six and several months. That Sunday morning Miranda had told him, with feigned casualness, that Dr. Rose would be meeting them at the game and that he would be coming back to the house with them for dinner. Cray picked up the feigned part and said nothing. He knew that something was up with his mother, and now it turned out that the something was this Dr. Rose and he didn't like it one bit. In his four years growing up on the edge of Columbia, from time to time he'd seen men come through the house. Most seemed thumpy and loud and smelled of weird soap, or beer. They always started with dinner. During dinner he always watched TV in the other room. Often they were still there when he went to bed. Seldom were they there in the morning when he'd awakened. None had lasted more than a few weekends. That was fine with him. It was hard enough having a hollow where a father should be. It was harder having a man who his mom's attention would turn to even when he was there, too.

"No, I don't," Miranda answered. Her hands clenched the wheel.

"Good."

"Be nice to him anyway, okay?"

Orville got there on doctor time—late, just before halftime. The early-December day was strangely warm. The field, set in a grassy bowl next to the gym entrance at Columbia High, had thawed enough to produce child-friendly mud. He stood on the rim looking down, spotting Miranda's red hair on the sidelines. On the edge of the beehive of boys swarming after the ball—at this age they didn't seem to have grasped the concept of "the pass"—was another redhead, who, he thought, must be Cray. Orville watched him.

The boy was lanky and coordinated, a fast runner. As he chased the ball his straight hair flowed this way and that like a bowl of red water on his head. But he seemed reluctant to get into the pack and mix it up. He would kick at the ball only if it squirted free. Long ago, as manager of the Fish Hawk hoopsters, Orville had learned that you can tell just about everything about a person from the way they play a sport. Here was a boy who was timid.

Orville walked on down the steep grassy slope to the sidelines. As he greeted Miranda, his heart did a little twist in his chest. For the first time, their greeting was more loving than apprehensive.

The boys on Cray's team all wore shirts for Schooner's Spa. Henry was the coach. He waved gaily to Orville. The whistle blew, ending the first half. All the boys ran to the sidelines and clustered around Henry in a huddle close to Miranda and Orville. Cray ignored his mother and Orville. Schooner distributed quartered oranges, reminding Orville of himself, as manager, doing it at halftime for the Fish Hawks.

Casually but carefully, Orville studied Cray, his doctor's eyes searching for the penetrance of his mother's genes and clues to those of his father. The red hair, surely, was hers, though a lighter, younger red, more orange-red than her strawberry—reminding him of ripe persimmons in the summer sunlight in a market in Lago del Orta. His eyes, too, were hers, that fresh green, and the lashes were long and dark—sweet. The pale skin betrayed a lack of melanin, and Dr. Orville wanted to rush up and tell him to *always*—even when it's not summer—use sunscreen. Freckled cheeks, a pert nose, lips less full than his mother's—giving him a cute, birdlike look—and a dimpled chin. The rest of his body seemed to come from the other genetic pool, for he was tall for his age, the tallest of all the boys, and his hands and feet were big. Get a basketball into those hands. From watching him on the playing field and watching him eat his orange wedge, Orville sensed a tight energy, a restlessness, shadowed by that hesitation about throwing himself into the game. A great kid.

As the kids slurped at the wedges, Henry kept on coaching. He pushed the ball gently ahead of him, calling out, "Happy feet! Happy feet!" and then, getting up on his toes, did a little dance of the happy feet—with amazing lightness for all that icebox bulk. Then he pushed the ball again. As it rolled, again he cried out, "Happy feet! Happy feet!" He put the boys into groups of two and had them push the ball back and forth to each other and cry out, lightly, "Happy feet! Happy feet!" and do the little tiptoe dance. As they drilled, he came over to Miranda and Orville.

"Howdy, folks. Great to see ya." For Orville there was the political two-hand clasp and for Miranda a hug. "Orvy, you played soccer, didn't you?"

Orville noticed what looked like a fresh bruise on Henry's cheek. "A little. We lost every game, until the Hungarian Revolution. Then Bruno Baloghy arrived. Our strategy from then on was 'Get it to Bruno!' We never lost after that."

"Great country, isn't it? We take anybody in. A true melting pot. Someday, Miranda, I'll tell you the deep, dark truth about old Orvy. A real redhot in high school. Kind of a Fish Hawk's Fish Hawk." They laughed. "Oh, and by the way, *great* photo of you guys marching for the Worth. Good to see somebody *else* doing something for our town. Little Amy's got herself a purpose and it's great. 'Course Milt's not happy, but maybe we can up his dose of Valium, Doc?"

"We're at the legal limit. One milligram more and he'd turn human."

Henry busted out laughing. He rolled his head in appreciation. "Now *that's* funny. Yeah, Amy's got herself a purpose, and her dad's upset. But hey, that's America, right?"

They said it was right and the whistle blew for the second half and Schooner headed back to coaching.

"It's ironic," Orville said to Miranda. "Right up there, up the hill where the path leads from the gym door down into the woods around Kleek's Pond to Sixth, is where I last saw Henry, after he'd been expelled for scalping tickets to basketball games. He flipped us the finger as he walked away into the woods. Looked just like his son does now. Funny, I keep seeing, in all these adults I used to know, the kids they were—as if it's a town of children. The town's shrunk, too. It seems like a child-sized town."

"I know. That's how it feels when I go home, too. What year was that?"

"Sixty-two. He was a thug, a bully. Joined the navy, never looked back."

"People change."

"Yeah, well, given the first seventeen years, he's changed too much. As a kid he was a monster—and not only to me, you can ask anybody. Then there's this gap—what, another twenty years? And now he's doing everything right. A pillar of the community."

Squeals came from the soccer field. The boys were clumped on the ground, rolling in the mud, squealing like happy piglets.

"Look, I'm sorry," Orville said. "I didn't mean to turn this nice day into—"

"No, no," she said, putting a hand on his arm. "I know what you're saying. It's a big question—maybe *the* question—of history: Are we who we once seemed to be?"

"Exactly. All of us, yeah."

"Yes." She squeezed his arm affectionately. "But I don't have your baggage with Henry. To me, he's a dad, a coach—a terrific coach. The boys are crazy about him. He seems to be a good dad. Cray and Maxie are friends. They get along great. They've had only one fight ever, on the day I met you—Cray hit Maxie on his cast—which was strange, because he'd never hit anybody before, that I know of."

"Why the cast?"

"Broken arm. Maxie's accident-prone. Both Schooner boys are—they always seem to have bruises or cuts. His older brother, Junior, is twelve—a rough kid. He seems to be influencing Maxie, and then Maxie influences Cray. It worries me, but all in all—"

Shouts from the mud. Two boys were squared off. The beehive was now two opposing beehives. A boy on Schmerz Drugs—whom Orville recognized as the adopted Korean child of Mouse and Faith Schenckberg—shoved Maxie, who tripped over Cray, sending them both down into a muddy pile.

Maxie bounced up, ready to fight. He was about to grab the Korean Schenckberg when there was a strange, high-pitched whistle from the sidelines, like a teakettle. Henry had two fingers in his mouth. Maxie stopped, as if shocked. He turned and walked slowly toward Henry.

The two coaches waded in, making peace. The game ended. The boys gave weak cheers for the other team and sorted themselves out with their parents, almost all of whom, Orville was surprised to realize, he now knew from his practice. He knew their private selves, knew them undressed, physically and emotionally. Knew their secrets. He often heard them in public lie about their health, their happiness, their sexual prowess. As Bill said, "In here we lift up the lid and see the truth." The Schooners didn't come to Bill and him. They went to Ed-the-Shyster-Shapiro, way out in Spook Rock.

Cray walked over to them, a muddy warrior, his bowl of red hair streaked with black. He did not look at Orville.

"Cray," Miranda said, "this is Dr. Rose. Remember I told you he's coming back to the house for dinner?"

Cray said nothing. He hid behind her. His head pointed straight down. His eyes pointed straighter down.

"Hi, Cray. Call me Orvy."

Cray said more nothing and ran up the hill out of the grassy bowl to the parking lot. Schooner was collecting the team soccer balls used for the 'Happy Feet! Happy Feet!' drill, stuffing them into a big mesh bag, and cleaning up the paper cups and sucked-out orange wedges—much as, Orville thought, he claimed to be cleaning up Our Nation and Our World against Dirty Commies. Henry waved cheerily at them as they walked off.

Orville helped Miranda up the slick grass slope. Soon his New Yorker was following her Country Squire north on Route 9 out of Columbia.

In the car, Miranda asked Cray, "Did you have fun?" From the backseat came a loud nothing. "You still seemed a little afraid, hon, to go into the bunch of kids kicking at the ball."

"Yeah, I like to wait for it to come out and then kick it."

"How come?"

A pause. "I don't want to get bumped and thumped."

In the past, thinking always that if he'd had a father he'd be more brave, she'd tried to push him to take more risks. But it didn't work. Not that she knew what did work. But for now, in her gratitude for his honesty, she said, "Uh-huh," and nothing more.

They took a left off Route 9 onto the rutted dirt road that ran parallel to Kinderhook Creek. Orville's big Chrysler followed, pitching up and down like a whale doing aerobics, past snow-packed fields guarded by broken stalks of corn to a sudden opening up of the vista where the creek flowed under an iron railway trestle—which cut the foreground like the bottom of a picture frame—and emptied into the partly ice-locked Hudson. In the distance the Catskills climbed easily up into unfathomable air. The sharp light of a lone streetlamp ventured partway out on the ice, making it seem rumpled, a white-gray quilt spread over the water to keep the life in it nice and cold until spring.

Miranda's house was nestled into the crook of the arm where the creek met the river. At the end of the road at the railroad tracks was a circular turnaround, blackened by old cinders. The house tucked itself snugly into the slope of a cornfield and was guarded by three tall pines. It had two stories, the first of massive stone blocks, the second of weathered wood, out of which peeked four dormers in front, and two on the side facing west, toward the river and mountains. The stone was that same buttery-gold limestone Orville had seen in the Cotswolds and the Dolomites and the Columbia Area Library. It caught the low winter sunlight in a way that softened it, making the dwelling itself seem soft, a house of gold. In front of the house was one of those blue historical markers.

STAATS HOUSE

HENDRICK HUDSON LANDED HERE SEPTEMBER 17, 1609

BUILT 1654–1664 BY COLONEL ABRAM STAATS

Cray ran up the grass and in through the unlocked door. Orville helped Miranda up the icy path, grass set intermittently with slate stones. Inside he noted the low-ceilinged small kitchen and living room, reminding him of centuries-old houses in Europe. The place was wonderfully cluttered, cozy. Papers were scattered on the kitchen table. Two zebra finches flitted around a complicated cage with rotating mirrors and a tiny bell on a dangling chain of colorful plastic links. He saw a half-filled cat dish, human dishes undone in the sink, which had a drip. There was none of the Lysol, Windex, and Murphy's Wood Oil that Penny, with Selma's maid Hayley's help, periodically showered down upon Selma's house. The Lysol never lasted—the house soon relapsed to what Penny called "pigsty." In his childhood, Hayley had been the warm body of the house, a child-sized black woman with a chipmunk face and enormous black-rimmed glasses, looking at the Family Rose with a certain bemusement. Her son, Whiz, had been a best friend of Orville's. Lately Orville hadn't seen much of her, not only because he was busy, but because Whiz was fighting another bad round of the addictions he'd brought back from Vietnam, and her husband Clive was having emotional issues at his job at Geiger's junkyard. Orville was delighted to see that Miranda's was a lived-in household. The woman running it was down in the trenches of the essentials: food, clothing, shelter, animals. No vinyl runners. No clean guest towels for clean guests.

"Mom, can I watch TV?"

"Not TV, a video. I got you *Jungle Book* again."

Cray hustled into the living room.

"But first, a bath," she yelled after him. "You're total mud."

"Aw, Ma!"

"You heard me. You can run the water and get in. I'll start dinner and help you when you're ready. It'll all be over before you know it."

"Not before *I* know it," he said, but he started stripping and moving upstairs.

Miranda lit the wood-burning stove, and it was soon sending out warmth in that way that reminds you of mortality—heat dropping off fast to that chill just behind your back. She and Orville started in on the Chardonnay he'd brought and got dinner going. Cray called down that he was ready, and she went upstairs to finish him up.

After what Miranda called "the shortest bath in history," Cray was back down at the TV. He popped in the cassette and sat an inch from the screen and yelled back over his shoulder, "Can I eat in front of the TV?"

"You know the rule."

"Yeah, but tonight's special 'cause there's a guest."

"A guest who'd like to have you eat with us, right, Dr. Rose?"

"Yeah, I really would," he said loudly so Cray could hear. "Call me Orvy."

"But mo-om, that's *why* I wanna eat in front of the TV!"

Miranda looked at Orville and shrugged. "Okay."

Cray shouted, "yes!" and became silent and still, but for his eyes.

At dinner they talked relaxedly about anything but themselves and their probable love, spending much too long on Hendrick Hudson.

"His name isn't Hendrick but Henry," she said. "He's English, not Dutch. He sails not under the flag of England but for the Dutch East India Company. The trip here is a disaster. He's trying to reach the Spice Islands. First, he sails in the exact wrong direction, due north up the coast of Norway. The ship freezes. The crew mutinies. He turns back and sails in another exactly wrong direction, west across the Atlantic, and finds the mouth of this river, thinking it will lead to something called the Furious

Overfall, and then to the Spice Islands. The Overfall, of course, is a total lie, a fantasy made up by a British explorer named Davies."

"I love the way you do that," Orville said. "How you always tell the past in the present tense."

"Oh. Maybe because the present is so tense sometimes. History's easier for me."

"For me, too, ever since I met you."

She blushed. "Colonel Staats, a surgeon and fur trader—" Their eyes met and she laughed. "Colonel fur trader—" Again, they blushed and laughed. "Oh, fuck Colonel Staats!"

"No, no," Orville said, in mock seriousness. "Colonel Staats is crucial." She grinned, dimpling her cheeks. "So, does Henry Hudson really land here?"

"How do you mean, 'really'?"

"I mean, is it true, then, that he lands here?"

"You think that there exists a 'true' history?"

"Sure."

"Oh. Well. When I teach history, in my first lesson I ask the class to write down a sentence describing the weather that day. I write down my own sentence. I read a few of theirs out loud. They're all accurate descriptions: 'It was a sunny day,' or 'The sun shone all day long.' Then I take out my description, 'The day was dark, filled with incessant, driving rain.' I hold mine up to them and say, '*This* is the one that will survive.'"

"So there's no true history?"

"The little histories can't help but be true."

"Little histories?"

"Of people like us."

"Ah," he said, nodding. "Little people like us, yes."

Looking at him, she got flustered, and brought in of all people Tolstoy. "If you believe Tolstoy, the big history—singular—the one that's written down in books and called 'history' is at heart a few crucial little ones. When someone asked Napoleon how he chose his generals, he said, 'I choose the lucky ones.' Apocryphal, but still."

"Sounds good to me, Miranda." The use of her name felt intimate. The glow and scent of the wood fire, the glow of the white wine, the first real easing of worry about how each appeared to the other—it was sensual, even sexy. They sat and talked for a long time.

"*Look for the bear-necessities, for Mother Nature's recipes, forget about your worry and your strife—yeah, man!"* interrupted the video from the next room.

Miranda watched Orville turn to look. He clearly was not used to having a child around, to attending to two or three or ten things all at once.

Orville was of two minds. He wanted to make contact with Cray but at the same time wanted Cray to evaporate for awhile so he could take Miranda in his arms.

"I'd like to try again with Cray," he said.

"Fine." She got up, feeling a little tipsy from the wine. "Let's make a little sally into Cray Country."

Cray was still frozen by the set, a few inches from the screen. A forkful of pasta was in his hand, a plateful on his lap. His straight red hair shone.

Orville made several attempts to engage Cray, starting with, "Hi, Cray."

Nothing. The boy wouldn't even look at him.

Miranda watched this, saw in Orville the clumsy overtrying of a man who never had children. She felt both sorry for him and more loving toward him for that lack. She touched his arm and said, "It's okay. Let it go."

But Orville persisted. He himself loved Disney's *Jungle Book,* having watched it years ago when he'd babysat Amy. His favorite animals were the elephants. At one point the elephant leader, Colonel Hahti, does something stupid with his own son, the littlest and last elephant in line, and the colonel's wife, Winifred, confronts him. Orville, knowing the line by heart, recited Winifred's line along with her, mimicking exactly her voice, that of a stern old Victorian matron, *"Oh shut up, you pompous old windbag!"*

"Shhh!" Cray hissed. "Now you made me miss it!" He hit Stop, Rewind, Play.

Miranda held out her hand to Orville and led him away, out of the reach of the TV.

"Bye, Cray," Orville said airily.

Nothing.

"Well, that was a big success," Orville said.

"Join the crowd. It's almost nine-thirty. He and I are gearing up for what I've labeled 'The Nightly War of the Bedtime.'" They laughed. "He's a night owl. He'd stay up until midnight if I let him. Lately it's a real struggle to put him down."

"I'd like to stay, but with Bill gone, I've still got to make rounds at the hospital."

"Some other time."

"I don't mean—"

"I do."

He understood and took her hand. "Is it that he doesn't like me? Or is afraid of me? Or just doesn't care?"

"I would guess—and it's just a guess, mind you—that he's afraid to care, 'cause he might just care too much."

Orville sighed, relieved. "Yeah, like us all." He squeezed her hand, feeling sad, sad to leave her, the boy, this cluttered coziness.

Saying good-bye on the doorstep, out of sight of Cray, they hugged. At first it was a we're-adrift-together-in-a-life-raft kind of hug, but then the physical space turned more friendly and they really hugged, he feeling her breasts against his sweater, she feeling his fingers on her back, then tracing light whorls on the nape of her neck, like phantom hair. Standing together out on the cold shelf of winter, just behind the boy's back, it felt illicit, sexy.

"Maybe I could stay?" Orville said.

"You will sometime." Turned on, she shivered—and then doubted. "Won't you?"

"Yes."

13

Howdy, partner,

Boca's great. Babs shops & we play bridge with a nice couple Wolfgang and Kenni Vista from Altoona, PA. ("If God'd wanted to give America an enema," Wolfie says, "he'd stick it in Altoona.") They're starting a trip around the world. Weather great. Starbusol working even at low doses. Be back a little later than planned. Keep the good virgins of Columbia happy—all three of 'em. Heh heh.

Yr frnd, Bill

This oversized postcard, picturing on the obverse side a glorious sunset framed by a palm tree swooping up from a beach like an exhaust trail from an exploding missile, was dated December 17. It had arrived the day before Christmas. When Bill's expected date of return to Columbia had passed, Orville tried to call him. There was never an answer at the condo.

Liberated from caring for the Columbians, Bill had no need for an answering machine.

The troubling thing for Orville was that Bill had mentioned no clear date for his return. And Orville was superstitious about dates. December 17 was a particularly auspicious one: at exactly 10:35 A.M. on Thursday, December 17, 1903, at Kill Devil Hill, Kittyhawk, North Carolina, Orville Wright took man's first flight, 120 feet in twelve seconds. Bill writing on the eightieth anniversary of this great day for mankind seemed ominous to the other Orville now. Even the headline in *The Columbia Crier*—BOARD TO DEBATE CHICKENS AT KINDERHOOK LAKE—couldn't cheer him up. His thought? Don't bet against the chickens. But who cared. He was in love.

Despite the holiday-season carnage in Orville's practice, he and Miranda were seeing each other as often as possible. They told each other their life stories—the censored versions that you tell to non-first loves. He told her about Lily and the hamster—the scientific proof of his sterility. He said nothing about his conversations with his floating mother and nothing more about Celestina, whom he'd come to realize was also a floater. Ever since the day in the freezing cold outside the library when he'd read Miranda a piece of a Selma letter and she'd said it didn't seem all that bad, he'd known that it would be a mistake to talk to Miranda about Selma at all. Lily had always despised Selma and maintained that one of the reasons their marriage had fallen out of the sky was that Selma was always *there,* always sticking her nose into things, trying to control them. After seeing Miranda's reaction to the letter, Orville vowed never again to let Selma into this love affair. He promised himself that he'd never talk about her, never even tell Miranda when he had gotten another one of Selma's letters. In his mind there was now a big KEEP OUT, MOM sign on the door. Selma would be his secret.

Miranda told him about her tragedy with her daredevil husband and about her move up to Columbia from Boca Raton. But she never talked about her polio and kept everything to do with Selma a secret—not only the letters but also how Selma had told her what a "saint" her son had been, staying by her side during that long summer of her hellish disfigurement and recuperation. As Orville and she got closer, each time she sneaked into Columbia to mail a new Selma letter, she felt a little strange. But what could she do? It was, after all, a good deed. While she thought it strange that he never again mentioned his mother, that was okay, too—it kept Selma out of it.

Every time they had been together, Cray had been with them. Orville's *Hi, Cray*s were still met with silence and downward glances. Now, on Christmas

Day as Orville drove out to Miranda's with Amy to exchange presents, he felt a sense of relief. He'd gotten coverage from a local surgeon until midnight, trading Christmas Day for New Year's Day, and Miranda had arranged a sleepover for Cray at Maxie Schooner's. Finally they would have time alone.

As the weeks went by, Miranda struggled with the romance. There was a physical fire between them, and she loved the way that, despite his shyness and doctor's cynicism, he had a remarkable energy, a real interest in and responsiveness to her, and to history, big and little. But with the blossoming attraction came doubt. Over and over she would hear a small voice inside saying, I doubt it, I doubt it. The doubt was about whether or not he was sincere, and about why he never brought up the fact that he was leaving in August. She knew from her past the risk of doubt, how her doubt isolated her from the person she doubted, from the person's world, from the world itself. It had happened with her husband, from their first meeting at the Gasparilla Inn on Boca Grande. He had courted her, reassured her. She resisted. Finally she had let go of her doubt. But now she was alone. In the four years since his death, she'd come to see that when he promised to stay safe for her and Cray, he lied. Stunt flying, *safe?*

With Orville she felt she couldn't just jump in. The voice inside kept saying, He's leaving, right? The cost isn't just to you but to your son. Eventually Cray will respond and say hi to him. Once you say hello, you face the terror of saying good-bye.

When Orville and Amy arrived that Christmas afternoon, Miranda felt a surge of happiness. "I'm so glad you came, Amy," she said. "You must be nervous about tonight, opening night and all?"

"Not really. Greenie Sellers says that if something goes wrong, it's right, and if it's too right, it's all wrong. Shakespeare's text doesn't count—'cause it's postmodern."

"Poor Shakespeare!" Miranda said. "This is my son, Cray. Cray, this is Amy."

"Hi, Cray. What a wicked-good tree! My parents don't believe in Christmas."

"They don't?" Cray asked, his eyes wide. "What are they, Grinches?"

"Jewish. We can't even like utter the name . . . um . . . Jesus Christ."

"But Jesus was Jewish, right, Mom?"

"Until he converted, yes."

"This is so neat, Uncle O. My first-ever Christmas. Show me *everything,* Cray!"

Miranda was delighted. Over the past several Sundays spent with Amy working for the Worth, Miranda had fallen a little in love with her. And Amy had responded to her with the full force of an eleven-year-old going on sixteen who's found an alternative to her mother. She told Orville, "Mom and Miranda are like two different species!"

The presents were presented. Orville gave Miranda a pendant on a gold chain, a gold whale with a diamond eye. She gave him a facsimile of a Shaker book published in New Lebanon in 1823, *Gentle Manners: A Guide to Good Morals*. Amy thought this a riot, snatching it and reading aloud in her stage voice a passage about "Life as a Moral Essay" and also from "Sixty Rules of Civility," by General George Washington.

"Scoff at none," she read archly, "though they give occasion."

"Scoff at none," Cray mimicked. "Scoff at none! Yuck!"

"And listen to this!" Amy said, turning to the inside cover. "To Dr. Rose, in gratitude for your gentleness walking with me in love. . . . Uh-oh. . . ." Amy stopped, mortified. "Sorry. It's personal, right?"

"It's okay, Amy dear," Miranda said, blushing. "Here's your gift from us." A first edition of Stanislavsky, Volume 1: *On Acting*. Amy squealed in delight and clasped it to her heart theatrically. Orville gave Cray a video of *Jungle Book*, "to keep for your own."

They sang a few carols and drank some mulled cider, and then it was time for all of them to go, Amy to the theater and Cray to the Schooners'. Cray gathered up his sleepover necessities—clothes and a teddy and a *Babar* and the *Jungle Book* video. He hoisted his backpack and a smaller wicker basket shaped like a duck. As they were putting on coats and boots, he pushed Miranda forward toward Orville, hiding behind her.

"Go on, Cray," Miranda said. "You give it to him yourself." Cray vehemently shook his head. "But it's from you, not me." Another no. "Okay." She handed Orville a card.

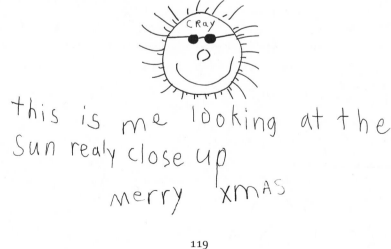

119

"Hey, thanks, Cray. It's beautiful. I love it very much."

Cray said nothing. But then he peeked from behind Miranda's pants and for a split second made eye contact with Orville, who was so touched that he made sure not to show any sign of it, so as not to scare the boy off. Miranda felt joy, then doubt, but was left leaning toward joy.

◊ ◊ ◊

Later that evening, as Miranda and Orville walked together down the aisle of the decaying Opera House on lower Washington, they created a stir. They were together in public for the first time. Penny waved them over to sit with her and Milt, greeting both of them warmly. Milt greeted them coolly.

"Unreal," Penny whispered to Orville. "Amazing!"

"What?" he whispered back.

"Maybe you're getting *socialized!* Mom said she'd die before she saw it, and she did. But I always said all it would take was the right girl."

"I thought you said Miranda's the wrong girl."

"To Milt, yes. Me, I'm agnostic. And hey—Faith Schenckberg she's not."

As the lights started to fall, the Schooners entered—grandly, smiling and waving. Both looked gorgeous, Henry in his crisp white naval officer's dress uniform and Nelda Jo in a silky red gown suspended by spaghetti straps, making her seem, to Orville, a live advertisement for whatever she ate or drank or did aerobics to or had surgery on. And was it patriotism or lust, he wondered, astir in the pants of the sturdy men of Columbia? The Schooners smiled deeply at each other, as if they'd just that day fallen in love.

Miranda bent forward and talked across Orville's lap to Penny. "Don't you feel great when you see two people smiling at each other like that?"

Penny thought hard about this. "No," she said, matter of factly. "I feel great when they both turn and smile at *me.*"

The lights went out. *Midsummer Night's Dream* went on. Sort of. The Fairies were Hell's Angels, the Lovers were Kabukis, the Rustics were gay. The play was cut severely, and it was hard to understand who was who and what was what.

But Amy was game, playing the Queen of the Fairies, Titania. She was the only child in the play, and Orville was touched to see her stand up so bravely and sweetly in front of the crowd. She seemed to have a natural flair and voice for it. When Titania caressed Bottom (dressed as an ass), somehow the innocent sincerity of her voice and her lines—for who of us, Orville thought, has not been fooled in love?—brought a hush to the audience.

Sleep thou, and I will wind thee in my arms.
Fairies be gone, and be all ways away.
So doth the woodbine the sweet honeysuckle
Gently entwist; the female ivy so
Enrings the barky fingers of the elm.
O, how I love thee! How I dote on thee!

Miranda, holding Orville's hand, caressed it, and snuggled into his neck.

At that tender moment, however, the action shifted to a biker entering on a real Harley, and the rest of the spectacle left the audience puzzled and disgusted.

But then the New York antique dealers "got it." A murmur sped through the crowd: "It's all a joke—on *us!*"

The play lasted forty-two minutes, which seemed to Orville and Miranda more like two hours. The New Yorkers leaped to their feet for a standing ovation.

Milt said to Orville, "Forty bucks an hour to that fucked-up dwarf Greenie Sellers for lessons in royal bullshit like *this?*"

In the receiving line, Amy asked them, "How'd you like it?" Orville and Miranda said that both the play and she were great.

"Yeah? *Really?*"

"Really," Orville said. Miranda nodded.

"Cool! And did ya hear? They're talking about taking it to New York!"

Orville shook the tiny Sellers's hand. He'd known Greenie as a boy, a misfit sent by his rich parents to prep school in Tokyo, and from his office—a man expert in phantom complaints, but for a menagerie of veneria to make a profligate Venetian proud.

"*Grazie, grazie,*" Sellers said, for some reason speaking only mock Italian. "*Por della granda apprecionissimo del'arte.* I am feeling so good, but not at all well, *dottore.* So overwhelmed, *cosi confuso!*"

◊ ◊ ◊

Back at Miranda's house they stoked the woodstove and sat together on the couch in the low-beamed living room, sipping brandy. They stared at the glowing grate and talked over the boneheaded production. Orville stroked her neck and shoulders, her face taking on a glow as he did. With both of them still dressed up, Orville felt like a teenager at a prom, wanting her desperately but worried about going too far too fast. She, too, now

121

that the physical was so present between them, felt shy. But she also felt that if they didn't get naked soon she would burst.

Their words took on the false tone that words carry when the sensual world starts to take over. As they finally kissed, a spark bit both their lips—the static electricity in the dry room—and they laughed together. Gingerly, like chastened but diligent students bent on completing what they had begun, they kissed again through the diminishing static, their alonenesses giving way to their hungers.

Miranda rose and took Orville's hand and led him toward the narrow stairway. Unused to drinking, she tipped a little. He, also tipsy, steadied her, his arm quickly around her waist. Face-to-face, bodies pressed together, they saw the yearning in each other's eyes and then their lips were on each other's lips, tongues on tongues, with a sudden tenacity. A bolt of excitement zinged up from his toes to his skull and bounced back down. He unbuttoned her blouse and slid it from her shoulders and, the stairs too much to think about, helped her gently down to the rug, his dim sense of her lameness bringing a nurturance to his passion. He took off his clothes, she her pants. Nuzzling her neck he reached around and undid the clasp of her bra and helped her shrug it off and was lifted by the swell of her breasts in the almost-dark of the neglected fire. His fingers felt the silky roll, and then his lips, as lightly as in imagination, the plumped-up tips. Putting his arms around her, his palms against the strong *latissimi* of her back felt a murmur—she was telling him that she was losing herself fast and wanted to prolong, savor, hurry.

Hands around his neck, Miranda felt the curly hair of his chest against her breasts. She felt him with her, the *with*-ness catching her up like on a curl of a wave in the Gulf. But then he stopped.

His hand was on her withered leg.

Under his fingers he felt the sharp shin bone and the wasted muscle mass, and couldn't help but sense the story of this person he was beginning to love and the sadness of that story and the anger at that sadness. He felt as if he were facing the juxtaposition of the body and the human, the doctoring and the loving, which he'd been trained to split apart from the first cadaver on. *God, this child's withered leg!* Despite himself, his doctor's mind attuned not just to the person but the patient, not just to the beloved body but its history: symptoms, diagnosis, treatment, years of bereft parents doing everything for her and her trying hellishly hard, brave beyond belief, the physical therapy and fear of never walking again, the electron micrographs of the virus itself and the photos of Dr. Jonas Salk.

Miranda sensed his shock. She took his hand, still resting like a question on her shin, and brought it gently to her lips, then to her breast—an answer, of sorts, to her first suffering. Her other hand caressed his cheek, sought out his lips.

"Shouldn't we talk about it?" he asked.

"No. Not yet."

"I want to."

"I don't." She nuzzled his ear, rolled his fingers on her nipple. She kissed him again, his mouth more hesitant now. She stroked his belly.

"I may, uh, need to," he said.

Her touch went lower, onto his penis. "Uh, well, Dr. Rose, I happen to know that you don't."

He laughed, and, relieved, clicked pretty much into the erect sexual, though her fragility stuck in his mind like an allergy warning stuck in the front of a patient's chart. He balanced between his sexual power and that brittle tibia and fibula passing in X-rays before his eyes.

But Miranda had spent a good part of her life living that X-ray and learning to gauge the limits of that fragility, learning to read the fear of it in others. So she took the initiative and tried to tell him by her touch that she was holding onto that X-ray a lot tighter than he ever could and that she wouldn't fracture anything—not a bone, not her son, not her soul—for pleasure. She took his hand and moved it over her good hip and down along her inner thigh to that moist pungent place so ready for him after all the weeks of foreplay. Then she straddled him and rose up and with a sigh began to move, riding that curling wave.

"Oh God," she whispered, "hurry!" She started to stifle a cry but then realized what she was doing and shouted, "Cray's not here! No one can hear us!"

"Yeah!"

She rocked on him harder and screamed happily, lustily. He, too, let go, screaming. They howled like two animals, the two caged finches answering. And then she settled down on him feeling as if she were settling into a warm bath of just plain love.

He felt her settling as if she were two people: one, on his chest, a strong, pliant, firm-breasted, vibrant woman; and the other, on his leg, a spare and fragile girl. With a rush of tenderness he had started to think he was too worn-out for, he took the woman and girl to his breast, to his life.

Just as they were dozing off, she spoke. "Great whales, eh?"

"Yes, sweetness, great wet whales."

◊ ◊ ◊

His beeper roused him at two in the morning—the delivery ward, something urgent. Miranda hardly stirred as he rose and searched out his clothes and nuzzled her good-bye. In the low glow from the embers his eyes made out her alabaster face and firm shoulder and he filled in that blaze of hair and the red grape nipple. He sighed happily and walked out into the icy night that couldn't touch him—not until his butt hit the ice cube seat of the Chrysler, making him cry out with shock, happy shock, because just then it was merely a part of being alive.

The nurse had paged him for a delivery of twins. He'd been tending the couple through the pregnancy, her first. They were poor and black, a man and woman he'd known vaguely as a girl and boy, friends of Hayley and her son, Whiz. They'd lived their lives smack up against the railroad tracks in the shantytown between the North Swamp and the Hudson River. Bill had never bothered with insurance, and by this time Orville had also given up dealing with that evil. This was charity.

As he arrived, the labor was stalling out. What was going on? He had delivered hundreds of babies in Dublin, at the National Maternity Hospital on Holles Street. A baby an hour, the whole year 'round. Get drunk with the other medical students in O'Dwyer's across the street, get pushed out the door tanked and cursing at the eleven thirty closing time, stand there wobbling in the night damp staring up at the building, and ask each other "Shall we pull out a few babies or just go to bed?" They'd take the rickety elevator to the top floor, deliver a baby or two, and bed down on the horse-hair mattresses on the first floor behind reception.

Orville understood births, but this one required thought. Should he use a pitressin drip, as they did routinely at Holles Street? Do a C-section? "You make 100 percent of the decision," Bill always said, "on 50 percent of the evidence." Orville made sure that the fetal monitor was working and left the delivery suite in the newly dedicated (by Henry Schooner) Maternity Wing of Selma Rose, Founder of the Women's Auxiliary. He got the chart again, lit up a Parodi, and sat in a room overlooking the town to think it through.

"Hi, boychik."

There she was, bobbing up and down gently outside the fourth-story window as if wearing a flotation device. Dressed in an Amelia Earhart khaki flight suit complete with leather cap with earflaps and goggles perched jauntily on her head. "Oh, God."

"Not God, *me!*" She did a peregrine swoop. "Second Lady of the Air!"

"Go away."

"I am away. You're not. I am. Happy Chanukah."

"Merry Christmas."

"Don't do that to me don't you dare. We're Old Testament, remember?"

"You're Old, I'm New. At most, New."

"Jesus? The Bible Lite?"

"You'd prefer 'an eye for an eye'?"

"You betcha. On this issue I stand with Penny and that cute Plotkin! Never again! I keep asking up here to go back down as a sabra. Those Israeli gals are tough. Chevy-truck tough."

"Not as tough as you."

"Me, hell, *you!* Have you cried for me? Have you shed even one teensy-weensy tear? I am your mother. I am dead, and you're too selfish even to cry for—"

"Dr. Rose?"

"We're boarding, honey-bunny. Catch you later."

"Yes?"

"There's something wrong," the night nurse was saying. "Come quick."

Wrong big-time, he realized. The tap of death on a baby's shoulder. He explained that he'd have to do an emergency C-section. The couple agreed. He scrubbed in fast and did the section. Twin boys. One was well-formed, robust, squawling. The other was microcephalic, its head the size of a doll's but with lips and nose and eyes crammed together and with no forehead—giving it a froglike look. Trunk and legs normal but for a remnant of tail. It was horrible to see, yet transfixing, like something you see in a bottle of formaldehyde in a medical museum.

The obstetrics nurse was more accustomed to seeing Columbian babies with a panoply of birth defects, at a rate soaring high above the national average, which everyone figured (and those responsible denied) was the result of the PCBs and other toxic shit dumped in the river by General Electric and sprayed on the fruit trees and soaking the rail bed with all the creosote of childhood. And the sempiternal cement dust. Abnormal APGAR scores were the norm. Orville wasn't yet used to this.

The nurse took the healthy baby to the father, leaving Orville to wait for the other to die. Luckily, and quietly, by the time he had gotten done with closing the groggy new mother's abdomen, it did. Orville went out to the father. He was still holding the healthy baby, in that awkward way that new fathers do. The nurse had told him the other had died.

125

"What happened?" the man asked, in shock.

"The other baby lived only a few minutes. It was deformed."

"Can I see him, Doc?"

Orville hesitated. The older doctor in him, the good old Doc Starbuck pushing Starbusol and paternal sense, would've patted him on the shoulder and said, "No, son, better you don't." The younger doctor applauded his wish, though knowing that once seen, it would be indelible.

Orville said, "You can, sure. I just want you to know that you'll never forget it."

"*Him.* I want to see him."

The nurse took the healthy baby, and Orville and the father went in together to see the other son. He had been cleaned up, so he looked better, less frightening. The father reached out a hand and touched the perfect shoulder, and then the squashed head. He bowed his own head and crossed himself.

"In the name of the Father, the Son, and the Holy Ghost. Amen." He looked up at Orville. His eyes were wet, sorrowful. He said, "Thank you."

"And you," Orville said, feeling in this man the power of facing into, in a world that as a rule turns away.

"I think she will want to see him, too."

"Fine."

The father picked up the dead baby to take him to his mother.

Orville got beeped away to tend to a drug overdose from the Bliss Towers Housing Project and a stabbing victim from a happy household and a car crash and several Christmas specials, including a shepherd from Austerlitz sure he was picking up Radio Free Europe through a metal plate recently placed in his skull.

Later during a break in the action, he walked out into the parking lot and searched in his pockets for the half-smoked Parodi and matches. The night was crisp. The little town was iced up and the air tasted like cold quarters and seemed stretched tight as an eardrum so it was like you could hear everything. He thought of the dead twin who would always be almost there, floating there like all the dead, and the live twin. He thought of Miranda, of her histories and of their lovemaking, and he whispered out loud, "This is the one that will survive."

14

By New Year's Eve, whenever Orville said, "Hi, Cray," the boy would look at him. Once, he might even have said something back, but too softly to make out.

Miranda and Orville were spending New Year's Eve at the hot social event in Columbia, the dinner-dance-swim at Schooner's Spa out at the mall on Route 9. They had arranged for Amy to babysit and sleep over. Cray liked having Amy around, and Amy liked being a big sister. And so Miranda and Orville bid them good-night and said they would see them next year. The kids were so engrossed with Amy helping Cray write his first novel that they hardly even noticed the adults were going and then gone.

Orville kept right on being surprised by Henry Schooner. Henry had done a similar party his first year back; this second one made the event a Columbian institution. Anyone who was anyone was there, and a few Columbians who were not really anyone were there too. The food—all you could eat from a room-long buffet—was a mix of Columbia and worldly: steak and fries, salmon and salad, pad thai and pork ribs, plantains and egg foo, Knickerbocker and Perrier, and Pepsi and Gallo. The ambiance was unheard of in Columbia: all glittering chrome and mirrors and a whirlpool with steamy water bubbling at one end of the near-Olympic-sized pool. In the separate locker rooms the saunas were scented with stuff from Sweden. There were not only free weights but sparkly exercise equipment previously unseen in Columbia—Nautilus and Stairmaster and high-tech pneumatic machines guaranteed against breakage that made weight training as painless as watching TV. Television seemed to be the leitmotif, not only the four TV monitors—one for each channel—suspended in a row from the ceiling and facing the stationary bicycles and treadmills but in the persons of their hosts, Henry and Nelda Jo.

Orville had gotten into the habit of what he called "Schooner Watching." Now he watched Henry, dressed in a dinner jacket with a pink carnation boutonniere and white hair slicked down tight, gliding as if on rollers here and there, filling glasses and egos, and doing that two-handed clasp and then in the same motion handing the person off so that he could handle the next—much like a TV game show host. He watched Nelda Jo, hair now platinum to match Henry's, in a lavender spandex top that scooped and stretched timelessly across her breasts and a short flowered miniskirt also stretching athletically every-which-rounded-way, smiling and coaxing lesser-toned Columbians of both sexes to give the machines a try. She looked like that woman on TV at six in the morning who showed you how to improve your body, your life, your world. Her Oklahoman good humor was infectious. She was clearly the hit of the party.

Orville and Miranda felt shy and out of place, their long histories as wallflowers at school dances pushing them out from the action toward the walls. For a brief moment they were alone.

"1984, imagine?" Orville said.

"Yes." She quoted Orwell, "We are living in a world where it is virtually impossible to be honest and remain alive."

But a small town won't allow that aloneness, not in the presence of a palpable new happiness, and people sought them out, dragged them over, enticed them in to try food, conversation, normalcy.

"I always knew you two were meant for each other, old buddy," Henry said, pumping Orville's arm, having given Miranda a European two-cheeked kiss. "Your mom would be so pleased!" With a hint of reluctance, Henry let go and ushered him off to Nelda Jo and moved on to the next guest.

"You two be careful not to behave," Nelda Jo drawled and winked.

Penny made a big deal of their being together, a more frank deal probably than she intended because she was champagne-drunk. "I can' believe it, little brother, how you're into *fun.* Y'know, Miranda, he never let himself go, never really got into just plain having *fun.* Cerebral, him. I never woulda thought it, especially not with you, Miranda, because if you'll pardon th'expression, you're every bit as much a character as himself." She left, Orville and Miranda rolling their eyes at each other. Then she came back. "And what you're doing with Amy is *unreal.* Keep that up too."

"Except for the socialist part and so forth," Milt said, munching a burrito. "What a spread, eh?" He watched Nelda Jo pass by. "And the food's not bad either. Haha." Laughter seemed to consolidate a thought. "Henry's a comer, Orv. A real comer."

The party got wilder. Columbians flopped and frolicked in the pool and pumped some iron and danced to ear-splitting oldies and newies.

"Sorry," Miranda said. "I can't dance."

"Thank God. I can't either. You know, it's amazing. Even people who hate each other's guts are talking, having fun."

"Yeah, it's small—"

The music blasted.

"What?" Orville shouted.

"It's small-town life!" she shouted back.

"Community?"

"Not really, no," she shouted. "Not since 1790—"

The music stopped suddenly and Miranda's "1790!" rang out like nobody's business. Everyone turned to look and then laughed and hustled to ring in 1984. As soon as possible Orville and Miranda left and were suddenly embraced by the arctic stillness of the night.

Orville held her arm firmly. "Careful, it's icy."

"Thanks."

At the car, Orville looked up at the stars, pointing out the bright jewels on the sword and belt of Orion—Betelgeuse and the smudged seven sisters of the Pleiades—and gave a sweet little lecture on the mythology. They hugged and kissed, and he held open the car door and helped her in.

When they arrived back at Miranda's house, they found Cray in his pajamas, asleep on the floor, clutching a large book. Amy was asleep on the couch. The TV buzzed white noise, the video having run its course long ago.

"Should we just let them sleep down here?" Orville asked.

"Yes."

He took her hand and turned toward the stairs.

"Wait, love. Look, just for a second. Look with me." Together they took in the beauty of the sleeping children.

"Momma?"

"Yes, dear. Orvy, too." Cray shot a sleepy glance at both of them. "C'mon. To bed."

"Wanna read this book." He held up an orange book with elephants on the cover, two adults and three kids, *Babar and His Children.*

"*Part* of it," Miranda said, readying herself for a fight. Cray hated half-measures. "It's so late, cute-heart, and the book's way too long—"

"Okay, but only if Orvy reads it to me."

Orville was delighted. "Okay."

Cray got up and climbed the stairs, the two of them following, and snuggled down in his bed. Orville, unfamiliar with fathering, perched on the edge. Cray motioned him to lie down next to him, which he did. But then Cray said, "No, no. Lion Army, Lion Army."

"Lion Army? I thought it was about elephants?"

"No, I mean lie-on-arm-ey. Lie-on-arm-ey." Cray raised himself up and turned around and took Orville's arm and put it under him so he could lie on it and snuggle in.

Miranda watched the two of them from the doorway, the awkward man and the sleepy little boy. She thought, Each of them is hungry for this.

Cray's freshly baby-shampooed head against his cheek stirred up such feeling in Orville that he could barely focus on reading. As if a father, he thought. As if a father. "Elephants are my favorite, too." As he read, Orville recognized this Babar book as one he had loved as a child. When he came to page 16—where baby Flora swallows a rattle and turns purple and Queen Celeste tries a pre-Heimlich slap unsuccessfully before the monkey Zephir pulls the rattle out—he found that he recalled every detail, even the position of the eight drawings on the page! It brought back the bufalo mozzarella and Celestina, but he was surprised and relieved that the memory held no hurt anymore.

Miranda leaned against the doorjamb. Seeing this man she loved make the move toward fathering, she felt her heart lighten, lift, her whole being lift so it seemed she had to hold onto the door to stay down on the ground. Her face flushed, her eyes teared up, her heart opened like a new tulip. Orville had crossed a line drawn like diamond on steel, a line between parent and nonparent, and at that moment she felt no fear, no doubt. There was nothing shy about him right now. She felt her good hip cuddle into the molding of the doorway of the old house that must have seen everything, and the voice inside her say, Maybe there's a God after all.

Lying on the man's arm, Cray felt the comforter of sleep cover him. He yawned and murmured, "S'nuff," and lifted his head and shoulders to give Orville back his arm. He turned over on his side and settled in under the quilt, riffling the edge of "Shirty," a tattered soft shirt, through the fingers of one hand.

Miranda went to him and kissed him. "Good night, sleep tight. Love you."

Orville said, "G'nite, Cray."

Nothing—except from under the comforter maybe a giggle.

Orville said, "Hi, Cray."

"Hi."

"Hi, *who?*"

"Hi, *Orvy.*"

"Oh, I *love* that word!" Orville said, happily.

Cray peeped out from under the quilt, glanced at Orville, then Miranda, the look on his face saying, Who is this nut anyway?

Downstairs, on the kitchen table, they found Cray's novel, each page illustrated with a drawing.

THE DOG
A novel by
Cray Braak

The dog livd on the strets
Becass he did not hav a
Homm

He etss grbg

1 day he cam to a prkk.
A man sied I will tac you homm

The man wkt and wkt into a
Car. The dog flold him

So the man toc him homm to
Hss hos.

Wan he plld into the drivway
The dog lokd arownd.

THE END

15

Two Columbian ice fishermen and their dog had a bright idea. It was the end of January. The Hudson was ice-locked. Even though they never caught anything much in the polluted river when it was free of ice, many Columbians imagined that when ice a foot thick covered it the fish would reappear. Their greatest difficulty in ice fishing was not keeping warm.

After all, they would drink enough beer so that it acted like antifreeze, and they would drag portable gas stoves out to their huts on the river. The difficulty was cutting through the ice. Many male Columbians had a love affair with internal combustion. They often seemed at a loss when their hands were not wrapped around the shuddering steering wheel of a car, truck, van, tractor, bulldozer, wrecking crane, or Bobcat. And one of the sweetest moments in this love affair was when their manly hands were caressing a chainsaw. Yet in the dead heart of winter, a chainsaw required just that little bit extra presence of mind from inebriated Columbians to cut through the ice without shearing off a toe or a foot or a leg.

At dawn on this viciously cold day, the two Columbian ice fishermen and their dog had the bright idea of using dynamite to blast their hole in the frozen river. They drove their pickup out onto the ice toward the neglected old lighthouse. They got out, all three. They managed to identify the fuse end of a stick of dynamite, congratulating themselves on their creative intelligence and hardly able to contain their excitement. One held the stick of dynamite. From his cigar, the other lit it. It sizzled, a fuzzy phosphorescence. The Columbian threw the lit stick a long way away. It sailed in a high sputtering arc out toward the decaying lighthouse.

They watched—first in drunken puzzlement mixed with a hint of satisfaction at the order of the world, then in drunken horror as their dog ran after the stick of dynamite, fetched it, and started barreling back toward them. See the dog run. See the Columbians run. See how fast the dog runs. See how slow the men run.

◊ ◊ ◊

At the time of the explosion, Orville was at Miranda's kitchen table finishing up "Egg Trickee" before driving Cray to Sixth Street Elementary School.

"How many?" Orville asked Cray, holding a square piece of Cray's morning omelet in the palm of his hand. The birds and the cats watched too.

"One!"

"Miranda?"

"Two."

Orville flipped the piece of omelet up in the air and tried to catch it in his mouth. He missed the first time. The second time he did it.

"Not again!" Cray cried. "I never win anymore."

"You won yesterday," Orville said, leaning over and making a great show of kissing Miranda on the lips. Whoever got the right number got kissed by Orville. If neither of them called it right, he kissed his own reflection in the mirror. Cray dawdled over his breakfast, reluctant to go to school. As they were all headed out the door, the call came in about the exploding ice fishermen and their dog. Orville said he was on his way.

The door of the Chrysler had hardly closed and the engine barely rolled over when Cray said, "Can we play the Animal Guessing Game?"

Cray had invented the game. One person thinks of an animal, and the other two have to guess it. After five wrong guesses there are clues.

"Orvy, you think of one first," Cray said.

"Okay."

"You got it?" Cray asked.

"Not yet." Orville was always amazed at the speed at which Cray's mind worked, compared to his own. A six-year-old brain versus a thirty-nine-year-old model. Growth versus decay. He paused, as if thinking, and then said, "Got it. But I warn you, Cray, this time it's a hard one. Real hard."

"I go first, okay, Mom?"

"Fine."

"Is it a . . . ," Cray stopped, finding out that he had no idea what was at the end of the sentence he had started. "A tree sloth?"

Orville feigned amazement. "Did you say . . . a tree sloth?"

"Yeah!" Cray was bouncing out of his seat with excitement.

"You didn't say . . . a tree sloth, did you?"

"I did, I did! Mom, you heard me, I did!"

"Unbelievable!" Orville said. "It *was* a tree sloth."

"I knew it!

"How'd you do that, Cray?"

"I *always* get it with you."

"You sure do," Orville said, nodding with grave assurance.

"My turn," Cray said. He thought. "Okay. Guess."

Miranda sat and listened with amusement. Orville connected with Cray by joking around. Cray loved it, mostly, but once in awhile he got a confused look on his face, not knowing if Orville was joking or serious. Amy, who Cray now called Big Sister, told him the other day, "The thing about Uncle O., Cray, is that he's a big joker, so you can't tell sometimes whether he's serious or not." Miranda knew the dangers of too much joking around. Orville didn't yet seem to realize that kids need to know where you really stand. She kept reminding herself that Orville had never been a father. He didn't have six-plus years in the trenches, hadn't felt the humiliation and ineptitude and, worse, the rage that comes with parenting.

He just plain didn't know how to do it. And Cray came with no instruction manual. To see Orville using the outdated manual of his own father was both touching and disheartening.

How reluctant he had been to join in with Cray and her and sing out loud in public, or even in the car. When sureness was needed, how shy he seemed, and when pliancy was needed, how sure. The worst, though, was how impatient he was with child-time, those moments when, needing to get somewhere in a hurry, Cray would suddenly discover a toy he couldn't leave the house without but couldn't find, or a book or a worm in the yard, and dawdle. Orville had trouble realizing that it isn't only what you do with a child but what you don't do, what you ignore, or even, after you screw up, what you do next.

Neither did he realize how having him around didn't make it much easier, because she had to take care of not only Cray but him. There was also the Cray-Orville thing, the Cray-herself-and-Orville thing, and the herself-and-Orville thing. And all the while she had to hide the constancy of her caretaking from them both.

But she loved how he jumped right in with Cray and when he found himself in over his head, how he thrashed around, fighting to break the surface. His energy had made some things better: there were fewer skirmishes in The War of the Wakeup and The War of the Getting Out of the House to School on Time. But The Great Battle of Bedtime had escalated. Cray was responding so intensely to this father-y person in his life that the Sleepytime Skirmishes were worse. Cray didn't want to shut off the world of Mom and Dad, and who could blame him?

◊ ◊ ◊

As they drove into Columbia, the day darkened. It was one of the bad cement dust days, the wind blowing in from the Universal Atlas. The buildings and bundled-up Columbians were gray, spectral shapes, and the vinegar scent was an acrid backdrop to a world of broken sunlight. Orville dropped Cray off at Sixth Street School and Miranda at the library down on Fourth and headed for the emergency room.

The dynamite had rearranged the life force between the two fishermen and their dog. The front half of the dog and the lower half of one man had been blown off. Both were dead. The other Columbian was okay, except for a hand and arm that looked vaguely like a leg of lamb trussed up by a drunken butcher, a silver belt buckle imbedded in his crotch, and a case of hysterical weeping.

"Nigel! Nigel!" the fisherman bawled. "Nigel!"

"I'm sorry. Your friend is dead, but you've got to hold still!"

"Friend? *Friend?* Nigel was my dog!"

As Orville sliced and diced and patched and matched, seeking to create an arm as useful as a thalidomide flipper, as he tried to reconstruct the scene on the Hudson. The dog must have been in the process of giving the dynamite to the dead Columbian when the live Columbian threw himself not on the dynamite to save his buddy but on his buddy to save himself. How else would a belt buckle with the name J. Rhodes get imbedded in the crotch of a man named Ulysses Stoiber?

Works of art are not finished but abandoned, he thought, as he walked downhill to Eighth and the Hendrick Hudson Diner for coffee. Along the way he noticed that the empty storefront next to the never-open Suttee's— where as a kid he'd bought long strings of rock candy, probably the same stuff still hanging in the window—was now dressed up in red-white-and-blue bunting and a new sign:

VOTE AMERICA

VOTE SCHOONER

"Happy Days Are Here Again" played from a loudspeaker. A crowd had gathered. Orville moseyed on over. It turned out to be the grand opening of the Henry Schooner for Congress Campaign Headquarters. The aging long-term incumbent, a Republican with old fascistic proclivities and a new young wife and Alfa Romeo, was retiring to become a lobbyist. The Republican primary in September was wide-open. Schooner was ready.

As Orville watched, a many-colored crocodile of children in their winter outfits, puffs of breath like cartoon blurbs above their heads, wended its way across the Seventh Street Park to the Schooner headquarters. A teacher escorted them. Orville recognized red-headed Cray bundled up, paired with Maxie Schooner. The first-grade class was getting a living lesson in democracy. Cray saw him and shouted, waving him to come over. Orville did. As he approached, he saw Henry and Nelda Jo and teenaged Henry Jr. standing bareheaded and without jackets on the sidewalk in the dusty, freezing cold. Maxie broke rank and ran to Henry, who lifted him high up in his arms. Catching sight of Orville, Henry smiled broadly and motioned him to come closer.

Why, Orville wondered, does Henry always seem so happy to see me?

The scene was chaotic, amateurish. Music was playing too loudly, kids were shouting and fooling around, mittened hands kept spilling the cups of punch or coffee or hot cocoa or dropping the cookies or doughnuts. Nelda Jo and Henry Jr. wandered aimlessly among the crush of Columbians and New York antiquers. No one was organizing anything. It was a mess.

Henry pumped his hand, shouting, "Glad you could make it to the opening, Orv—"

A sudden spotlight, fighting the dull gray cement dust. A TV camera from the Albany station had started shooting. Flashbulbs popped. Henry smiled at the cameras. The TV lights went off. Henry moved on to the next hand.

For awhile Orville stood there and watched what seemed to him a pathetic launch of Schooner's campaign. Even Schooner the Great, he thought, isn't immune to the Columbian Spirit. Yet walking away down Washington toward his office, Orville was struck by what had *not* happened: no breakage. And it wasn't until he was all the way down to the office on Fifth that he realized that he'd been had.

He turned around and ran back. By this time the music was off. The children were gone. Henry was alone in the office, sitting upright behind a metal-topped desk that looked like it came straight out of the war surplus at Geiger's junkyard. He was smoking a cigar, studying a neatly folded *Wall Street Journal.*

"Henry, you can't use . . ." Orville was unable to catch his breath and made yet another mental vow to lose the weight he was gaining by eating like the Columbians—and to stop smoking.

"Why, hello there, Dr. Rose!" he said cheerfully. "Siddown, siddown."

"Henry, you can't use me on TV."

"What's that, buddy?"

"That camera, that TV videocam that was shooting me shaking your hand?" Henry nodded. "You can't broadcast it. I won't let you give the impression that I'm supporting your run for Congress."

"Really?" His face showed such surprise and hurt that Orville winced a little. "Well, okay," Henry went on, recovering his good cheer. "If I'd knew you felt that way, I never would have let 'em ran it right then." This time Henry didn't catch Orville noticing his bad grammar. "No problem, Orv. I got the TV guy's number right here." Henry dialed. Waited. "Axel? Henry . . . Yeah, thanks. Hey, listen, you can't use anything with the picture of Dr. Orville Rose in it, okay? What's he look like?" Henry described him, in a flattering way. "You run that piece of tape, you never get an exclusive again, get it? Great." He hung up. "Done."

"Good."

Schooner eyed him. "Wait a sec. You think I set it all up?" Orville said nothing. "How could you even think that I would without your permission—"

"Easy."

"You think your endorsement of me, as town doc, means that much to—" He stopped. "Yeah, I see. It'd mean a *lot,* the town doc and all, yeah."

"Gotta go, Henry. Got work to do."

"Cut me some slack, Orv, 'kay? You know, we're more alike than otherwise."

"Bullshit."

"You'n me should sit down alone and chew the fat, get it all out on the table, get it over with and move on. I mean, we never did that, right?"

"Why should we?"

"'Cause we're in the same boat, bein' back in this shit hole town after bein' out in the wide, wide world! We both want to make it better, right?"

"Shit hole town?"

"Who said that?" he asked, looking around at the empty walls, chuckling. "Not me. You didn't hear that from me."

"Which is why we're not sitting down." Orville left.

Back at the office, he settled into Bill's chair. On the desk Orville saw a postcard among the mail—the Sphinx, a palm tree, a camel held by an Arab in a *jalabi* and ridden by two hefty Western tourists, a man and a woman. He flipped it over.

Howdy, partner,
Joined Wolfgang and Kenni Vista on their round-the-world trip. First stop, Egypt. Hot! Mosquitos big as small children. Babs bowels bad, but Starbusol working good, so far. Food foul, even at Cairo McDonald's. Good luck.

Bill

Orville raised his eyes from the postcard and found himself staring up into the dead eyes of the fourteen-point buck.

"I'm screwed."

◊ ◊ ◊

That night Miranda, Orville, and Cray sat at her kitchen table for dinner. It was the first time Cray was eating with them and not in front of the TV. Clearly unused to the idea of dinnertime conversation, Cray had to be coaxed into talking about his day at school.

"Well, today in class I started my new novel. It's called *CFIT*."

"Sea Fit?" Orville asked. "What's that?"

Miranda knew. She held her breath.

"C-F-I-T." Cray spelled it out. "It stands for Controlled Flight Into Terrain. That's how my dad died. He died in a CFIT. He crashed his acrobatic plane. I got a picture of him and his plane. Can I be excused to go get it, Mom?"

Miranda, startled both by his wanting to show it and by his courtesy, said, "Sure."

She and Orville barely had time to exchange glances when Cray was back with a framed snapshot of a stunt plane, gleaming all red and yellow, a man standing beside it, hand on it affectionately, as if it were a woman. Beside the plane he was small, his features hard to make out. A shock of sandy blond hair, ruddy cheeks, a strong jaw, a smile. Aviator sunglasses and leather jacket completed the picture of the flier, tough and confident.

"That's great, Cray," Orville said, moved.

"Yeah, but for my novel I need to know why he crashed. The problem is I can only ask him why he crashed if he didn't crash. But if he didn't crash I could ask him, but he wouldn't have. It's confusing."

"Very," Orville said.

"I wish I knew too, Cray," said Miranda.

"Okay," Cray moved on, "now you tell me about your days."

Orville told a funny story about a boy bringing his pet pig into the office because he wasn't oinking right. Miranda told them about Mrs. Tarr and her finding in the DAR attic a gigantic old map of Kinderhook County, the Penfield Map, as big as a two pingpong tables and drawn in an old style that showed orchards by drawings of rows of individual trees and farms by rows of corn.

"Cool," he said. "I'm finished. Mom, can I go watch TV now?"

"Sure." She was stunned by all this, and by Orville's presence bringing it out.

Cray turned on the TV but then came back. "I got an idea. I could ask his grave. Where's he buried, Mom?"

"Mississippi. Avalon, Mississippi." She had told him this several times.

"Can we go ask his grave?"

"Sure. If you think you're ready."

"I am. Can Orvy come too?"

"He sure can, cute-heart." Her voice was unsteady.

"All three of us? Cool." Cray went back to the TV.

Miranda, wide-eyed, said, "Do you know how incredible that is?"

"No, how?"

"A first. I just . . . I'm just amazed."

"I'd love to hear more about him."

Miranda took this in slowly, as if it were a hand reaching in toward the store of her secrets. A little war took place inside. A negotiated settlement came out. "Sometime, yes. I'm not sure I'm ready yet to talk about my . . . well, my pre-Columbian history."

Sensing her struggle, Orville offered her his own secret. "You know, this thing about asking his grave, well . . . not only do I get these letters from my mother, but from time to time I . . ." He stopped himself, unable to admit to seeing her flying around, and instead said, "I talk to her." But suddenly it seemed too intimate, and he regretted putting himself out there.

"Yes," she said, nonchalantly. "After my parents died, I'd have conversations with them. In fact a few times, in the year after, they'd come to me when I was, you know, half-asleep, as if they were in the room, and I'd talk with them. What do you say to her?"

"It's not so much what *I* say, it's more what I imagine she says to me, and—"

"Hey Orvy, look!" Cray was shouting. "You're on TV!"

They rushed to the set. There he was shaking hands with Henry Schooner. Orville had told Miranda about Schooner's promise, and now they watched his betrayal. In spite of himself, Orville's disgust was tempered with astonishment. What he had seen as a chaotic, pitifully amateurish scene with a *schlumpy* candidate and an unattractive crowd under a brooding sky had been transformed.

The camera had created a world of order and professionalism. Henry Schooner looked terrific—chest out, smile big, collar and tie snappy, white hair wind-blown, hatless and winter jacketless and impervious to the cold that had everyone else bundled up to their eyeteeth. All of this gave the impression of vitality, of an outdoorsy youthful candidate who those of a certain age could not help but associate with John F. Kennedy or Robert. In the segment they ran, Henry was clasping Orville's hand and elbow with confidence and conviction. "God Bless America" played subtly in the background. Orville, identified as "the town doctor," looked pale and tired and, yes, *schlumpy* but seemed in that video moment to be in the very process of being *transformed,* popped out of the worn, dull groove of his daily grind and uplifted. Clearly, one man's hand-and-elbow clasp was lifting another man up into the rare atmosphere of a seminal event in Columbian, perhaps even American, history. Other footage showed Nelda Jo and Henry Jr. and little Maxie held up high in Henry's arms—all as telegenic as their man. The background music was somehow muted yet hopeful. Strangest of all, the day itself had been fashioned anew. It was bright and cheery, lit with angel-rays of light streaming down through the clouds, a joyous, even biblical, illumination.

And when Henry spoke, it was magical. That voice! Where had they heard that voice before? It was a little husky, down-homey, honest, even authentic—a voice neither Orville nor Miranda could ever recall having come from Schooner in person. A leader's voice, a voice they could follow: The Voice.

"You asshole!" Orville shouted at the tube. "You slimeball!"

"Orvy?" Miranda said, squeezing his arm, motioning to Cray.

"What's wrong, Orvy?" Cray said, frightened.

An ad for acid indigestion came on. "Nothing, Cray. Sorry."

"But I *like* seeing you on TV. Why are you mad?"

"I said, *nothing!*" Cray's face collapsed. Orville felt terrible. "Hey, I'm sorry." Cray turned away, back to the TV.

"Why don't you and Cray play something?" Miranda suggested.

Cray turned around and looked at her, then at Orville. He seemed to be calculating. "Will you help me make my B-52?"

Orville stifled a groan. Sol's Toys—because of Selma's love affair with flight—had specialized in model airplanes. For years, on every birthday he was presented with a new model airplane kit to glue, decal, and paint. Orville grew to loathe making the planes. His finished products never matched the pictures on the boxes. But now, what choice did he have?

They worked on the bomber. But soon Cray was whining, criticizing Orville's technique. "No, you're not doing it right! Let me do it myself!"

"Cray," Miranda said, across the kitchen table. "Be nice, okay?"

They went on a while longer and then Cray, again in a whining tone, said, "No, you don't know how to put on the decal right. You *never* do it right!" He burst into tears, threw down the plane, ran upstairs to his room, and slammed the door.

In the heightened silence, Orville and Miranda stared at each other.

"Should I go up there?" he asked.

"Give him a little time."

"I feel terrible."

"I know. It's okay. Just wait."

They sat together quietly, straining to hear any sounds from upstairs.

There was a squeak, Cray's door opening. They held their breath. Was he coming down? Nothing. They went upstairs, Orville leading. The stairs creaked.

The door slammed. Harder. Taped to the door was a fresh sign.

PLEZ CAEP OET

"At least he said please," Miranda said.

"Yeah, but why's he writing to us in Dutch?"

She laughed, hugged him. They went into her bedroom, undressed, and got into bed.

There was a knock on the front door. Several more knocks.

"Who in the world?" Miranda said, suddenly frightened.

"I'll get it." He pulled on his clothes, went downstairs, turned on the outdoor light, and opened the door. Henry Schooner. He looked bad and smelled bad. Sweaty, boozy.

"I know, I know," he said. "Can I come in?"

"No. Get out of here!"

"I know you think I'm a sonofabitch but—"

"A lying sonofabitch—"

"—but you heard me call the fucker, and—"

"I don't think there was anyone on the other end of the line."

"You *don't?*" Henry seemed about to collapse. Orville instinctively reached out and grabbed his arm. Henry seemed to be trying to get into the house. "Can I come in?"

"No!" Orville closed the door firmly and went outside to face him.

A window opened above. "Orvy, who is it?"

"Nobody."

"Aw shit!" Henry cried out drunkenly. "Izz *me*, M'randa! Kin I come in?"

"No!" Orville said. "I'll handle it," he said to her. "Go back to bed."

"Okay." She closed the window and turned off the upstairs light.

Suddenly he was seeing Schooner up close. His doctor's eyes took in the tiny spider telangectasiae on his nose, a sign of chronic alcohol intake, the weathered skin older than his years, the little fatty deposits on the half-hooded lids that suggested a family history of high cholesterol. There was a strand of spaghetti and a red stain on his rumpled white shirt.

His hair was messed up, his mouth looked sloppy, his chin flabby—not only had the TV camera hidden all this, Orville realized, but it was as if in creating something more of Schooner, it had reached in and taken something from him, leaving him, in reality, somehow less.

"I came here to make retributions—no, reparations . . . razza razza roo."

"You were always a sleazeball, and you're still a sleazeball, so forget it."

"Here." He reached into his shirt pocket for a piece of paper. "I called the fuckin' station, sent this to them and *The Crier,* saying it don't mean you support me."

Orville took the letter and crumpled it up and threw it away.

"It's a free press," Henry went on. "I can't control the bastards. I'll make it up to you. We'll do deals together, play golf. I want to earn your respect."

"*Why?* Why in hell do you keep talking about earning my respect?"

"'Cuz it'd be like finding out my big brother loves me after all."

"Get a life, Henry. Get a damn life."

"I'm tryin' ol' buddy." His eyes were wet. "I really am."

"Go home." Henry didn't move. As if talking to a dog, Orville repeated, emphatically, "*Go. Home.*"

"I respect you so much, Orvy. I even dream of you, did you know that?"

"How the hell could I know that?"

"Nice dreams, where you're my friend." The Voice, the husky and kindly and sure one that commanded attention, had gone, replaced by just a voice, one like any other.

"Good night." Orville turned and went in, closing the door and shutting off the light. He listened for the sound of the Grand Marquis starting up and, for what seemed the longest time, heard nothing. Finally, there was the cough of the starter and the pebbly rush of the tires, fading.

Miranda met him at the head of the stairs and took his hand. They went in to check on Cray and then got back into bed.

Orville still felt terrible about how he'd acted with Cray. Miranda tried to reassure him, talking, holding him close, caressing him until his doubt and anger gave way to the electricity of touch.

And Cray? The boy had clicked off like a light switch, with no sense of having fallen asleep until the moment he awoke.

16

Honey-b,

How are you? I wonder how I am. What I really wonder is how I will have died. I hope quick. But it doesn't matter what I hope now because now it's over. Not now, you know, but *now.* The dead now.

By now you're probably still not over your resentment of my will. Of my grounding you for a year and 13 days. Well, Mr. Bigshot Stubborn, too bad. *Father Knows Best* is a joke. *Mother Knows Best* is God's Truth. It's a human thing for a mother to want her son to have a normal life, especially if he's gone off track. But not you, no! In *none* of Sol's beautiful Kodak family color photos are you smiling. Not one smile. This is saying something—"

"Why do I keep reading?" he asked the toaster oven. It didn't reply. He had gotten the letter that morning and had started it. It was instantly upsetting, though, and he had a hard day ahead, so he'd put it away. Now, at six that night, he felt he could face it.

You have no memory of your childhood. I remember every second. You were the most stubborn kid on the block, silent and sullen. Not like your old friend Henry Schooner. Delightful boy, and now quite the man! He's back, as you know, and a big success. A Pillar Of The Community. Married a nice girl. *Zaftik,* but Baptist. This morning—it's 3 A.M.—I want to chat about one eensy-weensy little piece of your global selfishness that hurt me very deeply.

You and Lily couldn't have children. Abnormal. SO *WHAT?* (To have you, I had to have my tubes blown by Bill Starbuck—talk about *pain!* Good man, bad doctor.) On July 24, 1981, Sol and I hop in the New Yorker—*Nice* car, isn't it? And the trunk space? You could die! (And I have!)—and drive down to Jersey to celebrate what you think is your 37th birthday. So hot you could puke. The Garden State stinks to high heaven. Your house is dirty. All this we endure. We go out for a meal. (Lily never cooks.) Chinx. We sing Happy Birthday—very difficult for Sol and me, since it really isn't. You pay. We appreciate.

In the car you look in the rearview mirror and tell us you two are thinking of adopting a half-Negro girl and have to decide by tomorrow and that you already asked Lily's parents their opinion.

Your father and I almost blow our Chinx. But we keep cool. I say to myself, WHAT NEXT? Sol tries to be constructive. He says of course being half-Negro she could not be Jewish, and of course when you visit us in Florida she could not stay in our condo so you'd have to rent a motel and so forth. But otherwise, Sol says, it's wonderful.

You start screaming. Lily pulls her crying trick. Shocked, we quiet right down. Arrive at your less-than-clean home. No one is talking. I'm biding my time. Finally after you've had two large scotches before bed, I catch you alone in the hallway and say, "I am deeply deeply hurt that you told Lily's parents *before* you told us." You go bananas. Scream a lot loudly. Given our family history, I worry you will make a suicide gesture. As usual when I invite you to converse, you run. Run right out of the house. I'm so tired my good eye is seeing triple, but do I go to sleep? No, I wait up. I stay there on my mother-vigil, sitting up like I did all those nights in high school when you were running around with Laurice the *shiksa,* 'til you come home safe and sound. Even after the horrible things you said to me, your mother. Why do I do this? *Well, who the hell else will?* I stay up.

Because I am a person who is loving and kind and who cares. For your information, a good mother. This may come as news to you. But just ask Penny or Amy or Henry Schooner. Do a little survey.

Love Mom

Orville looked out the kitchen window, into the yard, up into the trees, hoping she'd be there so he could crucify her. But no. The Columbian weatherman had predicted an unseasonably mild and sunny day; a vicious midwinter storm had arrived. An arctic air mass sliding down the Hudson had met a low pressure slithering up from the Carolinas and bingo!—heavy snow carried on gusting wind in which even dead mothers wouldn't fly. He was tempted to throw the letter into the garbage, but since he'd saved all seven previous letters, locked in a safe in Bill's office, he tucked it into his black bag.

Clack! The wind clapped a branch against the window. Better get out to Miranda's before I get stuck. Hayley came in, bundled up to leave. She stood beside him, so short that she was at eye level. She'd spent the afternoon cleaning out beer bottles, cigar butts, strewn clothes, and horrific Columbian junkfood. Hayley was a reminder of much that was good. They'd gotten close again, she cooking, they sitting and watching TV or listening to Mississippi John Hurt, her favorite Delta bluesman. Her favorite lines: "When my earthly trials are over, cast my body down in the sea. Save all the undertaker's bills, let the mermaids flirt with me." And his: "It ain't no more potatoes, frost have killed the vine. Blues ain't nothin' but a good woman on your mind." He was treating her arthritis successfully with Starbusol. Whiz was going to AA, and her husband Clive's mechanical and electrical genius applied to the salvation of junk at Gieger's had recently merited a raise. Hayley was happier.

"Dr. O.," she said, "will you check out this obituary I writing for the paper?"

He looked it over. "Terrence Jones Sr., Shiloh Baptist Church member. On February 18, God walked into His Garden and admired everything. With a great interest, God made a decision to give our Terrence a call. So family, may yesterdays memories, each and everyone, help you accept in sympithy that God's will is done. Terr is going home."

"Hayley," he said, "it's beautiful. I wouldn't change a word." She gave him that chipmunk smile he adored. "Tell me. You think Selma's gone home?"

"Not hardly. She buried here, but never was home here. She said 219 West Tremont Bronx was home once, long gone. I asked her about Heaven. She told me the Jewish way says they ain't no such thing! No *Heaven?* So I suppose she very *jumpy* up there now—"

The front doorbell rang. Hayley went to answer it. He heard her say, "Oh, Lord!"

"Hi, Hayley. Good to see you again."

Orville went rigid. *You never forget the voice.* And then she was in the kitchen, his ex-wife, Lily Wolf.

How different she looks—older, thinner. Richer. Richer because of her cute mink pillbox hat and mink-collared charcoal coat flowing elegantly to her shoes—and talk about shoes! Sleek, shiny high heels built up in gleaming zebra layers of hardwood that he knew from Celestina were Italian and cost a billion *lire* a pair. Over her shoulder was a black leather purse. In one darkly gloved hand she clutched a narrow paper bag scrunched up at the top—clearly booze. Her nails on the other, ungloved hand were scarlet, as were her plump lips. A diamond as big as a dime caught the fading daylight. Not daring to meet her eyes, he stared into the diamond and saw in its facets the falling snowflakes of the storm outside, flashing here and there like angels in flight from a serious dark. She looked good. Kind of gorgeous, really, in a new, sophisticated way. Meeting her dark brown eyes, he braced himself against the red Formica countertop. In the long silence he searched her older face for clues. Strange to feel a stab of love toward this woman who'd convinced him that he was profoundly unloveable, and unloving.

"Hello," Lily said. Her voice had deepened, relaxed down the chromatic scale. She took off her mink hat. Her black hair was shorter, styled back as if fluffed kindly by a breeze. Her scent read "expensive." Hayley excused herself and left.

"What are you doing here?" he asked.

"I was driving up to Albany for a deal, and the snow on the Taconic got worse and worse and here I am. The meeting's not until tomorrow morning." He wondered if she expected to stay over with him. "Don't worry," she said. "I'll stay in a hotel."

"That's okay. You can stay here. Plenty of room."

"We'll see. I heard about your mother, you know, through the grapevine."

"The Penny grapevine?"

"Yes. I would have sent a card, but . . ."

"You didn't want to trust the mail."

They laughed. After a year of their student romance in Dublin, Lily had gone back to NYU while Orville stayed in med school. The long-distance relationship didn't work. They fell out of touch. After a few months, Lily sent a letter that she was getting married in ten days to an older man who worked on "The Street." Orville was surprised to learn that this meant Wall Street. Heartbroken, on the day of the wedding he sat around O'Dwyer's getting shitfaced with his fellow med students. Weeping gallantly, Gaelically, into his Guiness. Two weeks later he felt better. He was done with her for good.

But then one night after midnight an emphysematous postman trudged into the med students' sleeping quarters on the ground floor of the National Maternity Hospital with a letter for him. It was marked "special delivery" but was postmarked the day of the wedding, ten days before. He opened it and read. "Disregard previous letter. Couldn't go through with it. Still love only you, forever. Forgive me. Love, Lily." Why had it taken so long to get to him? She forgot to send it Air Mail. It was the world's first Special Delivery Sea Mail letter. It had floated lazily across the Atlantic and upon arrival in Cork City had been rushed across Ireland on the Cork-Dublin Express and hurried up to him by the night-shift postman yearning for oxygen.

Now she was taking off her expensive coat, revealing other riches. A smartly cut pinstriped suit with two points of a hankie puffing up out of a pocket, and around her neck hung a lyric of gold and a few grace notes of diamonds. Flat tummy, wonderful boobs, visible cheekbones, sleek hair, perfume, and a friendly sparkle in her eyes.

"Everything looks so small!" she said. "The town, the house, the kitchen."

Orville was alarmed to realize that for him this was no longer the case. It all looked normal-sized now, even big. "Not to me. So, what's the deal?"

"There's no *deal*," she said, tightly, mistaking what he was asking. "I really did get scared driving in the snow and—"

"No, no, I mean the deal in *Albany*. Your deal?"

"Oh." She laughed, slightly less tightly. "Oh, well, it's an LBO, some company that makes plumbing fixtures. A hostile takeover."

How fitting, he thought. At the time he'd run off to Europe, she'd just graduated from business school and was job hunting. "So, you're in business?"

"VC." She picked up his puzzled look. "Venture capital."

"Ah. Funny, isn't it. Not so long ago it meant Viet Cong."

"I'm with Drexel," she went on, seeming not to register this, which made him a little sad, "junk bonds. The money's incredible. Reagan's amazing, as if he's giving us permission to *print* money. They say the market'll go to a *thousand* by the end of his second term. It's wild. Offer a junk bond, you have to beat away the money with a stick!"

All this seemed strange to him. When he'd met her in Dublin, she was majoring in English lit at NYU, focusing on criticism, which, when the marriage died, seemed fitting. She had strengths, but calculations were beyond her. Her checkbook read like a novel.

"I'm surprised," he said. "You never were all that terrific with numbers."

"I'm still not." She smiled. "The guys with the short pencils and the green eyeshades do all that. Business is relationships. Fear and greed. Who you know and who you . . ." She stopped herself. Picking up the brown paper bag, she said, "I brought us a present."

"Bushmills."

"What else?" She took out the square bottle, solid amber. "I've traveled a lot, you know, but I've stayed away from Dublin. Our Dublin."

"I went back once." Her face showed a flicker of hurt. "To see my old doctor friends, Tony and Noel. Remember them?" He held up the bottle. "Neat or on ice?"

"Neat. And if you happen to have a beer chaser?"

He did. They settled in at the kitchen table, drinking. She wanted to reminisce about Dublin. At first he was reluctant, the way you are reluctant when someone starts to tell you what you were like as a kid. But soon her insistence on nostalgia seduced him. It was easier than anything else in their past and far easier than the present.

He'd been doing obstetrics at the National Maternity Hospital on Holles Street. She showed up in the hospital's small old amphitheater one day for a lecture on James Joyce. Being the only Americans, they'd gotten together. She knew nothing about medicine. He knew nothing about literature. She told him that three chapters of *Ulysses* were set in the hospital, back then called Horne's House. He asked, "What's *Ulysses?*"

Soon they were inseparable. She hung around with the medical students. They went to parties at the Mater, short for the Mater Misericordia, the other maternity hospital, the one affiliated with the snooty Anglican Trinity College, and spent nights in all possible pubs. Joyce, too, she said, had been a medical student briefly at UCD. Orville read *Ulysses* and visited the sites with her, from Howth Head to Leopold Bloom's house at 7 Eccles Street in coal-smoke-scented-and-damp north Dublin, walked the high-arched metal footbridge over the Liffey and past Stephen's Green, and took a bus to Dalkey and Sandycove and the Martello Tower where Daedelus begins his day's odyssey.

The recalled high points of that part of their past matched, both of them remembering a weekend when they'd taken a train to Galway, bought a Jack B. Yeats pen-and-ink and watercolor drawing called *The Side Car,* and made love for the first time in a bed-and-breakfast overlooking Galway Bay. The next day they'd hitched a ride on a small scruffy fishing boat the twenty-some miles out to Aranmore. The captain insisted they share his lunch, which was Spam tasting of diesel. They walked the silent, stone-fenced lanes of the great last island before the Atlantic, both burping diesel. They crawled into the bee-hive stone huts of the early Christian hermits. They climbed to the edge of the sheer drop-off of the cliffs facing west, toward home. They fell in love.

"And Selma's really dead, is she?" Lily was asking now.

Well, he thought, glancing out the window, now *there's* a tough question to answer.

"I mean, I'm sorry," she went on, mistaking his silence for offense taken. "But to be honest, I hardly trust her even to be really dead."

"Dead she is. You want to, maybe, do a little sitting *shiva?*"

"After what she did?" she said angrily. "*Please.*"

"Still mad, eh?"

"Hey. The more I've thought about you and me and her, sweetie, and what went wrong, the more I think it has a lot to do with her. Sometimes I feel like I'd like to mop the floor with her! The relationship between you and your mother should have been protected under the Helsinki Accords!"

"Ha! I love it!" He felt a stab of attraction to her, to the whole thing, and immediately felt guilty. And yet Lily's Selma-riff was enticing, appealing. Here, maybe, was an ally. He sat back, poured another Bushmills for them both, and said, "Tell me more."

17

Miranda was worried. Orville was supposed to have been there for dinner two hours ago. She sat by the phone at the kitchen table waiting, wondering if she dared call. I shouldn't bother him, she thought. But that just made her feel more trapped in the deference that she, as a woman, had been brought up to show a man. What to do?

Something about the fingernails of the wind on the windowpanes of the old house, the snow squall building to a steady storm, made her more worried than usual. He must be busy, too busy to call, she reasoned. She drummed her fingers on the wood, recalling the first time she'd gone through a panic about her son being late.

A year ago or so she'd let Nelda Jo take Cray and Maxie to a fiesta across the river in Athens and then to dinner with one of Nelda Jo's friends. Cray was due back by six thirty. At seven she tried to reach Nelda Jo or Henry. Nothing. Nelda Jo was usually meticulous about calling if there was any change in plans. Something must be wrong.

Seven thirty. Seven thirty-*four*. When do you actually call the police, the hospital? She envisioned the car going off the Rip Van Winkle Bridge. Or a domestic explosion. A propane tank explosion. A breakage. A kidnapping. By nine, she had called the police and both Kinderhook Memorial Hospital and Catskill Osteopathic.

Tethered to the phone in the kitchen, she was shouting at it, sometimes crying, even once down on her knees praying. "Please, God, Cray is all I have. If he dies I'll kill myself, and you don't want *that* on your conscience, do you?"

Finally the phone rang. She snatched it up, clenched it. "Hello?"

"This is the Columbia police." Her heart stopped. "It's about a Memorial Fund for—" She almost fainted, until she realized that the policeman was soliciting money for dead Columbian officers and their families.

It wasn't until after nine thirty that the phone rang again. Nelda Jo. Cheerily, she said, "Just lost track of time, honey, 'cause they were having such fun."

Miranda exploded in tears and said over and over, "Thank God! Thank God!"

Nelda Jo was apologetic, puzzled, and a little annoyed. "Why honey," she said, "I'm never late. Don't you trust me?"

"It's *because* you're usually so trustable that I was scared!"

Now, thinking of that wait for Cray calmed her. This wait for Orville was nothing like that. Cray was right here, safe in the next room. End of comparison.

But another hour passed, and Cray was getting ready for bed and asking where Orville was. With the storm building, she got more anxious. It was unlike him not to call.

The last time she'd spoken with him had been that morning, on their daily check-in call. He had seemed down. She'd asked about it.

"Got another letter from my mother. It's not easy for me."

"I know." She was surprised. He hadn't mentioned Selma in a while. "Do you?"

"Do I know what it's like to lose someone you love? I sure do."

"Yeah. Dinner tonight?"

She offered to cook. He said he'd try to be there early. She said fat chance but do your best. They wished each other nice days and hung up.

Now, still waiting by the phone, Miranda was concerned. Whenever he received one of Selma's letters, he was in a foul mood. It would come out as a shortness with her or Cray or in the way he talked about his patients—a cynical, even contemptuous way she found disturbing, at odds with what she loved most about him, his compassion. She was all too familiar with the ups and downs of grief, of the mourning process. She wished she could help. Sometimes she'd ask about how he was doing with his mother's death, but he wouldn't talk about it. Maybe it was for the better. Maybe not.

"Mom," Cray was saying to her, standing at the kitchen table. "I want to go to *bed*. Where's Orvy?"

"I don't know, honey. I'll call him." She picked up the phone and dialed.

◇ ◇ ◇

Orville and Lily were still in the kitchen, drinking and talking, when the phone rang. On the second ring, Orville looked at his watch. *Shit!* He let it ring again. He felt embarrassed, as if he were betraying Lily, not Miranda.

"Excuse me." He hurried upstairs to take it in his turret bedroom.

"Hello?"

"Hi. I was worried. With the storm. Are you okay?"

"Yeah, fine."

"I was waiting. Dinner and all. Why didn't you call?"

"I got, you know, busy. Lost track of time. Look, with the storm, there's no way I can get out there tonight."

"What's wrong?"

"Um . . . nothing. Nothing's wrong."

"Are you still upset about your mother's letter?"

"No, no, that's not it. I'm okay with that."

"Then what is it?"

He paused. "My ex-wife showed up, out of the blue."

Her heart slipped. She tried to hide her pain in silence.

"Miranda? Hello? Hello? You still there?"

"Sort of."

"Look, I'm really sorry. She just arrived, you know, after two years she happened to be driving up to Albany, got caught in the storm, came here."

"Fine," she said coldly.

"Wait—it's not like that."

"I'm not calling just for me," she said. "It's Cray. He won't go to bed until he talks to you."

Orville's heart slid somewhere awful. "Put him on."

The phone, passed down two feet, crackled.

"Hi, Orvy."

"Hi, Cray."

"Aren't you gonna say 'Oh, I *love* that word!'?"

"Oh, I *love* that word!"

"Can we do Animal Guessing Game?"

"It's late."

"Just one? You think of the animal and I'll guess. Please?"

"Okay."

"Got it?"

Orville counted silently to five. "Got it. But I'm warning you. It's a hard one."

"Is it a . . . a . . . a peregrine falcon?"

Again, Orville counted to five. "Did you say a . . . peregrine falcon?"

"Yeah!"

"You didn't say a . . . a . . . a peregrine falcon, did you?"

"I did, I did! You *know* I did!"

"Unbelieveable. It was a peregrine falcon."

"I knew it."

"How do you *do* that?"

Cray was silent for a few seconds. "Orvy, was it really?"

"Really."

"I mean really, really?"

"Really, really, yep."

Cray yawned, saying through the yawn, "I always get it with you. G'night."

"Good night. Sleep tight." Orville heard the phone, rising back up two feet to Miranda, crackle.

"Get your sleepies on, Cray, and I'll be up to read to you." The boy went up to bed. "One of these days," she said to Orville, "he's going to find you out."

"And?" She said nothing. "You mean I shouldn't let him think that he has magical powers?"

"When he finds out the truth you're going to have a hard time getting him to trust you again.

"Hey, c'mon, it's just a game."

"Good night."

"Wait. I love you. I'll call you later."

"Thanks." She hung up. Shaken, she made sure to take care in climbing the stairs.

Orville, feeling all torn up, went back down to Lily.

"What's her name?" Lily asked.

"Miranda."

"Do you love her?"

"Yes. And no."

"Meaning?"

"Yes, as I'm able now. No, as I'm unable. Disabled."

"Disabled in love?"

"I'm sure you'd agree."

"Don't be so sure. It's been two years. A lot can change." She smiled at him. "It's okay. I've got a banker. Net-net, we're both taken."

He looked at Lily. An old warmth had come into her eyes. He could have sworn he saw a wetness there, as if something harsh and hard were melting. She looked back down into her Bushmills.

Their reminiscing about Dublin and their talking about Selma had stirred him up. They had avoided talking about the marriage and the divorce. It had been a clean break, fiscally. At the time, he had felt so guilty at his oafish behavior that he'd given Lily everything. He figured that his only hope lay in letting go of whatever was dear to him. He ran off with only his black bag, a backpack with a panda on its back proclaiming *World Wildlife Fund,* assorted toiletries and tranquillizers, a deluxe Swiss Army knife, and a bunch of credit cards.

If their shared nostalgia about Dublin had spread a little magic around the sorry kitchen, their talk of Selma had spread a little spite. Lily and he had shared a foxhole in the Selma Wars. Selma had won the war, but you never forget the buddy you lost it with. Orville knew that what they were saying about Selma would be intolerable to her and wondered if she would fly in for a guest appearance. Maybe Lily would be able to see her, too. From time to time he peered out the large old windows in the kitchen and up into the snowy sky. But no, weather conditions must have been too severe, even for Selma. The only spirits present were their own younger ones—and for him, Miranda. He felt terrible about how he'd been just now to her.

"It *is* remarkable," Lily was saying, "what we had. For awhile."

"Yeah, it was," he said, the past tense shooting out.

She didn't seem to notice and went on in a warm, almost whimsical way. "I mean, the dreams." She sighed, less sadly then, as if comforted. "Bottom line? I wonder if *I* would try again."

The Hamster. Suddenly for him the hamster was the elephant in the room. The damn thing had sealed his sterility, crushed their dream of children. There it was, looming large, being ignored. Lily was looking at him expectantly. Was she serious? He felt trapped. With Lily it had all too often felt this way—the pressure on, he pinned at her sharp edges. Trapped in just this kind of moment where the room gets real still and the feelings are so intense that it seems you could reach out and run your fingers over them, but you dare not because if you so much as graze them

153

the whole room—hell the whole house—will collapse with all the comic breakage of a Columbian civic souffle. In such hopeful and hellish moments everything carries such intense meaning you dare not look away or toward, shift in your chair, even breathe. Everything hangs in the balance of a glance, a move, a word, a sound. It had been exhausting.

"C'mon," she said, cheerily. "I just want to have some fun." She rose, came over to him, bent down, and kissed him on the mouth. Then she sat on his lap. "It's great, after all these years, sweetie, to see your eyes. No more thick glasses! I forgot what a beautiful blue. *Good* move, contacts. Eyes are such a turn-on for me."

"You look great, too. You're gorgeous. In great shape."

"Yeah. I work on myself. Hard."

She kissed him again, mouth open, her tongue exploring. Then she unbuttoned the top two buttons of her white silk blouse and took his hand and put it on her bra. He slipped his fingers under the satin, searched out the small, pointy hardness there, thinking, of all things, *Cork City.* He was getting aroused but trying to fight it. *You're in love with Miranda, you jerk! Cut it out!*

But drunk and turned on, he felt a driving curiosity about Lily now. The old love was churning in his gut, and lower. Despite everything, he was opening up again to her, to this woman he'd loved longer and harder than anyone else, the first woman he'd let in under his shyness. He shivered, reminding him of how, at first, he used to shiver as they would begin to make love, a sympathetic nervous system response.

"What's wrong?" Lily was looking at him expectantly.

"Nothing." He disentangled himself from her embrace.

"It's okay, you can tell me. What are you feeling?"

He was feeling dread, which prevented him from telling her what he was feeling. The little voice inside said, *Nothing good can come of my going into this. It's just a matter of how bad it'll be before it's over. And it'll never be over.* He said nothing.

"Can you tell me?"

"I'm thinking of the hamster. About how it finished us off."

"*Hamster?*" She blinked, as if to clear her sight. "The hamster was a symptom."

"Of what?"

"Neurosis. Mine, yours. Early childhood shit. I'm taking care of mine. On the couch. I'm in psychoanalysis. Taking care of business. I know where it comes from in me. I know who I am, what I want. Look how I initiated. I *never* did that before, right?"

"Right."

"One thing I learned is that I don't need a kid to know who I am."

Her statement, her being so strong and sure of herself, rocked him back on his heels. It made him wonder if *he* needed a kid to know who he was. Cray. He loved Cray. He knew that. He could tell her that, but she wasn't asking.

"—To be perfectly honest," she was saying, with a conspiratorial wink, "I'm surprised at my cathexis to you tonight."

"Cathexis?"

"Id to id, kid." She laughed. "Early childhood attraction." She put her arms around his neck and smiled. "I know who I am now. I know all the little corners of myself. And not just the clean ones, either. I'm ready."

"I'm not."

"Of course you're not, sweetie," she said, reassuringly. "You're running on fumes. It's called Jewish mother guilt."

"You're over that, are you?"

"Worked it through on the couch. My banker, my new sweetie?" She paused and then went on proudly, "He's a German."

"Ah." Lily had always loathed Germans. "Amazing."

"Very. Show's where I've gotten. Tonight, hearing you talk about Selma, I know you're not done with her. She's still hanging around, isn't she?"

If you only knew!

"Poisoning your *self*. *I* worked through mine. You have to work through yours. And we'd be all set. Two strong selves. Win-win. Analyzed, the sky's the limit."

Orville felt cold. The century-old radiators banged the pipes, taking their time catching up with the thermostat. *Like I never seem to catch up with my life.* He yearned for that sensual motherly warmth as a bird in late autumn, stalling migration, yearns for imagined sun. But he knew from his doctoring how far the actual falls short of the yearning, like the gap between a flight and a fall. He remembered something that had happened last summer with Celestina Polo in the hotel overlooking Lago del Orta. A sparrow had flown into their room. A small sparrow, a fledgling. Even, perhaps, on its first flight. It fluttered frantically about the room searching for a way out. Finally, exhausted, it landed on the marble ledge over the fireplace. He reached for it and gently took it in his hand. It was tiny, remarkably light, as if made all of feathers. Ghostly but for its trembling. Its eyes glittered like black ice. He took it out onto the balcony, raised his hand palm up to the sky, as if offering a sacrifice from the realm of Good Human Beings to the Gods of Flight, and released it. It lay there on his palm, dead. It had died of terror.

"This may sound strange," he said to Lily, "but I'm moving in another direction."

"Which is?"

"I feel I've gotten too much into myself. I'm trying to get out of myself, looking for something else."

"Ohh . . . kay," she said, clearly suspicious. "What 'something else'?"

He didn't know but said, "The spiritual." This was Celestina's word, but he borrowed it like you borrow a friend's car when yours breaks down.

"Oh, boy."

Her obvious contempt brought back a memory of his own contempt, at first, for Celestina's talking about spiritual stuff. And then brought back something Celestina had said in one of their long talks after making love. "Freud is a joke, a cruel joke. Just another tight-assed *patriarca* putting evil energy out into the world, *caro,* the energy of the ego, the self. The self is the past. If you focus on your past, you live your misery. *Allora,* always comparing yourself to someone else and feeling better than them or worse than them. Always into becoming, while our freedom is in our very being."

"Never mind," he said now. "You wouldn't understand."

"Try me."

"Not getting into myself or my past but getting out of it."

"Running away?"

It was like a punch in the gut. This was her old accusation, and Selma's, too. "I was thinking," he said, trying to breathe, "of being in love."

"With?"

"Now, with Miranda and Cray. When I first met you, with you. We were so in love. Then, we forgot ourselves. Remember?"

"Cray?"

"Her son. He's six."

She sat quietly. Her eyes pooled with tears. He felt a rush of old love for her—more, felt for all she'd been through and come through. She was, after all, a fighter.

She reached for a tissue and her arm hit her drink and spilled it and she said "Shit!" pretty viciously. Faster than he thought possible she got up, snatched a roll of paper towels, and wiped up the spill, cleaning the whole segment of the cherry table, then the whole table. She faced him again.

"Bottom line?" she said. "I stayed, you ran. Where do I sleep?"

"Wait a minute—"

"Where?"

"Upstairs. Four bedrooms. Take your pick."

"Where will you be?"

"Down here. On the couch."

"Very funny."

"I didn't mean it to be."

"Exactly." She gathered up her things. "I'll find my own way."

"Upstairs?"

"That too." She turned away.

"Lily?"

"Yes?"

"I'm sorry."

"I'm not."

"This is all so, so incredibly sad!"

"Yes, it is," she said. "But I don't expect happiness anymore."

"No?"

"No. Just a liveable level of neurosis."

"Good night."

"Good-bye." She started down the hallway. He heard a sob. She came back and stood in the doorway. Her voice trembled as she spoke.

"My big mistake was not that I let you into my life, no. I loved you with all my heart, and we helped each other escape from our families, mostly, and that's a big deal. No, my big mistake was letting your mother into our lives. You want to know what did it, what screwed us up? It wasn't me, and it wasn't you, and it certainly wasn't any goddamn rodent. It was your mother. And it still is. Good-bye."

He had a rough night on the couch. Awakening at dawn, he heard Lily come downstairs. He lay there in the living room, squinting through his banging hangover down the hall toward the kitchen, pretending to still be asleep. She stood at the kitchen counter, pen in hand. She glanced at him to see if he was awake.

There was no sound. The snow had stopped. The wind had died. Sharp reddish light was starting to dice up the dark. She was leaving.

He lay still, in turmoil. An old part of him was desperate to open his eyes, a new part unwilling.

Lily finished her writing. She glanced at him again, seemed to shudder, or shiver, and, he sensed, even move toward him a step or two. Quickly she turned way and, without looking back, walked out the back door, forcing it open against a significant drift.

He sat up. A car door slammed. An engine started. She'll never get out, he thought. I'll help her. He walked to the back door, hesitated. Ah, the hell with it.

He heard her car wheels whine, trying for traction, and then he heard them getting it. Despite himself, he felt a wave of regret. Wait—there's more to say! He walked out the back door into the high drifts of the back-yard, his bare feet landing in her footsteps. Standing in the driveway he shouted, "Hey, Lily, wait!"

Too late. Somehow she had gotten out without a hitch, her big new Saab blasting through a drift where the driveway met Coffin.

She was gone. He stood there in the clear space where her car had been, as if at a barren fresh grave in a snowy cemetery, surprised at how sad he felt now that it was finally over. Then he realized, from the fierce bite of the cold, that not only was he barefoot and bareheaded but wearing only his underpants. He went back inside.

On the kitchen table was her note.

Dear O.,

I feel all torn up. I'm not as tough as I came across. I made a vow "'Til death do us part" and it's still down there in my unconscious some-where. I still love you but I know now that it's over. Because you have changed, and because you're so deeply involved with your "Miranda." And your "Cray." Finally I have closure. I'm crying but that's it. Love,

Me.

He was staring at the letter—at the stains of her tears that had fallen on it—when the front doorbell rang. Hope shot up his spine—and fear shot back down. He put on his clothes, went down the hallway, and opened the front door.

Henry Schooner. Bundled up beautifully, head bare, dazzling white. Be-hind him was his mammoth army Jeep, a snowplow hung from the front. It was revving rhythmically, like an animal growling, ready to spring.

"Hey, old buddy. Need any help gettin' out?"

"No thanks."

"Y'sure? I mean, you got that bare patch there for traction where your ladyfriend's car was parked, but that darn Chrysler's hell's bells in the snow. Can't have our town doctor socked in, right?"

Orville stared at him, stared into that cheerful good citizen's dark eyes, until he had a weird feeling that brought to mind how the boy Mowgli had been hypnotized by Kaa the Snake's eyes in the *Jungle Book* video, and the only words that came out, and from what seemed a long way off, were, "Right. Thanks."

"No charge," Schooner said happily, and tromped down the porch in those oversized no-nonsense boots worn by the astronauts walking on the moon, tromped through the four-foot snowdrifts where the walk used to be, and got into his indomitable moonbuggyish Jeep. Rolling down the window, from which came the optimistic strains of Copland's great symphony of the West, Henry called back up to him, "And don't worry, old friend. I'll send my man right over to do your walk."

18

Miranda was up in the attic of her house. She sat on the floor. The rusted lid of her aunt's old steamer trunk yawned wide above her. As if, she thought, to drive home the indifference of things to human history. They rust, we die.

The attic ran the length of the house, from the small gable window looking out at the two lone pines to the matching window facing the river, through which came the slanting sun of the February afternoon, settling in four trapezoidal sheets on the wide floorboards—much as it had, on and off, for 320-odd years. It was a Saturday. She was alone in the house. Cray had gone off with Amy to watch her rehearse *West Side Story* at her private school, Spook Rock Country Day. Penny had picked him up at one and would drop him back at three. Miranda had arranged all this carefully. She needed to be alone for a few hours of nostalgia. Her mother's satin-and-lace wedding dress, which had also been her wedding dress—floor-length, it had hidden her leg that day—flowed out of the trunk onto her lap. It was the fourth anniversary of the day her husband had died.

She saw now how deaths echo deaths. For the first time since his death, her time with her grief was not pure. Next to the trunk was the cardboard box emblazoned with Scomparza Moving and Funeral that contained Selma's letters. The slant of light on the floorboards reminded her not of Florida sunlight but of that autumnal light through the library window falling on the slab of Becraft limestone pocked with trilobites, the afternoon that Orville and her love had coalesced. She felt split between the memory of the man who had died and the little death of sorts, two nights ago now, of the man she had come to love. Both men had let her down. The worst was the false promise each had made to her son.

Maybe it was just her fatigue. Cray had caught the inevitable February cold, and his coughing and sneezing had kept both of them up most of the last two nights. Between her exhaustion and her grief, she felt as if she were in an altered state—quick to snap, slow to forgive. Cray had been the target of some of this. When he left with Amy and Penny, she thought she caught a hint of relief in him at getting away from her. Which also broke her heart a little. The weird thing now, she thought, in the fuzz of being overtired but not sleepy, is that of all these things in the attic, the Orville stuff is more vital to me than the stuff of my dead husband. Am I avoiding the pain of my marriage and its end?

She hadn't yet gotten together with Orville after the awkward phone call when he told her that his ex was with him. He called the next morning, said he would come out and see her after work that night. His voice sounded different—distant, filled with what she took as unfaced guilt— and she felt herself falling, spiraling down. At the end of the day he called from the hospital, shouts and sirens in the background, saying that he was overwhelmed. He sounded tired and sardonic. He called again after midnight. The sound of ambulances and horrific screams filled the phone line. People were dying, he said, but, "just my luck, not fast enough for me to leave." He couldn't get there but would see her the next day. Given the impending anniversary of her husband's death—which she'd kept secret from him—his easy cynicism about death didn't sit well with her.

His last phone call came an hour ago, his voice raspy with fatigue. He was in his office, hadn't slept all night, and said he'd be there within the hour.

"Don't bother," she'd said.

"At all?" He sounded worried.

"No, no—I mean that soon. Take a nap, get yourself together. I've got something to do. I'll see you for dinner. Say, six?"

"Is Cray around?"

Miranda felt a surge of resentment. Orville had lured Cray in and was reaping the benefits of a son without doing the true work of a father. She saw all this as her own fault, and instead of screaming at him, said, "Should be, by then."

"Great. I miss him . . ." a millisecond hesitation, but long enough, " . . . too."

You fucker, she'd wanted to say, but hung up.

She turned to the trunk again, to Joe. Studying their wedding photo, reading his love letters, her heart felt it all over again—the love, the tenderness, the hope, the spilling out of her secrets for the first time ever to a man.

She wept softly. But the sobs deepened, became angry. She pounded her fists on the dusty floorboards, screaming, "What an asshole you are and maybe you did it on purpose, you jerk! You couldn't stand our happiness, was that it? Too little risk?" The forlorn stupidity and aloneness of it all tore at her heart. "What about your son, fuckhead? Look what you did to your son! Do you know he goes around even at his happiest like a kid who's had a hole blown through his heart? That I can see in his hunger for the other asshole, the Great Doctor Rose, the questions he has to live with every single minute of every single day—'Why, Momma, why? Who was he, Momma, who was he?' You think I can tell him? I don't think I ever really knew! *Our* son. He's gonna walk around the world looking for you, Joe, and what do I say to him? Were you too much of a goddamn boy yourself to share him with me? And now I'm doing it again? Shit!"

She stopped. The attic seemed to have become small, a dollhouse attic. The trunk was a dollhouse trunk. The dress was made of paper, not satin, not lace.

Desolate, she wrapped her arms around herself and rocked gently back and forth, remembering now—finally!—the way he hugged her, how they fooled around and were foolish, and so young, and a wave of grief hit her and knocked her off her feet, surprising and inevitable like grief always is, and she was weeping quietly, calming, riding out the long ebb of her sorrow, feeling it start to turn to just sorrow.

"Hello? Miranda?"

Startled, she checked her watch. Of all days to be early, he chooses today? Damn.

Orville's head poked up through the open trapdoor.

"Miranda?" he called again, in a worried voice, his eyes searching the dim attic.

"Yes?"

"You okay?"

"Yes."

"Your car was out front, but there was no sign of you and . . ." He caught sight of the wedding dress and then the big cardboard box from Scomparza Moving and Funeral. "What's wrong?"

"What time is it?"

"Almost three."

"I thought I said six. Dinner."

"Two patients went quick, and I managed to arrange some coverage."

"No nap?"

"Nope." His eyes were accommodating to the dimness. In her eyes he saw distress. "You look horrible. Can I come up?"

"No!"

"What's wrong?"

"Nothing. Go away. I'll be down in a few minutes."

"I want to help."

"Please. Go away."

"I'm sorry about not seeing you sooner. It's all my fault. I wanted to, I tried my best to, but—"

"Goddammit it's not about you, it's got nothing to do with you!" She saw his face fall and felt awful. Reaching out a hand toward him, she said, "C'mon. I'm sorry. Listen." She took a deep breath. "I . . . well . . . today's the day my husband died." She saw his surprise, and then felt his shame.

"I . . ." He paused. "I'm so sorry . . . really, really sorry. I'll leave you to it." He started to climb back down the ladder.

"No! Come here." He hesitated. "Come here."

"I thought you wanted me to go away."

"Now I want you with me." But suddenly she remembered Selma's letters and, as he climbed up, gave the Scomparza box a push further back into the darkness. "Watch your head."

He crawled over, feeling like a big dog. Still on all fours, he asked, "You want to talk about him?"

"No, just sit here beside me." She smiled. "Sit! Sit! Good boy."

Breathing a sigh of relief, he did. They had just settled down side by side in silence when a horn honked outside, and then they heard the door open and slam and several voices call out for both of them.

"They're back," she said. "Let's go."

"No, no, you stay. I'll go."

"Cray will wonder—"

"I've been dying to see him. Let me."

"Amy's with him."

"Even better. Come down when you're ready."

Orville clambered down the ladder and met Cray just as he was running up the narrow stairs. "Hi, Cray!"

"Hi, Orvy!"

"Oh I *love* that word very much!" Cray jumped up into his arms and gave him a cross between a hug and a choke hold. He sneezed into Orville's ear and sneezed again. "Here," Orville said, taking a fresh tissue out of his left pants pocket, where he always kept a supply. "Blow."

"Uncle O.?"

"Amy babe!"

Orville carried Cray downstairs to Amy and Penny. Penny fingered her key ring. As usual, she seemed to him to be one step ahead of where she was. On a tight schedule.

"I'm on a tight schedule," she said. "Gotta hop."

"Okay. How was the show, Ame?"

"Great!"

"Were you good?"

"Way!" She looked him over. "You look bad!"

"You should see it from this side."

"Are you taking the vitamins I got you?" He nodded. "You're not! I told you—"

"C'mon, Amy," Penny said. "We're late." They left.

Cray, coughing, pulled at Orville's leg. "Orvy, I wrote you another novel." He put a piece of paper in Orville's hand.

MY FRIEND ORVY
By ***CRAY*** age 6 and 1

You are my frend I am yor frend
We are both frends together
Even tho we are apart
We still can be together in on way
That way is
If Im alon you are with me
If yor alone I am with you
Thats it!

"Hey, that's great! Thanks."

"Can we watch a video together?"

"Until your mom comes downstairs, sure."

"Why only until then?"

"'Cause I have to talk to her."

"You always talk to her!" He sneezed more stuff onto Orvy.

"Here, blow again. Hey, that was a great novel."

"Yeah, but my imagination isn't too big anymore."

"It isn't?"

"Nope. When I was little I had a big imagination. It was real big—this big!" He spread his arms wide. "And when I grew bigger it got smaller."

"It did?"

"Yeah. It's big 'til you get to school. Then there are all these things they teach you and it fills your head up so it gets smaller and smaller and then it's really small. Like this big." He put his fingers close together. "So now it's small."

"I don't think it's so small. I think it's still very terrific."

"Not as small as grown-ups, but it's small. When you're really really grown-up it goes away. I'll put on *Bambi*. You stay with me for the scary part."

But Orville couldn't. Bambi's mom was still alive when Miranda came down. Cray demanded that he watch with him since he was too afraid to see the hunters kill his mom. Orville felt a pull to Miranda, needing to attend to unfinished business. Miranda, too, needed to talk. Cray sulked and turned back to the TV. Miranda suggested they go out for a walk by the river.

The late February afternoon was cold, the sun mostly down. The dark trees and bushes and railroad trestle over the creek stood out as sharply against the shiny white fields as a photo negative. Both Miranda and Orville were exhausted, their perceptions awry and jagged. He offered her his arm. She took it. Through their puffy winter coats, touch was muffled.

They inched along the icy snow-packed road toward the turnabout where the road and the creek and the tracks in front of the river all met. The snow was deep. Only a few black flecks of cinder, disturbed by the snowplow, freckled the white. The wind was from the west now, from the mountains. The creek was iced over and silent, the river iced mostly over and silent. No boats were in sight, and no birds. But for the wind circling their chilled ears, there was no sound.

Orville kept silent to give Miranda a chance to talk. She said nothing.

He tried to clear the air about Lily's visit, telling Miranda pretty much what had happened.

"But she *is* in fact gone?" Miranda asked coolly.

"Yes."

"Not about to return?"

"No. She's in love with herself and her analyst—in that order." He considered. "And a German, too. She views the German as progress."

"How old is this woman anyway?"

"Chronologically, thirty-eight. Psychoanalytically, I think three or four."

"And you have no plans to get back together with her?"

"No way! What is this? It wasn't my fault she showed up."

"It was your fault not to see me for two days—"

"All I saw for two days was bits and pieces of Columbians." He took a deep breath. "Okay, okay. Okay. Look, she threw me. And ever since, I've been in a funk, a total funk. I'm a creep. I said I was sorry and I am. Can't you just let go of it?"

"You oaf! You expect a woman who cares not to care?"

He thought about this. "You got me."

Feigning a prosecutorial tone, she said, "Now. You didn't talk to her about the whales, did you?"

"Are you insane? Of course not! The whales are ours alone."

"Okay. I've got the information. It's history." She gripped his arm in the old friendly way and, balancing on him, led him slowly further into the iced air next to the river to the railroad tracks. The dry cold air brought the Catskills closer. The mile across the iced-up river with the ridged small channel kept open by the Coast Guard cutters seemed much less.

"You must be in a lot of pain about his death," Orville said.

"Yes, I am."

They took several more steps along the tracks. The rusted steel diagonal beams at the mouth of the trestle dwarfed them.

"Want to talk about him?"

"He was a daredevil. I've come to think that, deep down, he hated himself. Couldn't stand being loved." She hesitated. "Or maybe being loving . . . or . . . no, no." She stopped talking. "Let's walk."

They picked their way carefully onto the trestle and started walking through it along the bare ground between the rails of one of the two tracks, the one nearest the river. In the crisp air the scent of creosote was strong, making Orville think back to that field of childhood where he'd caught a glimpse of something else.

"What's really getting me isn't you and her," Miranda said, "it's you and Cray." Through his coat she felt him brace himself. "I'm worried about him. You saw how he was with you just now—after not seeing you for only two days? He's hungry for a dad, and, for better or worse, now you're it. It's scary, terrifying, really. I don't know how he'll survive when you go, in—what? Five months?"

"Five months is a long time."

"With a child, five months goes like nothing. You blink, and he's six. You blink again, he's ten—twenty!"

"In five months anything can happen."

"But if it's five months more and *then* you disappear?"

"Five months? I'm barely making it through a day! How can I plan that far ahead?"

"But I have to. I'm his mom." She stopped and faced him.

"You want me to stay, but—"

"Started to want it, yes, but maybe not. I don't know—"

"You don't want me to stay?"

"I want you to bring it up. You never bring it up."

"Do you?"

"I am. I am and all I'm getting is that I'm wrong!"

"Wait, wait—"

"I have waited, and—"

LROWWWWWWWWWaaaa!

A terrific blast came up from the earth around them. They snapped to attention as if slapped and saw a train speeding upriver from Columbia rounding the curve and coming onto the trestle straight at them, the sound rising up the chromatic scale as if running faster and faster to get at them or to overtake its own echo off the drumhead of the mountains. Another blast seemed to rise up from the throat of the trestle out at them and it was clear that the train could never in this life stop in time.

They froze, side by side on the edge of the ties between a steel rail and the girders of the bridge. Time slowed and sped. Orville knew there was only enough time for them to take a single step. Which way to go? Across to the other track? Jump from the trestle down a long way onto the icy creekbed?

Bodies are malleable. Orville grabbed Miranda and, as if she suddenly weighed nothing, pulled her hard against a rusted strut of the trestle, his arm pinning her there as he tried to mold their chests and faces into the diagonal spaces.

The train was upon them.

Orville tried to envision how much room they had between the edge of the track and the girder and started cursing "Shit no, not now not by a fucking train!"and praying, Please, for us and Cray and Amy!

They were buffeted hard by the outrageous sound and wind that seemed to last forever. But in an instant it was over. The train was moving fast away, wailing down the chromatic scale as if sad at missing its chance, rounding the bend upriver toward Albany.

They pried themelves off the struts, flakes of rust on their palms and under their nails. The air was filled with the edged scent of diesel. Trembling, their breaths coming in gasps that made little clouds in the air, they stared at each other wide-eyed, seeing the flecks of rust on each other's forehead and cheeks.

"There are better places," Miranda said, trembling, "to talk about the relationship."

They walked back slowly and stood at the door of the house.

"Don't tell Cray," Miranda said, her hand on the doorknob.

Orville heard this as yet another example of her hypercaution with her son and wanted to say something, but knew he'd better not. His exhaustion, the stupid close call with death—he knew he was on the edge of sending out something contemptuous, but he couldn't quite say nothing. "Why not?"

"I don't want to scare him."

He managed to say nothing, barely managed, hoping she hadn't sensed it.

"Come on," she said, sensing it but not doubting herself on this one, not after the close call. "Come in."

Cray was fractious. His worsening cough and cold (which made Orville think he ought to dig in his bag for antibiotics), his hour of video watching, the tension he was sensing between the two of them—all of this had wound him up. He glommed on to Orville, demanding that he pay full attention to him. Every bone in Orville's body was aching and yearning for sleep. But as a doctor he was used to making the normal superhuman efforts, and so he put himself on autopilot to try to do the same as a kind of father.

Cray first wanted to go outside and play soccer in the snow. Orville vetoed that because of his cold. Cray insisted on setting up a goal in the living room and, yelling "Happy feet! Happy feet!" tried to boot the ball past Orville. Miranda soon put a stop to indoor soccer. They then played knock-hockey, then checkers. Orville lost at hockey but won twice at checkers, which prompted

167

Cray to swipe the checkers off the board onto the floor. Orville picked them up, patiently, wordlessly. Dinner couldn't come soon enough.

The adults finished a bottle of wine. By the time eight o'clock rolled around, Orville was yawning incessantly and Miranda was trying to keep her eyes open while sinking deeper and deeper into the soft old couch. Cray, sneezing and coughing, was still going strong. He refused to take Tylenol or go to bed unless they played one last game.

"Okay," said Orville, "one more—" he yawned long and hard "—and that's it."

"Animal Guessing Game. You think of an animal first."

Yawn. "Okay."

"But don't let me get it."

"Okay."

"Got it?"

"Yep." Another run of yawns. Miranda, too, started yawning. "Guess."

"But tell the truth, okay?"

"Right. It's a hard one, a very, very, very hard one."

Cray squeaked with delight. "Is it a . . . a bottle-nosed dolphin?"

"Did you say a . . . a bottle-nosed dolphin?"

"Don't! Don't do it if it's not it!"

"I mean," Orville yawned again, feeling a perverse wish to string the boy along, "are you really guessing a bottle-nosed—"

"Is it or isn't it?" Cray asked, not smiling anymore.

"No," Orville said. "It isn't a bottle-nosed dolphin."

"Then why'd you say it was!"

"I never said it—"

"But you made me think it was!"

"I was just kidding, just fooling around."

"Cheater! You big cheater! I hate you! I'll never let you read to me again!" Cray started upstairs. Orville got up and took his arm to try to stop him, but this just made Cray fight back. He hit Orville in the belly and then, in a fit of coughing, fell on the stairs, kicking him from above.

"I'm sorry, but I didn't say—"

"You were just kidding me around, you big shit!"

"Cray!" Miranda said, getting up.

The boy ran up the stairs and slammed the door. Twice.

Orville looked at Miranda and felt ashamed. In her eyes was a question, which he read as, Why in the world did you do that? Crumpling up, he said, "I was just trying to entertain him, keep it going . . ."

"You don't have to. All he wants is you *here*."

"Okay, I've had enough for one night. G' night."

"Wait—"

"No, no. No. No matter what I do, it's never enough." He grabbed his coat and walked out the door, tripping on the stone doorstep in the terrific dark.

He walked out to the Chrysler and then past it to the cinder bed on the edge of the river. It was pitch-black. The north wind hit him. He started to shiver but made no move to put on his coat. *Is this the end?* He felt hopeless, standing there seeing nothing. His shivering felt right—in all the deadness, a sign of life.

But then he started to really shake, his teeth chattering, his whole body vibrating, as if his bones were clattering against each other—the response of the body to bone-cold, and to terror. The harder he tried to stop himself shaking, clenching down with all the power of his will, the harder he shook.

Convulsed with cold, bent almost double, he tried to put on his jacket, shaking from his knees to his gut to his chest to his chattering teeth. Bursts of little cries escaped his lips. Bent low to the ground he made his way back to the Chrysler, an inch at a time. He tried to straighten up, his spastic fingers searching his pockets for his key. His eye fastened on the light over Miranda's front door. One of those bug bulbs, invisible to bugs so that in summer they're not attracted to the light. It glowed in the clear air, glowed golden over the old door.

In that house are the two people I love most in the world.

◊ ◊ ◊

Miranda tried to comfort Cray, but he wouldn't open his door to her. Downstairs, as she passed the front door, for some reason she turned on the outside light. She sat at the kitchen table for what seemed a long time, listening to the wail of the north wind, feeling its cold fingers work their way through the chinks of the old house. She shivered, less from the chill than from the heartache that seemed to be all that was left of her.

Will he come back? Do I want him to?

◊ ◊ ◊

He knocked, gently, on her door.

19

The public hearing on the Worth Hotel took place several weeks later in the Council Chambers of City Hall at Fourth and Washington. City Hall was a brick structure built by the Quakers in 1805, during the first term of Mayor Caleb Starbuck, one of Bill's Nantucket ancestors. The ceiling was remarkably high, probably twenty-five feet. The row of windows facing the street was also high and narrow, and set much further up in the wall than in later styles. The standing-room-only crowd was restless.

Miranda and Orville sat together in the front row. Penny was beside Orville, and next to her were Henry, Nelda Jo, and Henry Jr.—the teenager in a white button-down shirt, red tie, and blue blazer and sporting a fresh, ugly black eye. Cray was with Maxie, back at the Schooners'. From Henry's direction came a faint scent of toasted oats and barley, of hearty and delicious breakfast cereal. Henry and Milt had recently moved their offices into the old Gadicke Feed and Grain Building, and after a day at the office the enticing aroma clung to them. Amy and Milt sat in a row with the other scheduled speakers, behind the low railing separating the audience from the council members and the mayor.

Orville was in a foul mood, preoccupied. The practice now was, as he had told Miranda earlier that day, "beyond belief." March had been a month of prolonged cold. Columbians were hanging on to the year by their fingernails, waiting for warmth, waiting to let go—and mutilating each other's bodies and minds and pets and livestock and cars and TVs and homes and churches (yes, two churches up in flames and no one caught)—in the process. The countryside was sere and bare, the clumps of fruit trees looking less like orchards than like pegboards for an abandoned game, the leafless maples and oaks and beeches strung out along the windblown fields like broken power lines.

Today, driving back to the office from an emergency call to try to save two farmworkers who'd fallen into a manure tank and who were dead by the time he arrived, Orville found himself stuck out in the middle of nowhere behind an errant Wonder Bread truck, staring at its two bumper stickers: JESUS IS COMING, LOOK BUSY and KEEP HONKING, I'M RELOADING. Back in the office, in his mail was a postcard of Mount Fuji.

Hello, son,

Fuji crowded. Sushi mushy. Tokyo jammed so there's NO parking (get it?). Wolfgang and Kenni wearing thin. He's a dope she's depressed and a real yakker. Babs back is bad. Starbusol working okay, but supplies low. Best,

Bill

It was clear to Orville that Bill had no intention of returning to Columbia anytime soon, if at all, and that he couldn't care less what Orville did with the practice. Orville made a mental note to start looking into whether he himself could sell the practice before he left in August.

Mayor Americo Scomparza was the first speaker and proceeded to set the scene. The building had been vacant for many years and posed a hazard. The cost of restoration was hundreds of thousands of dollars; the demolition fee, $18,000. Five years ago the U.S. government, through HUD, offered to pay two-thirds of the demo cost. A contractor had been hired. The Worth Saving protests had begun. The venerable Helen Hayes, who had stayed at the Worth during her heyday, and Mabel Mercer and Harry Belafonte, both of whom had homes out in the county (Belafonte bought his after filming a B movie in Columbia, *Odds Against Tomorrow*) sent telegrams. A judge signed an injunction against proceeding. The Department of the Interior proclaimed that every effort should be made to preserve the Worth as part of our national heritage. Recently, Worth Saving had succeeded in placing the hotel on the National Register of Historic Places. This meant that Columbia could still demolish it, but they would get no money from HUD to do it.

"You mean those jerks lost us twelve grand?" said someone angrily.

"Uh-huh," said mayor Americo.

The crowd erupted in angry shouts and name calling.

"Bottom line," the mayor went on, "we either leave it as is, or spend your tax dollars to tear it down or fix it up, or sell it to someone else to do it. It's zoned for any damn usage." Leaving the podium, the mayor glanced furtively up and around to check out if anything was about to fall. Without incident he sat back down behind the railing in front. Columbians relaxed. The mayor had spoken and nothing had broken.

Next came the other scheduled speakers, alternating between pro and con. First, for Worth Saving, Mrs. Tarr of the DAR who, despite her tight dry cough, did well with her brief biography of Columbia's most famous son, William Jenkins Worth, and her personal reminiscences of organizing fashion shows and Junior League Balls and other charity events at the hotel over many decades. Next, against saving, Gus Clinton of Whale City Savings representing SPOUT. Then came Mrs. Clive Follywell, owner of Quite Dear Antiques, founder of CATS—Columbia Antique Traders Society—for saving the Worth, who also reminisced but went on at Melvillian length and soon lost what, if any, ground the spunky Mrs. Tarr had gained from the majority of the crowd—Columbians dead set against preserving Columbia in general, and the General Worth in particular. May Carter, representing the hastily formed PALH—People Are Living Here, an alliance of poor people who lived "Downstreet" and who were against having to deal anymore with "that rat-trap hotel" and "want a Price Slasher of our own."

The final speaker was Amy Plotkin. She stood front and center at the podium and began. "The quality of mercy is not strained, it droppeth as the gentle rain of heaven, upon the place beneath . . ." As she went on, color rose in her cheeks. She ended with a simple plea, "But mercy is above this sceptred sway, it is enthroned in the hearts of kings, it is an attribute to God himself, and earthly power doth then show likest God's when mercy seasons justice." She bowed her head.

Silence. Then a shout came from the back—"*Bravo, bravo, bravissimo!*" Greenie Sellers stood on a chair and in Italian words and gestures was encouraging the New Yorkers and antiquers to rise and join in, which they did. Amy bowed to their applause. Even Columbians rose and applauded. After all, she was one of them, Milt's daughter.

Flushed, Amy went on, "Please show the Worth some mercy. I'd like to close with a prayer." She closed her eyes, bowed her head. "Dear God, please protect the beautiful old hotel where my dear grandma Selma was in fashion shows—from my *father!*"

It was Milt's turn. He got up and said he was representing Plotkin and Schooner, Developers, who would buy the property "in a flash," pay for a safe demolition, and erect not just a Price Slasher Supermarket but a whole mini-mall, called the General Worth Mini-Mall, an architect's rendition of which he would unveil in a moment.

"Even my dear late mother-in-law, Selma Rose, declined to take part in Worth Saving. She wouldn't even drive past the place these last few years. We need to remove the infected tooth and put a gold bridge in there," he said, glancing at Basch the dentist, "and so forth. We have to destroy the

Worth to save it." Many in the crowd nodded. Milt introduced his state-of-the-art computerized projector with which he would show slides. "Blinky, could we dim the lights?"

The lights dimmed.

Milt clicked on the computer and there was a soft *poof* and the chamber went black. Nervous laughter, then catcalls. It was a definite breakage, and in the dark the anxiety rose. The janitor lit a butane lighter and opened the fuse box. Luckily there was a spare fuse. He replaced the fuse and the lights went on—to cheers and applause. But Milt had forgotten to turn off the computer, so there was another *poof* and the same thing happened again. Milt called out that he'd turned off the computer, but the janitor called back that that was the last fuse. Someone shouted that they should use a penny, but that was shouted down. They were in the dark.

After some scurrying, and a lot of shin banging, a few candles and flashlights appeared on the speakers' table. The eyes of the crowd began to adjust to the dimness. An argon streetlamp outside threw in some light—pleasantly harsh, as if from a UFO—filtering down through one tall window. Soon, people could see well enough for the meeting to continue.

But as Milt went on—badly, without his slides—the crowd realized that the problem with the meeting wasn't the light but the heat. For several days there had been a bizarre warm spell. Now the air conditioning, which had kept the room cool, had been knocked out, and the ancient radiators were still on, blasting heat into the crowded room. The janitor went down to the basement and, in a desperate act, disconnected the boiler, but he told everyone that it would take an age for the old radiators to lose their heat. The room was stifling. Folks suggested opening the windows, but even with the long gaff and with the strength of heavy Columbians, the windows remained stuck, as if nailed shut.

Milt sat down, sweaty and defeated, and the mayor said the meeting was now officially open to discussion.

Things got ugly and then dangerous. One problem with having light only at the front was that the audience was in darkness. No one could tell who was shouting at, or cheering on, the speakers. Supporters of the mini-mall, who talked about how much it would mean to them to have their very own mall to shop at, and how it might lead to other business coming downstreet like, say, McDonald's and Taco Bell, were cheered. New Yorkers, who tried to point out the priceless historic legacy and pledged to form a citizens' committee and hold benefits and hire consultants and look into urban renewal, were shouted down, despite the mayor's attempt to keep order. Mrs. Tarr, trying a rebuttal, was verbally attacked.

"Hey, lady," someone shouted from the dark. "You don't even live here. You and your historical ladies are out having tea at Spook Rock, and I'm tryin' to keep my kids out of that dump, away from the drunks, the drug dealers, and the perverts. And rats. When's the last time you saw a rat?"

Before she had a chance to speak, someone else shouted, "Yeah, it's our taxes, not yours. You don't pay taxes in Columbia."

"I pay my taxes in my public service. Given time, we can raise money privately to save the hotel. Fixed up, it can be a centerpiece for the whole downtown, the antique stores and homes—all of it, as well as for our bicentennial celebration next year. And the last rat I saw was two days ago."

"But *I* pay taxes," said Mrs. Follywell, founder of CATS, "and I and my antique store colleagues want to pay *more* taxes if it'll save the Worth. And I would propose, for the first time here a special levy to do so."

"Yeah, 'cause you can afford it."

"Order, order," shouted the mayor, banging his gavel.

Orville stood up and talked about the Worth being an important landmark in his growing up. "It was a place Dr. Bill Starbuck used to take me for lunch. That was when I first decided to become a doctor. *Your* doctor, and—"

"'Til August!" someone shouted.

"Shut up!" someone else shouted back. "He's a good doctor, so far."

"He ain't no Bill Starbuck!"

"Thank God for that!" Everyone laughed.

Orville was startled. It was the first time he'd been ridiculed by Columbians. He sat down, shaken and then angry.

Greenie Sellers rose and, in his dashiki and green hair, gave a fiery speech peppered with Italian and German words. He was passionately on both sides, supporting "the grand old lady hotel and my New York *antico negozianti*" as well as "my oppressed proletariat, my fellow downstreeters. *Ich bin ein Columbian!*" He was shouted down most cruelly.

The meeting spiraled crazily out of control. The heat was oppressive. Breathing was tough. Body odor took over. The obese, the pink puffers and blue bloaters representing Columbians With Emphysema, and the claustrophobes, left in droves. From the dark came shouts and accusations and muffled racist and sexist and homophobic jibes and whispers, all of which Americo tried to control with his gavel. The threat of new taxes, and the notion of a brand-spanking-new not just Price Slasher but in fact a *whole new mall* led to the portrayal of the Worth Saving crowd as "outside agitators and hippies." The crowd started to feel like a mob.

Orville watched Amy, sitting up front, and saw how terrified she looked. He stood and motioned her to come back and sit with them. As Amy stood up, a familiar voice rose from the front row.

"Your Honor? May I have the floor?" Henry Schooner was on his feet.

"Uh-huh."

Rather than stay in his seat like the other speakers, Henry moved to the center aisle and stood before the small gate in the low-railed barrier. He turned to Amy, who was standing on the other side of the gate, trembling.

"You've got nothing to be afraid of, dear," he said, and then held open the gate, took her hand, and led her back to his own seat, next to her mother. He returned to the aisle, stood facing the crowd, and said nothing for a moment. Then he took off his sports jacket and laid it across the railing and meticulously rolled up both shirtsleeves, smiling at the crowd.

Orville was rapt. Schooner had positioned himself just where the argon rays from the streetlamp were highlighting his white hair and round face. His sleeves were rolled up casually, but his regimental striped tie was still knotted crisply around his thick neck. He looked cool, in both senses of that word. The crowd was still. *How does he do it?*

"My fellow Columbians," he began. "Our lovely little lady there, Amy Plotkin, has the right idea in her choice of words. Mercy. *Mercy.*" He paused and then said, once again, "Mercy. Justice and mercy."

The Voice, Orville thought. Husky. Mature. Sure.

"Let's show a little mercy to each other. It takes all kinds to make a world."

The crowd was still, as if transfixed. To Orville, to Miranda, to Penny, to the others, it was as if Henry were speaking only to each of them and paying attention only to each of their reactions, as if each were the most important person in the room. As if each were a TV camera.

Remarkable, thought Miranda. *Truly.*

Orville wiped a runnulet of sweat out of his eye. *He's not even sweating, how come? His tie's cinched tight and he's not even sweating?*

"Let me begin with a pledge of my neutrality. I am not for saving the Worth and am not for destroying it. I am for us, all of us. For Amy and Milt, for my family and yours, for Columbia, for America, and for the world."

"Oh, yeah?" came a contemptuous voice from the dark. "What about Plotkin and Schooner puttin' up the Slasher?"

"And the mini-mall. Don't forget the mini-mall!"

"I'm glad you asked that question. As you know, I'm running for Congress. As a candidate to represent *all* of you, I do not want to be beholden to any special interest group, any monies."

Orville was amazed—had he really said "monies," not "money?"

"Thus Milt and I have agreed that, effective today, I am resigning from Plotkin and Schooner. I will put all my holdings in escrow. If I lose the primary in September, or win that and lose the election in November, I will rejoin my firm. I'm sorry to leave my dear friend and partner, Milt— he and I have batted this around in great depth—but I need to devote my full-time effort, 150 percent, to serve my country in peace as I served her in war. I want to now publicly offer a hearty 'Thanks, partner!' to Milton Plotkin." Henry applauded Milt. Others joined in. Milt looked like this was news to him too, and not welcome news either. He sat there, waving limply to the crowd, and despite the wan smile on his face he seemed to be saying, *I'm toast.*

"And so, my fellow Columbians," Schooner went on, "we have to learn to live together and to work together. This isn't about I or you, it's about we and us. We Downstreeters, like my friend May Carter, representing PALH. We antique sellers and lovers of antiques working our best to rejuvenate downstreet through CATS. We SPOUTers, working for basically the same goal with different means. And we parents of terrific kids like Amy Plotkin, who can give such a stirring rendition of Shakespearean poetry. Not I or you, but we Columbians, we Americans, and, in this world where we are constantly threatened by dark forces with nucular weapons, *we* human beings. And so, my friends, I humbly propose the following solution. I make a motion we employ what my dear old friend the good doctor of Columbia, Orville Rose, calls 'tincture of time.' My motion, to the council and to this gathering of goodhearted citizens and friends all, is that we give the hotel a stay of execution, challenge our friends in Worth Saving to come up with sufficient monies to renovate within nine months, until the end of the year. If they fail, then at that time, we as a community will have no choice but to sell the rights to others. That's the American way, through private-sector efforts, to raise the funds for the public good."

"Ain't they had enough time already?" someone shouted out.

"No, they have not," Henry said firmly. "Tonight is the first night that we finally addressed the issue as a community. Together. We are processing this together. I have been informed that they require nine months, minimum, from tonight."

"We wasted enough time on this!"

"Yeah, let's just get it over with!"

"Let's not rush anything," Henry said, so softly that it was hard to hear him, but everyone strained to hear, so what he said next, though said even more softly, was heard by all. "Once destroyed . . ." Henry held up a closed fist, paused, and then opened his fingers like the *poof* of a magician making a live dove disappear, "gone forever." He paused, letting this sink in.

Death, the crowd thought. He's talking about death.

"Gone. Forever." Schooner sighed, as if thinking of all the deaths he'd seen in war. "I make a motion we give the Worth Savers until the end of the year to make the hotel the centerpiece of a revitalized downstreet. If they fail, Milt or other developers can extract it and make the Price Slasher— and the mini-mall—the centerpiece. Either way, we all win. Second, I propose we organize more police protection—if we can afford it—to ensure the public safety of all those who live near the Worth. If we can't afford it, I propose we form a citizens' patrol for safety, to make sure the undesirable elements don't continue to inhabit the hotel, which, despite her rich history, has fallen so low. I for one am volunteering here and now to take the first patrol, tonight."

He turned to the low railing, picked up his sports coat, and slung it over his shoulder, looped around one finger, an ordinary guy ready to fight the good fight against evil until he won. He turned back to the crowd.

"*We need to pull together.* We need to have our differences add, not subtract and divide, us. We can be an example—and not only for our children, but for each other, and for others. We Columbians, we Americans, we who inhabit our dear planet Earth for a brief moment of . . . yes, mercy under God. God bless you all, and God bless America."

Henry bowed his head. There was thunderous applause, stompings, and full-throated cheers. Henry made his way back to his seat, squeezing into a remarkably small space between Amy and Nelda Jo, who put her arm around his shoulders and kissed him.

Henry sat looking straight ahead.

"Do I hear a second to the motion?" the mayor asked.

"I second it!"

"I third it!"

Laughter.

The vote wasn't even close.

Everyone left the meeting feeling up, high.

Orville and Miranda got into the Chrysler. They were due to pick up

Cray, but they found themselves just sitting there, not moving or talking, stunned by Henry Schooner.

20

"He even *smells* good!" Orville finally said. "Smells like breakfast cereal—'Schooner Flakes' or something. The most compassionate of the Columbians, Henry Schooner?"

"Amazing," Miranda said. "I've never seen him do that before. Something's happened. Whether we like it or not, the boy's got it. He's launched. He's on his way."

"Smooth as puppy shit. A total fake."

"Maybe not."

"That smarmy, patriotic God-goop, are you kidding? C'mon, I know the guy—he's a bully, a brute, a fake. At best a fake."

"You knew him a long time ago."

"I know what I've seen since, too. Look, I don't mind fake, if I know that underneath the fake is more fake and more fake—but not evil."

"What?" She was stunned. "Wait a second. How can you possibly know that?"

"You know right here," he said, tapping himself on the sternum, "in the center of your chest. You know when you're a kid and you wake up in the middle of the night in terror and realize you're seeing his face in a nightmare. He was a bad kid, he's a bad adult. A total phony. He doesn't really care about anything. Nothing."

"So?"

"*So?!*"

"What difference does it make?"

"A lot. I've seen the damage. When I went around the world trying to patch people up, I'd run into guys like Schooner—I'm sensitive to them, the hollow ones, the ones who don't care. And one thing I learned. People who don't care about anything can *do* anything! Suppose, under all that fakery, instead of nothing, there's really bad shit? Suppose, deep down inside he's so vacant and . . . and untethered that he'd do *anything?* Suppose he makes it look so good that you buy it? That everybody buys it?"

"And?"

"And look at the effect! Look at the town, the country! Come spend a day with me—no, no first, spend a night watching TV, seeing what Reagan Inc. is putting out as 'normal' American life, *then* come spend a day, come see what I see—the poverty, violence, racism, gay hating, the fear of commies, of bad guys with bombs! You saw it tonight—they hate these antiquers not because they're rich or successful but because most of them are gay or Jewish or 'liberal.' It starts right here!" He tried to cool down. "So when I see it happening on a small scale here, people falling in love with Schooner, I get very wary."

"So do I. But the country's tired. People want a rest. After the sixties—civil rights, Vietnam, the assassinations, Watergate—people don't want to face things, they want to believe. So they believe in Reagan, they believe that 'America's Number One.'"

"Reagan's screwing them, emptying their wallets and handing it to the rich, and they're saying, 'Oh, thank you, Mr. President, for screwing us and handing the money to the rich. Thanks for the denial—and thanks for giving us permission to hate.' Think I'm crazy? Where did he kick off his first campaign? Philadelphia, Mississippi, where the local Great Americans tortured and murdered the three civil rights workers. It was a clear racist message, sent subtly—brilliantly disguised. He's given them license to hate."

"I guess it's just human nature," she said. "History—American history, anyway—seems to go like that, in thirty-year cycles—the sixties were like the thirties, the eighties like the fifties. Watch—in the nineties, when Cray's in college, kids will be activists again." She paused. "Americans want a rest. Reagan's a rest. And so's Schooner."

"Terrific."

"The other day I came across something in Emerson: 'The great lesson of history is the good that comes from evil.' As governments go, this may be as good as it gets."

"*This?*"

"Look how hard it is even for us—two people who . . . who love each other—to see eye to eye. Look at the thousands in this town, at the mob at the meeting. Magnify that up to millions, hundreds of millions. It's the way things are. It's the way people are."

"They can't do better?"

"I don't know. They haven't much, historically." She watched as his face turned sad. She felt a sense of doom.

"Yeah, well," he went on, somberly, "I feel like we've failed."

"Us?" she blurted out, panicked. "You mean you and—"

"No, no, we humans. Nothing as grand as us. Like the Quakers and their utopia. I keep imagining that we can do better, that people can change, grow. I've seen it."

How, she wondered, with all his cynicism, is he still so innocent? Is it because he's never been really sick or disabled? Is he so idealistic that everything winds up being a disappointment, his innocence fueling his cynicism? She asked, "But not Schooner?"

"No, not Schooner." He shook his head for emphasis—and felt energized. "Look, I can't accept things as they are. It can't be this shitty. It's not enough."

"I never said accept things as they are—"

"You're the one who's so cynical about the possibilities."

"*I'm* the one walking the picket line," she said hotly. "Remember?"

"Okay, okay, but why picket, when you have such a dim view of human nature? Why not just give up?"

"Because if you don't get on a picket line," she said, her voice fiery, "then the great imbeciles of history that you're ranting and raving about, like all the people back in there who hate people like you and me and Amy—they'll tear down your dear old hotel, and if—" She stopped herself. "Forget it. We're late for Cray."

"No, no, tell me."

Miranda glanced at him, then away. At him again. "Because if you don't bust your butt trying to move the muscles of your leg, it'll atrophy and you'll never walk again."

Silence, but for the wind cutting across the half-open windows of the car.

He reached for her hand. "I'm sorry."

"Me too. I don't do outbursts well."

◇ ◇ ◇

Orville parked in front of the Schooners', not feeling up to seeing Henry. Miranda went in to fetch Cray. Henry came out, still in the white shirt but the tie now loosened, giving him a homey, paterfamilias look. He stood under the amber porch light and waved heartily. Orville waved back, feebly. Henry ambled down the steps and over to the Chrysler.

An audience with Saint Henry? Have I died and gone to heaven? Orville hit the window's UP button by mistake, shutting him out, and then hit the DOWN. There he was, face-to-face with the town savior.

"Great to see you there tonight, Orvy."

"You did a good job with the crowd, Henry."

"Democracy in action. It's a great country, isn't it?"

"Sure is, Henry," Orville said, feigning sincerity and wondering, Why is it that when I'm talking to him *I* sound fake?

"Damn," Schooner said, shaking his head in wonderment. "Maybe, old friend, one of these days you'll say that and mean it. Don't matter a damn to me, but, as they say, 'If you don't feed the teachers, they'll eat the students.'"

"Huh?"

"Cray-ballistic!" Henry shouted suddenly, straightening up as Cray ran fast toward the car. "Did you have a beautiful time with Maxie?"

Orville was glad when Cray gave Henry the response he used to give him: none.

"Glad to hear it," Henry said, chuckling.

"Hey Orvy!" Nelda Jo was calling him from the porch. She had changed into a silky bathrobe, showing a lot of curve and a little skin. "Why don't we see more of you? Y'all come see us, ya hear? Say 'okay.'"

"Okay." Miranda and Cray got in the car. Henry moved back out of the way, smiling and waving as if they were all embarking for a year on a trip around the world with Bill and Babs and Wolfgang and Kenni.

Cray was in a foul mood. He didn't respond to their questions about whether he had a good time with Maxie and about what they did and what they ate. When Miranda persisted on the eating part, Cray said, "I don't want to talk about it."

Miranda knew that Cray hadn't pooped for three days and was worried that he wasn't eating because he didn't like pooping. Although she knew she should just leave it alone, she asked, "Did you poop?"

"No! Don't ask me anymore!"

"Okay, I won't ask you anymore if you tell me one thing you did with Maxie."

They were out on Route 9, heading home. "He showed me some pictures, sexy ones, you know, sexy. He said it was 'fucking.'"

"What?" Miranda cried out. "Who said that?"

"Maxie. He showed me pictures."

"Where'd he get the pictures?" Miranda asked.

Cray said nothing.

"Come on, Cray, where?"

Cray said more nothing.

"Was it from his dad?" Orville asked, remembering how Henry, as a kid, had shown them all a set of Mexican playing cards with couples fucking.

"Nope. From his brother. From Junior."

"Does his father know this?" Miranda asked.

"Dunno."

"Well, he will tomorrow!"

"No! You can't tell him."

"Why not?"

"Maxie'll beat me up."

"Oh God, did he say that?" Miranda asked.

"Can't tell you."

"I'm calling his father as soon as we get home."

"No!"

"He'll take care of Maxie, don't worry. And you're too young to be seeing things like that and talking like that. Don't ever say that word again."

"You do. Orvy does."

"We're grown-ups," she said, with a glance at Orville, "you're not."

"Don't I have any rights?"

"Some."

"No, I don't! Damn and fuck!"

"Stop that right now!"

"Fuck."

"Or you lose TV for a week!"

"I never get my way!" He started to cry.

Back at the house Miranda called Henry, who said he was "Shocked, just shocked!" and he'd take care of it right away. Cray overheard the conversation and, though sullen, seemed okay. They did the normal things with him, Orville reading to him and Miranda lying next to him rubbing his back until he was asleep, and then they went to bed, too.

As they lay together they both sensed a slight shift. They had said things without love and had survived a scare, had sensed themselves a little out of their depths, just that inch or two, which, in novice swimmers, can drown them. The close call had brought them back in to where they could touch bottom, stand, and breathe.

"I'm glad you're here," Miranda said, snuggling into his neck.

"Me too. What a day."

"Maybe, given what Junior did, you're right about Henry."

"I've had enough Schooner for one day, okay?"

"Me too. But not of you." She traced a circle on his thigh and brought his hand to her breast.

"Well, sweetness," he said, feeling that merciful release of being excited and relaxed both, "I guess we'll find out, eh?"

"Hmmm?" She was letting go of the pain of the day, easing down into him. "Find out what?"

"Whether the humans can do better."

"How'll we find that out, Doc?"

"From us."

◇ ◇ ◇

At four in the morning, called out into the precarious dark, Orville sighted Selma flying in low off the Hudson from Athens, banking sharply overhead so she was facing due south, floating a little as if getting ready for a final push down the tracks down into Columbia. Hair permed, she wore a silky black dress with a scarlet scarf billowing out behind. She was moving fast, riding what looked like an Electrolux.

"Can't stop to chat!" she said, zooming off. "I'm on my way to something else!"

21

Several weeks later—at three in the morning on May Day—Orville sat at the nursing station in emergency, ear-sitting. In iced saline before him was a human ear, female, midfifties, waiting to hear if the surgeons at Albany Medical Center wanted it and its owner shipped up for reattachment. It was yet another medical event in the long story of the family Scomparza that seemed to be at the heart of so much disease, breakage, and death among the Columbians. Fiesole "The Bomber" Scomparza, the mayor's older brother and barber/bookie to the town, had taken a straight razor and sliced off his wife's ear "in some heavy love-play, you get me Doc?" His wife, Lovely, wasn't talking about how the ear came off, except to say, "If youse can put it back on okay, elsewise I'm goin' home I got another, don't I?" Both were "knee-walking" drunk. By that time, Orville had been awake on and off for two days and kept falling asleep between emergencies.

Since the hearing on the Worth, the medical practice had made a significant shift, from "beyond belief" to "beyond beyond." Orville couldn't fathom how Bill managed it. Bill—and now he—was on call for thousands of Columbians, day and night, in solo practice. Sure, he could call in help if he needed it, but he couldn't count on any standard rotation of days off. Orville kept trying to arrange coverage, without much luck—there were few doctors who had time, and to send anyone to Dr. Edward R. Shapiro was a death sentence. Often the flow would go the other way, a Shapiro disaster landing in Orville's lap. One of them, two days ago, had been Mrs. Tarr.

Orville got a call from her via the nurse in intensive care in Albany Medical. She was on death's door and wanted to see him. He drove up at once. Besides their contact around the Worth, he knew little about her life—she was of old Nantucket stock, which had over many generations distilled the quality of WASP-reserve to a nutty essence. He knew that she lived with a spinster friend in the family's grand old house in Spook Rock, dangerously near Shapiro's office, and used him as her doctor. In intensive care Orville found her flat in bed, breathless, getting oxygen and IV fluids. She had gone to Shapiro with breathlessness a month ago. He did tests that he said were normal. Unfortunately for the unsuspecting Mrs. Tarr, to renew his medical license Dr. Edward R. Shapiro had taken a ten-day mail-order course in Freudian psychoanalysis. Lying her down on his examining table and analyzing her ruthlessly by rote, Shapiro found out that the breathlessness had begun around the fifth anniversary of her husband's sudden death when his chest was crushed by a hay baler; drilling deeper, he learned that when she was six she had almost suffocated when a feather pillow had burst in the night. Diagnosis? He told her she had "penis envy and depression" and sent her to Germantown Asylum. There her breathing worsened, and she was sent to Albany. The only abnormalities the Albany doctors found were decreased lung function, a diffuse X-ray with no specific diagnosis, and increased eosinophelia—blood cells indicating an allergic reaction. They tested her for every known allergenic substance; they treated her for infection; they even cut her open to get a morsel of lung for the hungry pathologist. Nothing. They had more or less given up, planning to send her home with a tank of oxygen, to die.

When Orville saw her, he was astonished. Thin and white and blue-lipped from lack of oxygen, she could barely talk. What to do? After months of treating Columbians, he had come to value Bill's long-held belief that taking a good history is the doctor's best tool, and that if you could trace the history back through generations, you might not find the disease, but you'd usually find the truth, and the treatment. Orville led her through her history, and that of her family, and while it was a historian's dream, nothing seemed medically significant. Finally, he gave up. They just sat and chatted—about the Worth, Miranda, Amy, her concerns about her garden, life, death, and if she died what would happen to the poor magician.

"Magician?" he asked.

"Why, yes. The one I took in last fall." She said that at the Malden Bridge flea market she'd met "a destitute magician with a good heart" who was looking for a room. She felt sorry for him and took him in. He came with pigeons for his act. She let him keep the birds in cages in the basement.

"Where in the basement exactly?" Orville asked.

"Over the washer-dryer." It turned out that whenever she ran the dryer the exhaust launched an aerosol of pigeon droppings up into the air, which she had been inhaling for months.

Orville rushed to the medical library, looked up "pigeons," and there it was—"pigeon breeder's lung disease," an allergic reaction to inhaled pigeon shit. Treatment? Get rid of the pigeons, and a course of steroids. Prognosis? Excellent.

As the Chrysler flew from Albany back down to Columbia, Orville felt part of one of those rare moments when the spirit of good medicine comes alive, when sustained attention, and listening without an agenda or decision tree, saves a life. How rarely do we really listen, and think! She would live to picket again. He basked in the glow.

It didn't last. His afternoon out of town had produced a backlog at home. Mrs. Tarr was a bright spot in a long shadow of cruelty and carnage and horrific breakages for the next two days, ending with him sitting, staring numbly at that ear in that ice. In the blur, there were the ordinary cases: drug and alcohol and rage-filled car crashes and clubbings and beatings and attack with "shod shoe" and knives and guns and the crazies and psychopaths and of course the normally walking worried with diagnoses of mental illness that were so common among the Columbians that the adult assessment scores, like the consistently abnormal Apgars at births, had to be recalibrated to a fallen normal. But some cases stuck in his mind.

Sigmund Basch, the town dentist, was a meek, obsessive, and scared man who looked like a mouse and loved golf to death and was known around town for always going up a set of stairs or down counting the steps to make sure he landed on the last one with his right foot. He had just come out of the bank counting and landing when he noticed a pit bull had broken from its leash and, canines bared, was coming at him. The dentist took off, the pit bull gained quickly, the dentist thought he saw a cavity in the traffic and ran into the street and was hit by a ten-ton truck hauling cement from the Universal Atlas. By that time Orville was so tired he was seeing two dentists, but with a little superhuman effort revived Basch and shipped him up to Albany for reconstructive surgery.

The leitmotif through the violence was the sudden surfacing of a suppurative trail of venereal disease that had begun a month ago in a furtive visit from Mayor Scomparza, and that had since wended its way through that family and their playthings, all over the city and county like a bunny-hop at an Italian American wedding. The latest among those appearing at the emergency room were an odd duo—with a "third member" hiding in the waiting room—Greenie Sellers and Blinky the Clown. Greenie was high on coke and spouting what sounded like Norwegian but what a nurse said was Latvian, and Blinky—an alcoholic ageless refugee from Barnum and Bailey who marched in all the parades and entertained at all the school shows and private birthday parties—was low on quaaludes, and they both stayed histrionic even when Orville, using the double-gloved technique, milked their *putzes* for pus. At two in the morning, prescriptions in hand, they left gaily as if leaving a party or a show and Orville, with a morbid curiosity, went to the waiting room to check out the third member of the sexual ménage. Faith Schenckberg, of the sunburnt-offering Schenckbergs of the summer.

At least these provided comic relief, but fleeting relief, as he went back to a heroin-addict mother delivering a premature baby. The newborn was tiny, skin sallow, pupils pinned, sclera jaundiced, twitching all over in withdrawal as every cell in her body cried out for the narcotic. Just as Orville was trying to recall the correct dosage and schedule for managing withdrawal, his old friend Whiz, Hayley's son, a recovering addict in AA, brought in another Vietnam Vet named Timmo Schaffran, who was dying from agent orange and, half-crazy from the cancer in his brain, had attacked President Reagan on TV with an ax. Whiz helped Orville figure out the dosages for the withdrawing preemie. Afterward, Orville jumped at the chance to get out of the hospital on a house call. Relishing the privacy of the Chrysler, he drove to a hovel in the armpit of the county where he discovered an old woman who'd been dead for a while and was partially eaten by her trapped dog and whose pony was so neglected that its hooves curled back under its legs and it looked like a rocking horse but couldn't walk. He turfed the pony to the vet.

Just after the ear and its owner left, in came Seraphina Robb, the seventeen-year-old daughter of one of the hospital nurses Orville had known since grade school. Seraphina had been fished out of the Hudson River at dawn by a coal barge near Catskill, ice cold, dead. Her belly was ripped open, she was badly broken up—she'd jumped from the Rip Van Winkle Bridge, a distance he knew from his toll collector days to be 157 feet plus or minus 3 for the tides. A desolate sight. Her intestines had exploded out of her bright-red prom dress, a gold bracelet still sparkled on a horribly contorted arm. Orville called her mom, a widow.

"I have terrible news, Pam," he said. "Your daughter is in the hospital."

"Oh my God! Is she all right?"

"I'm afraid not, dear. Please come right away." He heard her cries and hung up.

Yes, he thought, it's true what Bill says, that as a doctor to the Columbians you get to lift up the lid and see all the secrets. Okay, and just *how* is that good for the world?

As he waited for Seraphina's mom to come in, he tried to get ready for the rest of the Saturday. Having gotten coverage, he was spending the day with Miranda, Cray, and Amy. He was feeling apprehensive. Ever since the close call on the trestle, Miranda had seemed mopey and, as he had gotten more swamped with work, moody. On the surface everything seemed pretty okay, and when he tried to ask her about it she'd always said she was fine, just a little tired. But he felt a slight distance opening between them—even when they were making love—as if a part of each of them was not really there. He was worried about it, wanting to get back to the seamless "we" that they'd had, that energized them both. But he didn't know how to do it, and he didn't have much energy to try.

He finally left the hospital at noon, feeling only half-alive. But in the parking lot he blinked in the hazy warm sun, and, being back in contact with the ongoing natural world, he felt a touch better. He lifted his face to a spring drizzle, soft and promising. The time of year when the river is flowing freely and an evening surprises you with its lingering light.

When Amy saw him she said, "Your eyes are bright red. You look terrible!"

"Terrible, right now, would be good."

On the drive out to Miranda's house, over and over the white lines started to wobble, and he had to stop for more coffee, figuring he'd find a way to catch some sleep during the day. Seeing him, Miranda, too, looked startled. Cray asked how he was.

"Happy as a dog's nose in spring!" he said. What the hell was he supposed to do, start the day off by telling them he felt like shit?

They drove a long way out to the edge of the county, a historical site in Lebanon, the grave of Samuel Tilden. Tilden, Miranda told them, was the ill-fated Columbian elected president of the United States in 1876 by a majority of the popular vote, but who had suffered a breakage in American history: the presidency was taken away by the corrupt electoral college, which overturned the people's choice. On his rowboat-sized granite memorial was carved a final nostalgia: I STILL TRUST THE PEOPLE.

From there they went to lunch at the diner—four "Whaleburgers and French fries"—and then to the new film at the Half Moon Theater, *A Passage to India*—featuring great scenes of festive elephants. Cray glommed on to Orville the whole day, which was fine with him, given Miranda's gray mood, but Cray was nasty to Miranda and even to Amy. At one point, refusing to walk down the street next to Amy, he announced that "girls are radioactive—you can't get too close!" Amy was hurt by the rejection but took it with her usual resiliency and high spirits, saying, "Hey, a lot of boys I know feel that way, but it's *their* loss, not us girls'."

Cray even turned on him once, during Animal Guessing Game. Orville's first guess was "a Himalayan snow leopard," and Cray, mimicking what he had done to him, taunted Orville, then pretended to think it over, and said, finally, "I *was* thinking of a Himalayan snow leopard!" Miranda gave both Cray and Orville a look. Things got tense.

Orville stopped off at home to change and pick up the mail before going back out to Miranda's for the night. Big mistake. There was another letter from Selma.

Hi, flier!

I'm in a good mood—I'm always in a good mood coming home from someone *else's* funeral. Today's was Sam Schenckberg, Faith's father. (Jewish, but horrid.) We all sat there at the service and no one would speak, no one could think of anything nice to say. Even Rabbi Werlin—he's *such* a pro at funerals—zilch. Finally somebody in the back stands up—I think one of the Athens Rosenblatts—and he jabs his finger up at God and shouts: "His brudder vas vorse!"

I can't wait to hear what they say about me. (Make that *said.*)

For some reason I'm remembering your hands: those long fingers, those soft palms. You always disappointed me in your choice of medical specialty. A GP? *Bill* is a GP! With hands like that, you could have been a gynecologist.

Which brings me to the question of your being normal. In a lot of ways you seem to be. Fine. But all in all I vote no. Your sister and your father and even your niece lately—and of course Milt—have voted no. There is one big way in which you are abnormal: your total selfishness. (Penny, who's had oodles of therapy, asked her psychiatrist about you once and he said that you fit the diagnosis of a "narcissist.") Oh sure, you're saying, who isn't selfish? Why, no one isn't, no one isn't at all. Even I have my moments. My dream was always to have my photo, with me smiling, on the front page of *The New York Times.* So instead of the *Mayflower,* we came over on the *Jewflower*? So *I* should settle for *The Forvitz?*

But listen: I'm talking about how you were always so focused on yourself that you were never focused on *me.*

Not even after my operation. I was normal, some said beautiful in fact. I was the star of those Junior League fashion shows at the Worth you don't remember, and then I was butchered by that *goyishe* neurosurgeon up in Albany your father met on the golf course. I came home dead from the face up, and did you take care of me, even once stay with me?

Nope.

Do you now what it's like to cry out of only one eye? Hear out of only one ear? Smile out of only one side of your face? To have to scrunch up your shoulder to blink your eyelid?

I'll bet that whatever girl you've chosen here it's going badly. You're about to fail again. You may ask yourself: "How do I know this?" Oh, I *know.* I know because I know *you.* Like you failed with *me!*

Be well, from your

High Flier

How *does* she know? It's uncanny. Could she still be *alive?* Hiding out? Wandering around town in disguise like in a witness protection program? Up on Cemetery Hill with binoculars watching all this? Could she somehow have faked her death? He made a mental note to ask Penny if she in fact had ever actually seen Selma's dead body and to check on Selma's death certificate. But Selma had faked his birth certificate, couldn't she have faked her death certificate too?

With the perverse thought that the letter might serve as an "exhibit" someday somewhere, he folded it as carefully as a love letter and slipped it into its envelope. Feeling heavy and light both, he drove out through the strangely portending May Day dusk to Cray and Miranda.

◊ ◊ ◊

Lightning flashed and sudden thunder rolled from Rip Van Winkle land across the river onto the roof of the old house. It was Cray's bedtime and he was putting up a fight, wanting to play yet another game of Clue with Orville.

"Come on, Cray," Miranda said, "bed."

"No!"

"Come on. This is a fuss-free zone. Brush teeth, change into sleepy clothes, and get into bed."

Another flash of lightning. Thunder blasted down sooner and harder.

"Only if Orvy reads to me alone."

"Hey, Crayboy," said Orville, "we both read to you, you know that."

"But the thunder scares me so much I should get what I want."

"Don't give me that scared stuff, kiddo."

"It's okay," Miranda said, sighing, giving in. "Just for tonight."

"Yay!" Cray ran upstairs to the bathroom.

Miranda went into her bedroom to change. Orville followed Cray. There was a terrific crack of thunder. The lights flickered and, enfeebled, went out. They all shouted to each other and tapped their way along walls and downstairs to cabinets and found candles and a tiny flashlight and went upstairs again.

With the flashlight, Orville read Cray Kipling's *How the Elephant Got Its Trunk*. Cray asleep, Orville extracted his arm and headed into Miranda's bedroom, which was pitch-dark. Turning off the flashlight, he felt his way into bed with her. Thunder crashed hard just above their heads, like a fist coming down on the roof, shaking rafters and joists, traveling down the backbone of the house so that they could hear the tinkle of plates and cups in the kitchen.

In the dark they devoured each other with touches and kisses. They were hungry, as if their passion could fly in the face of their recent clashes at the edges of love, could lift their moods back to good. Mouths open, noisily, kicking covers off, they let go.

Settling into each other's arms and down into sleep, they heard the fists of thunder open to long fingers of rain, and caught the clean scent of sulfur whooshing up from the lowering layers of the downpour and in through the slit of a west window left open, a cooling echo of the storm.

All the lights snapped on. There they were naked. On the coverless bed in the glare of the cheap overhead bedroom fixture that Miranda had vowed for years to replace.

It was, remarkably, the first time they were seeing each other naked in bright light. Miranda had always insisted that they make love in the dark or by candlelight, and under covers. Orville found himself staring at her shriveled leg.

The muscle mass was scarcely enough to fill out the form of a leg, with the warped bone prominent. At the knee were the scars of its many reconstructions. At the ankle the tissue was scarred in a different way, perhaps from her orthopedic shoe or even from, in the past, her steel brace. Orville flashed on anatomy, the dissection room, the sudden cadaver. His medical training had leached out the shock from the bodies he saw. He had learned to put a lot of bleached white—white coat, white bandage, white pages of doctor logic—between his heart and his job. But this was different. He was naked too—no white coat, no job to do. Stunned by the sight, he was more stunned by being stunned, shocked at being shocked. He saw far worse, day in, day out.

In the moment before his medical mask came down, Miranda saw his shock, even a flicker of revulsion. Exposed, humiliated, by reflex she did something that may have been brave. She touched his cheek to turn his head toward hers, away from her leg so that he was looking into her eyes as she questioned what she was seeing in his. He fought her questioning. She sensed his fight. He sensed her sensing. She too.

It might have been a moment of profound connection. It had that chance. But they couldn't hold it. They looked away.

"You all right?" Miranda asked.

"Yes."

"Turn the light off."

"No, no, it's okay," he said. "Let's face it."

"I don't want to."

"I do."

"No, you don't," she said. "Turn it off."

"You don't know what I want."

"A little discipline," she said firmly, "is required. Please, turn it off."

He did so, and lay down again beside her. She spread the light blanket over them.

They lay there in the dark. The lightning was over. The thunder was over. Only the snare drums of rain persisted.

The silence seemed, to Orville, to go on a long time. For Miranda, the silence was moving terribly fast—in a second a chance would be lost.

"We have to talk," she said, "about your leaving."

He stiffened. "Fine."

After he said nothing more, she asked, "You *can* leave in fifteen weeks. Are you going to?"

"I don't know."

"When *will* you know?"

"I can't tell you. I wish I could but I can't."

"At this point—now—what's your best guess?"

"I'm sorry, but I really have no idea. I wish I did, wish I could decide now. I want to stay, want desperately to stay—I'm totally crazy about you and Cray—but I'm not sure I can stand it here, stay alive here. Not just the town, the ghosts. Selma. You don't know how much it hurts."

"I'd like to know."

"Yeah, well, maybe." He sighed. "I'm sorry, but I guess we've both just got to live with it a while longer, until closer to August. Maybe we just try to live with the faith that it'll all work out for us, for all of us." He paused. "There are all kinds of options. Maybe you and Cray could come with me?"

"You have options, I don't."

"Maybe you do."

"Easy to say, but no. If I were alone, fine." She couldn't keep the sarcasm out of her voice as she said, "You may have noticed that I'm not."

Orville felt jolted by this, like when you step off one step expecting there to be another and there's not. "Are you saying that because he's not mine?"

"'Mine'?"

"Biologically."

She stared at him in disbelief. "I'm going on the assumption that on August 27th you're gone."

"So he'd be mine if I stayed?"

"Careful, Orvy," she said, trying desperately to be careful herself. "We've got a lot at stake here, and history's not on either of our sides. Take care."

He tried to take care, but it was like trying to take care with a current pushing you further out and at an angle so you knew that if you didn't strike out for shore right away and with strong strokes and taking into account the angle, you'd never get back.

"Look," he said finally, "I know you're afraid of what's happening. I am, too. But the way you've been lately, kind of mopey, and really tense with me and Cray? Maybe it's because Cray is so much into me lately. Maybe that's what's bothering you?"

"Maybe," she said. "Maybe not."

192

"Yeah, well maybe your fear about what might happen is bringing about what you're afraid of. Maybe your fear's provoking what you fear."

"Thanks a lot," she said, really hurt. "Like your contempt does?"

"What? You're saying I'm contemptu—"

"Damnit! I'm saying stay or go—but don't poison everything!"

22

One Wednesday morning about five weeks later, when the fleeting Columbian spring had already given way to Mosquito Heaven in the surrounding swamps and citizens were already sweating and slapping and scratching and cursing the pestilential Columbian summer, Orville sat in his office staring at Bill's latest postcard, thinking how thrilled Cray would be to see it. It was from southern India and showed elephants carved into cliffs, "Elephant Cliffs, Bay of Bengal."

> Howdy, doc!
> Having great time but boy the grub is hot. Riding elephant all day a mixed bag. Babs got sick but is OK. Hot as hell. Starbusol running low. Wolfy and Kenni a pain. Their son Glenn joined them today. Divorced, out of work, nose hair.
>
> Yr frnd,
> Bill

A call came from the hospital. In broad daylight just outside the CCC (Colored Citizens Club) on Diamond Street, a kid had shot another kid for a leather jacket.

Orville had just finished saving the kid and was signing out to his coverage for the rest of the day when the nurse rushed in with a telegram.

WOLFY AND KENNI AND GLENN GONE AND SO IS ALL OUR
CASH AND BABS DIAMONDS STOP PLEASE WIRE FIVE GRAND TO
ADDRESS BELOW STOP OTHERWISE OK STOP LOVE BILL STOP

Dismayed, Orville recalled how Bill, distrustful of checks and credit cards, always carried a big wad of cash around town with him. But had he been carrying big wads of cash around the world with him too? Never trust a young guy with nose hair. He tried to wire money through the Columbia post office. Despite the clerk's shock at attempting a new task, it seemed it might just work. But then there was a breakage.

Orville had promised Miranda he'd pick her up at 10:30 to help her set up for the gala benefit luncheon for the Worth. It was to be held at noon at the Joab Center house, a historic Nantucket whaler's house shaped like a ship, moored out on Harry Howard Avenue just beyond Penny and Milt's ranch. He'd arranged coverage and had been all set up to get there on time until Bill's telegram. Knowing he would be late, he picked up the phone to call her, surprised to find that he was fearing her reaction.

◊ ◊ ◊

Miranda, rushing to get ready for the benefit luncheon, felt sick to her stomach, headachey and light-headed. All her senses seemed hyperacute. Cray had a summer cold with some of the same intestinal symptoms, so she figured she'd caught it from him. Orville had said that there was something going around, but he *always* said that there was something going around. Her period was three weeks late. She half-thought pregnancy but given what he'd told her about his medical condition, dismissed it.

As she packed up the brie and Jarlsberg and English water crackers and cups and plates for the benefit, she felt on edge. Mrs. Tarr and she were supposed to have done the event together, but Mrs. Tarr's beloved cat Randolph had died and she was paralyzed with grief, listening to old Mabel Mercer records at home. Cray, too, had loved Randolph. He and Miranda had helped her bury the cat in her backyard the day before. Miranda was left to run the benefit herself.

As she worked, she tried to keep her mind off what had been going on with Orville and her, and with each of them and Cray. She realized that the two of them had been kind of limping along and that Cray was feeling it. With just a couple more weeks to go in school, her son seemed to have drawn back from her even more, and even from his god, Dr. Rose. The other morning when Orville had gone to wake him up, Cray, half-asleep, had shouted at him.

"You can't just dive right in! You have to do it gentle-gentle, like Mom!"

Miranda sensed that Randolph's death was stirring up Cray's feelings about his father's death. She felt a secret sadness in her son and wished Cray would just bring it out into the open. She felt it, too, late every spring, when the Columbian weather started to remind her of the sultry heat of the Gulf of Mexico. She wished they could grieve together. Not only her and Cray, but her and Orville, too. To her, Orville's grief over his mother's death seemed to be coming out as impatience. Lately, Miranda had noticed that her sadness irritated him. A big worry—his loss of patience at sadness.

And her work to finish her thesis had stalled out. She couldn't seem to find consistent time to work on it, and when she did she couldn't focus. As if the Columbian Spirit, watching itself being documented, was casting its spell of breakage.

◇ ◇ ◇

"Sorry I'm late," Orville said, coming into the kitchen. "I got jammed. But it's only 10:42, so we still should have plenty of time." He pecked her on the cheek. "How do you feel?"

"Lousy."

"Sorry to hear that. Symptoms?"

"The same. Same as Cray."

"Yeah, there's a lot of that going around."

"He's better. I'm worse."

"Sure you're up to this?"

"With your help, yes."

They pitched in together packing up the wine and cheese and munchies and utensils and napkins and soon found that they were way behind schedule. They couldn't be late because Miranda was the only one with the key to the Joab Center house. Amy would be waiting for them there.

Orville carried the heavy cases of Chardonnay and Beefeater gin and tonic and limes and armloads of Jarlsberg and brie and Stone Wheat Thins and Korn Kurls and Planters Peanuts from the house down the slippery, wet bluestone-and-grass path to the Chrysler's famous trunk space. After several sweaty and buggy trips he took a break and leaned against the hood, staring blankly out over the fetid river to the barren-seeming mountains, starting to feel as he had all those years shopping with his mother in stifling department stores in Albany as she tried on hat after hat, shoe after shoe, dress after dress for some family function like a bar mitzvah or yet another cousin's daughter's wedding or an endless number of ferocious Selma and Sol anniversary parties. In those stores he felt that his heart would stop with boredom or even had stopped without his knowing it because his brain had gone dead first without its knowing it either.

Up that river, he thought, Henry Hudson had sailed, duped into the fantasy of being on his way to the Northwest Passage to India, duped into imagining that the Furious Overfall was just around the next bend. Maybe it had even been right here, 375 years ago, right at this very spot that Hudson realized the shallowness of the water meant he had made a terrible mistake.

Glancing at his watch, Orville realized that now they were late. The Worth Savers and Amy would arrive finding a locked door and no Jarlsberg. He looked back up the walk to the door. No sign of her. His irritation grew.

◊ ◊ ◊

Miranda rushed into the bathroom and threw up. Looking at herself in the mirror as she rinsed her mouth and washed her face, she wondered, Is it possible? After what he had told her, no. Should I tell him what I suspect anyway?

Leaving the bathroom she was overcome with a confusion of strong feeling—worry and fear, hope and happiness. The power of it all—all at once—staggered her. Maybe I will tell him. Yes, right now.

In the kitchen she saw that Orville had forgotten the punchbowl and cups. She picked them up and walked with difficulty to the door. She suddenly felt flushed and then light-headed. She leaned against the doorjamb. Looking out from the darkness of the old house into the bright noonday sun, she was stunned by how just plain yellow the forsythia looked, finally, just now, in bloom. *Roses are pruned when forsythia blooms.* Mother, when I was a girl, told me that, in her garden in Boca Grande—and with such kindness!

"Dammit, Miranda, can't you hurry up!"

Smacked to attention, she looked up, seeing him standing at the car, his impatience obvious. She still felt faint, scared suddenly about falling. She heard, as if from a distance, the glasses go *clink clinkclinkk* against the punchbowl. She tried to keep standing, to hang on.

"I'm coming," she said firmly, and started walking carefully down the flagstones slippery with rain and mud from his repeated trips back and forth to the car, the slap of her bad foot muted by her taking care.

He rushed up the walk to her, a pained look on his face.

"Sorry, I didn't see you in the doorway—I thought you were still inside."

He took the punchbowl and cups and offered her his arm.

She didn't take it. "Let's just go."

◊ ◊ ◊

196

They were late. Amy was in tears. Some of the Worth Savers had already come and gone. Not many stayed. Fewer gave. The benefit was a bust.

23

It was a few days before they got together again. All week long Cray had been revved up, champing at the bit for school to end, summer to begin. Miranda was still reeling from the encounter. She still felt sick and had gone into her "survival mode," trying to do the necessities of food, clothing, shelter and (barely) tolerating a revved-up Cray. Orville, too, was overwhelmed, by summer accidents and real and phantom diseases. He had tried hard to show Miranda how sorry he was. He'd talked with her on the phone as often as possible, sent flowers twice with cute notes, and, once, one afternoon dropped by at Sixth Street School when Cray was getting out to say hi to them both.

Orville went to Miranda's for dinner later in the week. Cray latched onto him, hustling him into a soccer game and then running races and then to the river to skip stones and then back to the yard to dig worms for fishing. Miranda watched for a while before going inside to make dinner, putting on the water for Cray's millionth plate of pasta.

Eight months ago, when Orville was plunged into a sort of fatherhood, he'd noticed that being with the boy sometimes made him feel younger, sometimes older, sometimes both at once. Younger because he became a kid again to play with a kid. Older because clearly here was a member of the next generation, someone who could do things you could no longer do—from running with intense effort all day long through remembering everything down to the smallest detail to effortlessly pulling his legs up into a full lotus and walking along on his hands. Here was someone who would dare. The nostalgia, sometimes, was intense.

Today, Orville felt older. Tireder. Is that what older is? he asked himself, living tired? Miranda, too, had sounded tired and gloomy over the phone, weak and worn, her spirit down.

Orville detested worms and disliked putting hooks through them and throwing them to their deaths. So he told Cray he didn't want to dig for worms. Cray argued. Orville held firm. Cray threw dirt at him and called him "Dr. Dickhead!" Orville asked where he got that word, was it from

Maxie? Cray answered by chanting in an obnoxious singsong, "Doc-tor Dick-head Doc-tor Dick-head! Doc—"

"Cut it out, Cray!" Orville shouted, fed up. "Just stop it!" Cray stomped off, but then came back to tease him some more.

Miranda heard the chanting and came out. She told Cray to go in and eat his pasta while she and Orville took a walk. Cray refused and walked to the river and sat on a big rock—Miranda noted it was her "Promise-to-Selma" rock—elbows on knees, chin on hands. They left him there and walked up the dirt road beside the stream.

It was late afternoon. The mid-June sunlight was casting the same low slant of light on the blades of grass as it had in mid-November. Same light, different expectation. It had rained on and off all day. The washboard surface of the dirt road was pocked with puddles. The June air was thick and portending, almost loamy, as if carrying trillions of tiny fistfuls of wet earth. To their right as they walked, Kinderhook Creek roared toward the trestle, ducked quickly under and out into the seeming freedom of the river.

At a sharp bend in the stream, a soaring catalpa was in bloom. A rough-hewn bench sat underneath it. They were drawn to sit there too. The wet grass was a good green, but slippery. The footing down to the bench was treacherous. Orville took Miranda's arm, and they walked slowly together. To both of them it felt like a pretty good start—the feel of the support, the feel of supporting. Promising. They sat under the catalpa.

Catalpas, Miranda knew, had been planted all over Kinderhook County in the first celebrations of Arbor Day in the 1920s. This catalpa seemed to her even older. Every year it was so late with its leaves that Miranda worried that over the winter it had died, many of its banana-like seedpods from the previous year hanging there dead. But it always bloomed in time for her birthday, three days from now, and—yes, it had. The white, lily-like flowers with their lavender insides and their single streaks of gold perched on the end of long stems in groups of six. The blossoms would fade quickly, lasting only a week. Orville stood on the bench and picked a bunch, handing it to Miranda. They smelled the flowers. The bouquet, held afloat in the moist air, was a mix of jasmine, orange, and rose.

Their eyes were drawn to a shearing sound at a bend in the stream, where a knife-edge of moving water, hurrying along to make more river, had cut a scallop into the far bank, creating a ledge which looked, to Orville, like a miniature version of what the river had done to the bank of the Hudson at Columbia, leaving the high cliff of Parade Hill flanked by the two deepwater bays by the time the Quakers sailed in.

"An escarpment," Orville said. "You taught me that word, remember?"

"I do." The word had come up the day in the schoolhouse, the day they'd met. She did not offer this.

"It was the day in the schoolhouse," he said. "Remember?"

"I do."

They sat still, listening to the rush of water, the light breeze on their skin rustling the new leaves of a weeping willow nearby.

"I said I was sorry," he said, turning on the bench to face her.

"Accepted." She did not turn to face him.

"Why so down?" he asked. No answer. "You still feeling sick?"

It was a perfect time to tell him that her period was late, and that she'd been living with the impossible fantasy that she was pregnant—sometimes full of hope that she and he would somehow stay together and Cray would have a brother or sister, and sometimes dreading that it would just lead to more grief with him. She thought to tell him, tried, a little, to bring herself to tell him, but no. Given the mess they were already in, to add *that?* No way.

She took a deep breath in and let out a long sigh. "Some."

"Why so gloomy lately?" She didn't answer. "Everything I try—I said I was sorry."

"And I said I accepted it. You did everything right. You were good."

He felt the jab. "And?"

She turned, faced him, and said, bitterly, "You don't yell at a person with a handicap to 'Hurry up!'—"

"I said I—"

"Listen to me. You don't yell out at them 'Can't you hurry up?' Because you know what? They can't. You don't yell at them at all. You wait for them. You help them along."

"Guilty."

"I don't want your guilt. I want to understand. How could you *do* that?"

"You're being a little unfair. I wasn't even thinking about your handicap—at that moment I lost all sight of it, and—"

"Okay. Maybe unfair. But. There's something else going on here."

"How do you know? It was nasty but, I swear, innocent."

"After a lot of years of this, I've gotten to be a world expert on how people react. I can feel—in how people take my arm, my hand—what's going on. What's *with* you and my handicap? With handicaps?"

He took this in. "Maybe I've gotten so close to you I've stopped seeing you as handicapped at all. I treat you as normal, as a physically able person."

"And you stopped loving me?"

"Whoa! I love you *because* of your handicap? Come on!"

"I keep wondering why you wanted me that rainy afternoon in the schoolhouse. I ask myself, What was it that day? What attracted you so much to me? Was it when I stood up and walked away from you across the room? I felt your eyes on me. Like sunlight on my back, on my bare shoulders. When I came back, you'd changed. Such love in your eyes! What was it, then?"

"Just this incredible outpouring toward you. And yeah, it was something about your limp. Maybe your courage, your lack of shame, the contrast between your beauty and your disfigurement?" Why in the world, he asked himself, did I use *that* word? He went on, "It surprised me, too."

"Oh." She looked away. "Too bad. Seeing you so vulnerable at that moment, I imagined that, maybe, it was that our wounds matched."

"Maybe, yeah." He felt puzzled, then sobered. "You know, ever since that day, I keep feeling that you're looking at me in—I don't know—expectation? As if . . . as if you're searching to find something in me that's especially kind, open to helping you, helping my patients. Something endearing. As if you are always expecting the best of me. Expecting something that I don't feel I really have. It's weird."

"You took my arm on the ice outside the Quaker meetinghouse. You do take care of patients, good care, Orvy. I've seen you. Though you dismiss it."

"But it's as if you're expecting to find even more caring in me, like I'm hiding it from you, like you're asking yourself, 'Where's that caring guy?'"

She was about to respond but suddenly felt flushed, then chilled, and fuzzy, so that as he went on talking she tuned him out, hearing only the tail end of what he was saying.

"—because I'm a doctor?"

"Because of what she told me about you."

"She?" He saw her go pale. He stared at her, stunned. "Selma?"

"Yes."

"You told me you didn't know her."

She bit her lip, trying to focus. "A little."

"And?"

"We were both on a committee at the library. That's about it."

"Why'd you tell me you didn't?"

She looked away.

Orville had never seen her like this—unsure, embarrassed, as if she'd been caught in a lie, a secret. All at once he remembered the day he'd surprised her up in her attic, she at the steamer trunk with her wedding dress. He'd noticed how she quickly shoved a cardboard box away, back into the dark. Scomparza Funeral and Moving.

"Oh my God!" He felt a rush of humiliation, then anger. "You've got her letters. In that box in the attic. You're mailing her letters to me."

She weighed her chances of escape. None. It was over. "Yes."

For a long moment he couldn't speak. "Unbelievable! I mean this is unbelievable. You and she—you were that close?"

"No. We had a couple of heart-to-hearts, that's all. After she died, the box arrived on my doorstep. No one was more surprised than me."

"You . . . You're mailing me these letters, and I'm going crazy . . . I even read one to you . . . and all along you *know?* Why didn't you tell me?"

"I do *not* know what was in them. She sealed them all, wrote instructions for when she wanted each one mailed. I just mail them on the appointed dates."

"Great, great." He shook his head. "But why keep it secret from me?"

"I wish I knew," she said sadly. "She wrote me a letter—it came with the box when it arrived—and said it was her dying wish and I had to promise to do it. I looked up in the sky and promised. Your mother was not subtle, and she was very convincing."

"How could you?"

"At first I didn't know you, and . . . well, from what she'd told me, I imagined I was doing a good deed, helping her to tell you all the things she never got to tell you and that it was helping you to mourn her, go through your grief. And then I met you, fell in love with you, and I wanted to tell you, tried to get up the nerve to tell you, *almost* told you, in fact, but each time I tried, I was too afraid. I was afraid I'd lose you, more afraid the more I loved you. The deeper we got, the less I could risk it. It . . . it would be the end."

"Jesus." He shook his head. "I don't believe it."

Shamed, unwilling to show it, Miranda stiffened. The nail had been pounded in. The girl had grown around it to become a woman with a piece of steel in her soul. A voice inside said, *Never admit weakness. Keep it secret. Take care.* "The reason I look at you that way," she said, choosing each word as carefully as a step, "is that I *am* asking myself 'Where's that caring guy?' It comes from something Selma told me. She said that when she came home from her surgery that summer, when she was unable to care for herself, your sister and your father were not there for her. The only one who cared for her was you. You sat with her. Caring for her. She said to me, 'Orville stayed with me. He *stayed.*' So when the letters arrived, with her bizarre request—demand, really—I imagined that they were, well, love letters, from a mother to a son."

Orville was astonished, then awed, at this glimpse into Selma's real world, Selma vulnerable and scheming. She saw him as so inadequate a son, that to her latest little friend she made him into a saint. It was all so pitiful, so damning. He said, "She lied."

"What?"

"She lied to you. Big time. I ran like hell. Fast as I could. She never forgave me for it. Love letters? You want to know what's in those 'love letters'? Blame, ridicule, viciousness like you've never seen. And in every one of them, just about, she goes back to how I abandoned her." He stopped himself, thinking, What irony—I've just convinced the woman I thought I loved that I'm not worth loving. Thanks a lot, Mom.

"But why . . ." she could barely speak. "But why didn't you tell me?"

"Tell you what?" He felt himself sinking into a fogginess, a despair.

"Why didn't you tell me what was in the letters?"

"Too humiliating. And I'd be damned if I'd let her in to ruin things. And guess what?"

"Maybe if you hadn't kept it secret, and—"

"Look who's talking!"

They sat there. In all the movement of the water and the breeze and the willow leaves and the insects, they sat there still, as still as what the movement was arising from.

"So you didn't stay?" she asked.

"Nope."

"And now?"

"It just got a lot harder to. I'd started to think it was possible."

The word had been a touchstone for them—what was possible between them, what was possible for others and for the world. Each felt a flicker—'Is it possible now?' But a flicker playing on a scrim of anger.

"Mom!" They turned. Cray was on the road, straddling his bike.

"What?"

"Hi."

"Hi, hon."

"Hi, Cray."

"Hi, Orvy." Orville didn't pick up on it. "You *love* that word, right?"

"Sure do."

Cray had just learned to ride a two-wheeler and wasn't all that steady on it yet. Miranda asked, "Where's your helmet?"

"Mo-om. It's not a big road."

"The cars are big."

Orville said, "Big boys wear helmets."

"Okay. I'll go get it." He paused. "Can I ride back, I mean, without my helmet, to get my helmet?"

She appreciated his making peace with them. "If you take care, honey."

"Are you guys coming back soon?" They said they were. Cray shuffled the bike around, with difficulty got it moving, and bumped off down the pockmarked road toward the house.

The presence of the boy seemed a rebuke to their mean-spiritedness. After he'd gone, they felt drawn back toward an everyday level of kindness.

"I do love that in you, Orvy," Miranda said softly, "the way you hold out the idea of what's possible, how we can do better. It's a great thing, really. I admire how you still hold up the sixties that way—people working together, joining in—compared to all the self-centered stuff we have now." She turned to look at him, hoping. "I guess I just wish you would have walked with me." Hearing herself, she felt embarrassed. "I mean, like for the Worth. Since that first time, you haven't again."

"I carried the Jarlsberg." She nodded. "Look, I spend my whole life helping, trying to keep the people in this town in one piece. It ain't easy."

Suddenly she saw it. "Back then, did you actually join in . . . join in with people?"

"I . . ." he stumbled, feeling found out. "I was pre-med, in labs, and then I was over in Dublin—" Miranda looked down into her lap. He asked, "You?"

"I walked, yes, in the South. Alabama. Mississippi."

He felt awful. Sinking. Trying to stay up. "We each do what we can."

"But you're the one saying we can do more. Not just at our jobs, at our lives. Why waste time trashing 'the Columbians' when—"

"What would you suggest?"

"Cry. Cry for someone else."

He was surprised. "What? What has that got to do with anything?"

"When my mother died I cried for a year. Have you cried for her? Have you once visited her grave?"

"Jews don't. There's no headstone for a year."

"Fine." She tried to leave it at that.

"What?"

She shook her head, unwilling to say more.

"So this, between us, is falling apart because I'm a selfish guy who won't join a picket line for a hotel?"

"Damnit! This isn't about a hotel!"

"What is about then?"

"Staying. Walking the walk. With me and Cray."

"Maybe it's about risking, about your being so cautious, so scared to risk anything, you lose everything."

"Not my son. Not losing my son. I have to protect my son."

"From what, for Chrissakes? From life? From me?"

"From your not being there—*really being there*—for him. And for me."

"Fear is no protection."

"Running is?"

"You're never wrong, are you? You're never weak and you're never vulnerable and you're sure as hell never powerless and you're never wrong, ever! You're right, I'm wrong? Talk about pride!"

"You couldn't stand her handicap so for some weird reason you went for mine?"

"Let's stop," he said, stunned. "Let's go back. I mean, to the house."

"No. I'll stay here a while."

"Let me help you."

"No." She took a deep breath. "Good-bye."

A stab in his heart. "Wait a second—"

"We'll talk."

"I'll call you."

He stumbled up the grassy slope to the dirt road and walked toward the Chrysler.

On the bench she wept uncontrollably, alone.

◊ ◊ ◊

Numb, Orville went about his doctoring the next day as best he could. He missed Miranda and Cray terribly. That first night after their fight he picked up the phone to call to say good night to Cray. Cray was as he always was.

"Good night, Orvy."

"Oh I *love* that word very much!"

"Wanna talk to him, Mom?"

"No." Cray hung up.

The next day Orville picked up the phone but couldn't dial. Hung up. Picked it up again, a number of times. Once or twice dialed but hung up before it was picked up on the other end.

A day and a night later he was paged at dawn and rushing out the front door when he tripped over something on the porch. A cardboard box, Scomparza Funeral and Moving. Taped to the top was a sealed letter. He ripped it open.

THE DETH OF RANDOLPH
A novel by ***CRAY***
DedcassHUN

I dedcat this book to my mom and Orvy who love me very much.

I have a cat and he is a very nice cat and I was 6 and 2 when I wrote this novl in skool with help from Ms Simon my teacher.

My Godmothers Ms Tarrs cat died. He died. The name of the cat was Randolph. He was a nice cat and a clevr cat and he was a very shy cat becass my Godmothers friend she lives with Mss Beeslee had 2 cats and Randolph was ascared of them becuss they were both big cats and he was a small cat.

He had a lot of love in his hart becuss my Godmother took good care of him and Randolph lovd tuna and he lovd to sit on her lap and on his place on the reefrigator.

Randolph lovd me very much and one day he died. My Godmother and me bureed him in her bakyrd with his toy mouse and some tuna.

THE END

Orville looked inside the box. Staring up at him was a letter with a Post-It note in Selma's handwriting: "Number 14, to be mailed on the tenth month and first week after he's back." It was the top one of a packet of other letters bound by rubber bands. Also in the box were several large wrapped objects—by feel they seemed to be framed somethings, maybe photos—which he did not unwrap. He closed the box and put it away in his attic.

And called Miranda. A recording came on: "The number you have reached is not in service." He called the phone company. No new number. He drove out there. No one home. No car, no animals. House sealed up tight. He talked to the neighbors, all up and down the dirt road. No one knew anything. Mrs. Tarr. Nothing. Nelda Jo and Henry. Nothing. Penny. No. The school. School had ended the day before. Summer vacation had begun.

Orville worried about foul play. Hoped, in a way, for foul play, but of a minor kind soon brought to rights. Talked to Officer Packy Scomparza. Nothing. Filed a missing person's report. Nothing. Tried to find relatives. Realized she had kept any relatives secret. Called Boca Grande, Florida, and Avalon, Mississippi, her dead husband's home. Nothing. Realized she had even kept her married name secret. As it dawned on him, her core of secrets, he felt dazed and astonished—as if he'd been hit in the head with a brick.

He wrote her a letter. It was returned, "No Forwarding Address."

Amy was frantic. He tried to explain their breakup but couldn't.

It's as if they've fallen off the face of the earth.

Devastated, he sat alone in the ghostly house emptied out of everything but echoes. His mind filled with Miranda and that great little boy, Cray. And Selma.

"What hell!" he cried out. "Out of such love such hell!"

Part Three

◇ ◇ ◇

In Humility, we call forth the Divinity,
to be with us in living our Understanding.

—*Quaker (anonymous)*

24

"How can I help?" Henry Schooner was asking, one evening a couple of weeks later, framed by the front doorway of Orville's mother's house.

It was the endless finale to a feverish day. The house was not air-conditioned. Orville had come straight home from a house call—rather, a stable call, lured out by the false premise of dire human disease and then pumping a flaccid heifer full of antibiotics—grabbed the bottle of Dickel, a six pack of Knickerbocker, a bag of Korn Kurls, and a fresh cardboard box of Parodi cigars, and, shedding down to his underwear as he climbed the elegant walnut staircase, flopped down onto the couch in front of the Yankees. Hearing the doorbell, he put on khaki safari shorts he'd bought in Nairobi and a black T-shirt with no logo. In America without a logo, he mused, that sort of sums me up.

Since Miranda and Cray disappeared, Orville had been left alone in the house with his dead mother and a songless lovebird, stunned by the depth of his despair. Feeling really *down.* Too sick at heart to eat, too restless to sleep. By day, at work, exhausted and preoccupied. By night, lying in bed going over and over it in his mind, hollowed out by the knife of grief. As desperate as he'd ever been.

Facing Henry at the front door, Orville realized that, as usual, Schooner was more appropriately dressed than him. Ironic, he thought, that this ragamuffin kid who always wore hand-me-downs and mismatched colors is now the missionary of high fashion to the Columbians. Henry stood there in creased linen trousers, a crisp pink shirt with a button-down collar, and a jauntily loosened regimental striped tie—a costume you see in newsreels from the twenties of the upper classes at play. Across the red tie's blue and white diagonal stripes sailed a fleet of aircraft carriers, heading for deep water off the edge or maybe around on the other side.

Orville was sweating; Henry was not. Orville hadn't had time to shave for two days and was worn-out. Henry looked fresh and perky, his cheeks and temples shining a hairless pink. He gave off the ineluctable scent of baby shampoo.

Meeting Henry's gaze was always hard for Orville. It was as if Henry practiced how to look at you in front of a mirror. You felt he was looking only at you and in fact into you and more in fact through you to some more significant truth that, if he were lucky, you might just reveal. And when he was with you, you felt like you were the only one in the world who mattered. So far, in his run for Congress as the only Republican candidate in the primary, he'd been dynamite.

Orville found himself staring not into the Schooner eyes but into the Schooner forehead, into the pink flesh creased by a single worry line, and then higher up to his remarkable hair, which just could not be pinned down, so to speak, because it was neither the white-blond of the boy nor the gray-blond of the man. Even combed, there was always a cowlick in back. Henry's one sign of nervousness, Orville had observed, was to twirl his cowlick with a finger. It gave him a charming sense of boyish. And who could resist that? Even as a doctor schooled in reading bodies and, to a certain extent, minds, Orville had never been able to read anything in Schooner—except for this slightly revelatory twirl of the cowlick.

Fingering the nubbin of scar tissue on the back of his neck where Henry had put out his cigarette two blocks away and twenty-five years ago, Orville considered Henry's question. He noted that Henry hadn't asked "*Can* I help?" but "*How* can I help?" "*How* can I help?" assumed that Orville would be overjoyed to have the help of such a great guy and it was just a question of working out the details.

"With what?" Orville asked, finally.

"Finding 'em, and helping you cope."

Orville said nothing to this, staring down now, noticing that in Henry's hands clasped over the crotch of his creased slacks was a Panama hat, white straw, dark purple band—as if he were paying a visit to the recently bereaved, expecting even to join in sitting *shiva*, why not?

"They've vanished off the face of the earth," Orville said. "People have been looking for almost two weeks and there's nothing."

"Kinda awkward just standing here in the doorway, old friend."

Shit, Orville thought, a choice point: if he sits, he stays; if he stays, I've got to *relate* to the jerk. But if I turn him out, then I'm the shit, I'm the barbarian, not him.

"Come in."

They went into the kitchen. Orville cracked two beers and offered a jar of Planters Peanuts, salted. His doctor's eyes scanned the list of ingredients. He figured that the jar contained enough carcinogens to wipe out all the squirrels in the Courthouse Square.

Henry accepted, munching thoughtfully. "Sorry I haven't been more neighborly in your time of trouble. I've been in D.C. Takes a lot of money to run for Congress. Lucky I got contacts. You remember Beef Schweitzer?—*Food Solutions,* out on Route 9? Since '54 in Guatemala he's cooked for the CIA boys. Big success—third biggest food wholesaler around." Orville nodded. "And remember Larry North, lived just out in Philmont?" Orville shook his head. "Oh. Well, he goes by 'Ollie' North now, for some damn reason. I met him in the navy. Annapolis, him. Got to know him in 'Nam. He's on the president's staff, National Security. Last Tuesday I met with him about monies to help my campaign. In the basement of *the White House.*" Henry paused, seeming to be waiting for an awed response.

"He has money?"

"He *knows* money."

"National security by killing Nicaraguans? Death squads and torture?"

"'Freedom Fighters,' you bet." The voice was edgy. "Like the president says. Fighting the 'evil empire.'"

"Making the world safe for dictators?"

"There you go again!" Henry said shaking his head, as if in admiration for Orville's spirit. "But I'll die for your right to say that—seen my buddies lying facedown in the dirt of 'Nam, for that." Orville wondered why his buddies, in the navy, would die in the dirt. "But listen up." He leaned his elbows on the table, as if he were acting the part of someone in power telling someone not in power to listen up. "They can find 'em."

"Ollie North can?"

"And Beef, and their operatives. Find anybody, anybody in the world, in a day or two. Unless they're professionals, shaving off fingerprints, plastic surgery, you know."

"No, I don't."

"'Course you don't, and the less you know the better. Just give me the go-ahead and we'll find 'em."

"How much will it cost?"

Henry seemed devastated by this. His smile faded to disappointment. He averted his eyes as if witnessing a bad accident.

"Sorry," Orville said, worried that if he didn't stop the implosion he might have a puddle of Schooner on his floor and he'd have to spend even more time mopping it up.

"Accepted," Schooner said, brightening right up. "I mean, shit, Orvy, how could you know the drill? Civilian life is different." Cupping his hand around the peanut jar as if it were filled with gemstones instead of toxins, Henry asked, again, "Is it a go?"

Orville again felt trapped. If he said yes, what would he owe Henry?

Would Henry's methods intrude on Miranda and Cray's privacy? But he was getting nowhere trying to find them and had just about given up. His sense of loss and his frantic despair were unbearable. Every morning when he woke up his first thought was *They're gone!* It tore his heart out. All day long it haunted him—and affected his doctoring. Distracted, he was making mistakes. He would forget to order a test, to check it, to make a referral, to keep an appointment, and, worse, he would screw up with patients. There had been only one fatality—eighty-eight-year-old Mr. Targ, one of the Rope Alley Targs who Bill and he had been treating for prostate cancer, was hospitalized with an ominous tachycardia that, day after day, no matter what med Orville tried, wouldn't break. Finally, his heart gave out. Awake that night, thinking over the case, he realized he'd forgotten to consider hyperthyroidism. The next day he had the lab run a test on the saved blood. TSH, the thyroid hormone, was off the scale. Would he have caught it before? Maybe, maybe not.

"Okay," Orville said to Henry. "Go ahead. But nothing intrusive. I don't want them to know you're following them, or that you've found them. I just want to know that they're safe."

"Think I don't? They're dear to me, too. Tell you something, old buddy. Ever since I came back to this town almost three years ago now—my hometown and yours too—I feel like the town is part of me. This person, that person, this church, that synagogue, this soccer team and that, even the damn manhole covers and shi-shi antique stores!—all part of me. And if a building comes down or an antiquer gets sick with that gay disease shit or if a Nazi swastika is painted on that Temple Anshe Emeth of yours or even if there's a murder in Bliss Towers with the blacks? *I feel it.* Even the nameless blacks. And if I know the person who goes or dies *personally?*" Henry again seemed to crumple down into a depth of unfathomable grief. "I *take* it personally. It *kills* me. Like your dear mom's death. That great lady that was like the mom I wished I had. Like Miranda and that boy, um . . ."

"Cray."

"Cray, yeah—getting old, memory's not what it used to be."

"It's Reaganesque."

"Ha! Haha!" Henry slapped his cheek. "What a hotshit wit you got! *Still!*" Henry chortled a little more and then, sighing, went on. "I know you really love her and him, and I love her and him too. Hey, the boy spent a lot of time in our home with Maxie and Junior. And they disappear? Thin *air* into? Telling nobody nothin'? Not even sayin' good-bye? My Maxie is, well . . . devastated."

"Okay. See what you can do. I've got to go back to work."

"God, you work hard!" Henry said, shaking his head in amazement. "Why not relax a little?"

"Find me a doctor to take over until I leave and I will."

"You really leaving?"

"Nothing to stay for now."

"Oh. Oh, shit. That hurts, old bud. Right here." He placed a palm over what he thought was his heart but was his spleen. "Guess I personally never really believed you would." His face fell, his body sagged. "Talk about pain? Us and this town might never recover, the way you've dedicated your life here, modern medicine, and—"

"Not as modern as Edward R. Shapiro, though, am I?"

"Fair enough. But y'know why we go to him?" Orville said he did not. "'Cause we been goin' to him ever since we been back, and we're loyal. Loyal folk. Like I am to you." He rose suddenly and before Orville could get up Henry had plunked a hand down on his shoulder, man-to-man. Orville, in a man-one-down-to-man position, glanced up into those coal-black eyes and then away. "We got ourselves a growing relationship, Orvy, I know it. Takes time to trust and respect, but we're getting there." Without waiting for confirmation of this, Henry went on, "Why not come over to our house for Fourth of July? Hot dogs, burgers, beer, you'd be honoring us, as part of the family."

"I may have to work."

"Whenever. But come over anytime, day or night. Look, I know how shitty you feel—about losing your mom, losing your girl and that cute kid who was like a son to you. But two points: one, we'll find 'em, guaranteed; two, let the Schooners help with the pain. C'mon over anytime."

Orville thought he should say no but instead said nothing.

"Hey, hey! We got progress here! You didn't say no!"

Orville, puzzled by the pull of a sincerity he didn't buy, walked Henry back to the front door and out onto the porch. The evening was calm, recovering from the heat-stroked day. There was a hint in the air not of cool exactly but of lessening hot. Across the hazy park, the light on Schooner's front porch glowed golden, reflecting the gold-painted underside of the porch roof.

"So if not the 4th, come the 3rd or the 5th or whatever damn day you want. Come anytime. Drop in. No need to call first. Nobody much just drops in anymore, have you noticed? When we were young, we dropped in. Now, we don't drop in. Which is why I dropped in just now. Maybe, if you and me take the lead, in the 'drop-in' movement . . ." He sighed. "One more thing."

"Yeah?" With Henry there was always one more thing, and it was usually the one thing that underlay all the other things.

"The reason we haven't switched to you as our doctor is continuity of care. I mean, with you leaving. And also that Nelda Jo likes you too much to put it on a purely professional basis."

"What?" Orville's mind was flooded with those muscat grapes.

"Just jokin', Orvy." He popped him in the arm. "Laugh a little, okay?"

He turned away to go. Orville said, "One more thing, Henry."

Henry turned back. On his face was a listening look. "Fire away, old friend."

"Why me?" Henry seemed puzzled. "Why are you so interested in me?"

"You mean in addition to our just being old friends?"

"We were never old friends, Henry. You and I—"

"Well, what's a little difference of opinion among old friends?"

"Henry. Why am I so blessed with your friendship?"

If he caught the sarcasm, he hid it. "You want the truth?" Orville nodded, thinking, Here comes a lie. "Okay. I feel very deeply that I have to look out for you."

"What?"

"For some reason you hated me growing up. But I respected you. When I left Columbia, walking off into those woods with you and Whiz and Tommy staring at me, I was lost, a lost kid headed for trouble. I enlisted in the navy. It was rough. A year later I found myself in Seattle, facing a choice. A tour of duty in Vietnam, or run away, desert. I was supposed to ship out that night. I walked and walked in the rain. Found myself down at the harbor. Staring at a ferry coming in from Vancouver. *Toot toot,* it was goin' *toot toot.* Comin' in. I could get on it, go to Vancouver, save my ass. A buddy had done it. Said it was nice over there in Canada. Flowerpots hanging from the lampposts. Nice life. Or, there was 'Nam. I didn't have much time. But I couldn't decide. And you know what I did?" Orville did not. "I found a pay phone and called you up."

"*Me?*"

"You were the only guy I knew I could respect. And I decided that whatever you said I should do, I'd do."

"That never happened, Henry."

"Of *course* it never happened, Orvy. You were away at college. I got your mother."

"Oh, God."

"I always liked her and respected her. So when she said you weren't there, well, I asked her."

"You asked *Selma* what you should do?"

"I remember, in the background, the ferry was goin' '*toot toot*, I'm leaving for Canada now, *toot, toot!*' It was one of those moments, ya know what I mean?"

"And she said?"

"'Don't run away. Don't you *dare!* Stay. Do your duty to God and country. Like Sol did.' Great lady, your mom. She made me promise I would stay. And it changed my life. Your mother changed my life. Because I did the right thing. If I'd have gone to Canada, my life would've turned out crap. Going to 'Nam, doing the right thing, made me what I am today. The navy made me a man. Never looked back. Me, in the White House basement with Ollie North of the National Security Agency. Can you *believe* it?"

"Hard to," Orville said again. Henry didn't notice the dig.

"I owe it all to your mom."

The mosquitoes were at them. They both slapped for a few seconds.

"There's one thing I've been wondering, though," Henry went on, a slight hitch in his voice. "If I *had* gotten you on the phone, what would you have told me to do?"

"I'd've told you to run."

Henry busted out laughing, really laughing, starting with his square face, his eyes going slitty and his nose red and then his eyes tearing up and he holding his gut and then holding onto the porch railing. Despite himself, Orville joined in. "Well then . . . Orvy . . . it's . . ." he tried to catch his breath. "It's a good thing I got her! Ha! Haha!" He was off again on a spiral of guffaws.

Orville waited.

"So then . . . when I . . . when I came back, I got to be friendly with her. She was like the mother I never had. She wasn't in the best of health, so I kinda would look in on her. We'd talk about you. Rocky relationship, you and her." Henry held out his hands like an umpire telling two ballplayers to calm down. "Hey, understood. She seemed more depressed this time of year last year—actually toward the end of July, around your birthday. Didn't look healthy. I stopped in more. And she died. Alone. On the kitchen floor. Died alone on the kitchen floor." Henry seemed to wipe away a tear or two. He reached out, squeezed Orville's arm. "I figure she'd have wanted me to look after you."

Orville watched the refrigerator body walk slowly back across the park through the summer evening. At the midway point, in a cone of light where the path from the courthouse steps crossed the path linking the two houses, Henry turned and waved gamely. Then he turned away and walked on, off.

Don't believe a word of it.

And yet back in the spiritless house, Orville was startled to find that with Henry gone, he felt even more alone.

PhwweeeeeEEETT!

The lovebird saw him walking down the hallway toward its cage in the kitchen and let out a piercing shriek. It had been a Valentine's Day gift from Miranda and Cray. "You need a pet," she'd said, "and this one's low maintenance." "Can I name him Starlight?" Cray asked.

Starlight he was. Selma and Sol had hated animals. Penny and Orville had grown up begging for pets. In vain. Living out at Miranda's house, with her finches and cats and friendly raccoons, mice, squirrels, and deer, Orville had realized how suspicious he'd become of pets, how he'd grown up old. When they'd surprised him with the bird, it seemed to him the most beautiful thing he'd ever seen. Native to Africa, it was a peach-faced lovebird, its head peach and green and yellow and its wing and tail feathers the pastel shadings of blue-green that you see on a tropical coast. Taking a bath in a dish, its tail feathers moved faster than the eye could see. He was amazed by the seamlessness of the feather shadings, peach to gold to green to blue—the words pale and rigid by comparison.

And the miracle of flight! This little thing could fly! Well, sort of fly. With clipped wings, it flew only down. With fierce optimism it would leap, flutter frantically to gain altitude as it fell down to the floor, and then crawl, aided by its hooked beak, up the nearest pants leg to the highest point on the tallest person in the room, usually Orville. It seemed not to notice that it couldn't fly. When happily perched on his shoulder, it would chuff up—"Chuffbird!" Cray would call it—and then flick down its eyelid like a box snapped shut over a glittering dark jewel, and sleep.

As Orville stared at the bird in its cage now, it cocked its head and stared back at him in silence, and he remembered in excruciating detail how Cray, with his high-pitched child's voice, could imitate the high shriek exactly, Starlight answering in kind, in a kind of conversation. The bird would not only answer Cray, but the crash of plates, the ring of the phone, and the doorbell, but never Orville or Miranda. Once at breakfast it had fluttered down onto Cray's plastic placemat, a map of America. "It's walking across America!" Cray said, squealing with delight. "And pooping on Iowa!" Orville added. And on Orville. The bird could watch TV on Cray's shoulder for an hour without letting loose, and then the first instant he landed on Orville—jackpot. For better or worse the bird had arrived in his life at a level of love, and at first it could do no wrong.

A pain in the ass, he said to himself now, as he opened the cage door and let the lovebird clamber up onto his shoulder while he cleaned out the pee and poop and sunflower seed shells and feathers from the bottom. If two lovebirds are in a cage, they either tear each other to shreds or bond forever and tear anybody else who goes near them to shreds. And we call them lovebirds?

PhwweeeeeEEEETT!

"Owww! Not right in my ear okay?"

The bird made only one sound, this shriek, and when it let loose into his ear it rattled the ossicles horrifically, flooding the semicirculuar canals—an ear-splitting cry.

PhwweeeeeEEEETT!

"Can't you say anything else?"

PhwweeeeeEEEETT!

"Dumb bird," Orville said, looking it in the eye. As he reached for it, it bit his index finger hard. Reflexively he reached to hit it—but stopped himself in time. He bent his shoulder down to the cage door and in it went. A drop of blood the size of its eye surfaced on his finger. Great. I'll die of psittacosis, die right here in Columbia. Henry can cry for me.

They stared at each other, man and bird. Maybe, he thought, it misses them too? Lately it had been moulting and fretting. Whenever Orville would come into the room, it would race back and forth on the floor of its cage shrieking until he took it out. Every morning for the past week, he discovered that during the night it had knocked down its toy mirror onto the floor of its cage, and in the semi-dark under the cage cover he could hear it attacking the reflected bird viciously. The bird's irritation irritated him. It was an accusation. The bird was becoming a burden.

Figures, he thought. Lose what you love and your love for everything else fades. The bitter taste in his mouth was almost physical. Doctoring the Columbians, ill and injured and insane in the insect-ridden conflagration of summer, had brought out the bitter taste even more lately. He'd even started swigging Starbusol. Placebo, maybe, but the wintergreen taste helped.

And who do I give the thing to when I go?

The bird was off again on its pointless track meet, running back and forth on the floor of the cage, shrieking. Poor thing. I should apologize. He reached for the cage door, and then stopped. His hand lay extended, still as a wax hand, on the air.

A wave of grief hit him. *I've lost them.*

This is how it happened now. He'd be pretty much okay, going along with things as if life were normal, and then—*pow!*—like in the comics a fist would crash in from the frame of the picture and hit him in the gut and he'd stagger and try not to fall. All of a sudden, out of the blue, he would start remembering. He would recall to the slightest detail things said or done that he regretted, or things he didn't do or say but thought to and should have, that any normal person would have automatically—and he felt shocked, shamed, appalled. Haunted by it all. He heard again the last lines of the W. B. Yeats poem his wife Lily had thrown at him—literally—at the end, " . . . and not a day recalled, my conscience or my vanity appalled."

His hand stayed in midair. His mind flew down. I've screwed up everything, he thought, everything, everything! And when I go, where will I go? What's in Europe for me anymore? More nothing.

He got a glass and ice, poured some George Dickel and, taking the bottle with him, climbed the stairs toward the TV, his body made of lead.

The Yankees had won and the TV had turned back to men blasting away at each other with guns and women acting like cartoons and regular programming being interrupted by a news flash about Our Aged President threatening to drop a lot of nuclear bombs on something or other, itself interrupted by a commercial for a fabulous car. Unable to watch, he found himself heading up to the attic where he took down the Scomparza box with Selma's letters and photos and carried it to his bedroom in the turret.

When he opened it, a part-sweet, part-acrid scent filled the room. The scent of Old Lady—mothballs, musty cloth, baby powder, perfume. He picked up Letter Number 14.

Hi there, Earthling!

Nice to get mail, isn't it? The U.S. Postal Service does *such* a nice job.

I presume you're well. I'm not. (Is dead well?) I've had this damn indigestion again. Can't shake it. Took enough Maalox to plaster a bathroom, and no luck. Bill keeps pushing Starbusol. It was one thing when he put me on that junk as a salve for a muscle pull when in fact I had a hernia, another thing when he gave me a shot of it for my dizziness when in fact

I had a brain tumor, but to *drink* the stuff? What disease is he missing now? I'm not afraid of dying—just of dying alone. Not that you would care. This last time you left you didn't even leave your number.

I want to talk to you about love and hate. Of all of us you were the worst at love and best at hate. Penny was medium on each. Sol was bad at love but never got into hate. I myself am the best at love and the worst at hate. I just can't seem to help seeing the best in everyone!

So. You and love. Are you unloveable? When you were born, I was desperate. Twenty-two hours in labor, no dice, so they went in with the forceps. When they yanked you out of me you were long and skinny, your head shaped like a shoebox. The Air Force was awful, and your father greasing up the planes from below was filthy. (The only fun we had was trips from Fayetteville to the ocean, to the big dunes at Kitthyhawk where Wilbur and ***ORVILLE*** made their first flight. Flight—that's you to a "T.") When I came home from the hospital I felt blue. Sol was itchy to play golf. I said, "All I want from you are the 3 Cs: Care, Companionship, and Concern. Please, Sol, please!" No luck. It was wartime, but I decided then and there to divorce him.

I didn't divorce him and that was the biggest mistake of my life. I should have divorced him the day you were born. Even better, the day before you were conceived—what's one less Rose in the world? I'm sure this old world will keep (keeps) turning now with one less Selma. And to think I had to have my tubes blown to have you. Talk about pain!

You divorced Lily and you shouldn't have. (Despite the way she treated me.) I should've divorced and didn't; you shouldn't have and did—go figure. What kept me alive, you're asking? Why didn't I follow the family tradition of suicide? One *shabbas* in 1953 I had a religious experience, and I found my answers: Number 1: SO WHAT?, and Number 2: WHAT NEXT? I realized that for the Family Rose to rise, others had to fall. An eye-for-an-eye, dog-eat-dog, two-by-two world.

When you were five you ran from me and never looked back. Never gave me the time of day. Always off on your projects, trying to achieve things. One day we were driving along, you were telling me how great you were, and I lost it and said, "Stop crowing like a cock!" Did this faze you? Not one iota. You did achieve, some. But if Bill hadn't pulled some strings, you'd never have gotten into medical school—and he could only get you in offshore.

Your ongoing sin is being stiff-necked. I noticed at Yom Kippur services you never bowed down with the rest of us—too good for us, eh? Too good for G-d? You and your hifalooting love of Europe and how great Dublin was and how you preferred Paris to Columbia. Think *I* didn't like Paris? Sol didn't? (Okay, Sol didn't, but he came from a long line of short Polish peasants and don't let him or that stupid sister of his tell you anything different!) Every choice you made was a selfish choice and I've had it with you. It's not so much that you have a self-centered view of the world as a world-centered view of yourself.

No wonder I have a heartburn that would gag a vulture.

You ran away from me. You'll run away again in a few weeks, and good riddance. (You think it's bad for Columbia and good for you, but I've got news for you—it's the reverse.) You'll go through the money quicker than you think, and then what, Mr. Bigshot Doctor Without Borders?

It's like another rule I learned in life the hard way: If A Person's Feet Hurt, You Can Always See It In Their Face.

What's that got to do with anything? Lots. It means that by planning to leave again, to run away from your home and family after the year and 13 days are up, you're living proof that you're about as selfish as they come. Which means you'll end up about as lonely as they come. The bottom line? YOU LET ME DOWN.

All my love, Your Mother

Orville drained the bottle of bourbon, his chin to the ceiling.
"You know, mom," he said out loud, still looking up, "you're right."
"About what?"
There she was, floating at the level of the gold ball on the flagpole outside his bedroom window. She again wore the cobalt gown. Her hair was permed in the style of the 1950s, and again her face was strangely whole. She hadn't flown all that much when he was with Miranda and Cray, except toward the end when things had begun to fall apart. Now that Miranda and Cray had disappeared, she had flown more often. Once, floating overhead at Geiger's Junkyard as he tried with Hayley's husband Clive to rescusitate a Columbian who had put his finger into a live socket. Again one afternoon as he drove the Chrysler across the Rip Van Winkle Bridge, she doing aerobatic swoops from high up over the superstructure down almost to the water and then under the bridge deck and, waving gaily, up into the wild blue yonder over the Caskills. And most recently when he was at the county's newly christened Scrimshaw Airport to identify the remains of a flyboy who'd backed into a propeller, there she was in her Amelia Earhart outfit, practicing takeoffs and landings.

"Everything, Mom. You're right about it all."

"Good. So we're cool, and you'll stay. See ya later, alligator."

"Stay? Get real."

"Wish I could. Those days are over. Bye now." She was banking away.

"Wait!"

"Can't. Gotta *fly!*"

"Where to?"

"The Schooners'," she said enthusiastically, as if her flight were to a storewide sale at Macy's up in Ballston Spa. "That Henry's *such* a sweetheart. He was always a *zeesa boyala,* a sweet boy, and now he's such a caring, concerned, comforting man. Not like *someone* I know."

"You're going over to the Schooners'?"

"You bet," she sang out. "It's the place to *be!*" She turned away, hesitated, and turned back. "Oh, and by the way, Dr. Know-It-All—about your breakup with Miranda?" He stared at her, unwilling to respond. It was all too raw. "That'll teach you to try to keep *me* out of your love life! I was in the middle of it the whole darn time!"

"Where is she? Do you know where she is?"

Gone.

Dazed, he tried to follow her flight across the square, but she was lost in the parched oaks and maples.

Doorbell. He looked at his watch. Almost eleven. He stumbled downstairs and opened the door to Nelda Jo Schooner.

She was a vision from a certain heaven, blond hair swept back, eyes gleaming with what he could not help but see as mischief, lips the peach color of Starlight's face, and a body poured into her pink tank top and tan shorts.

"Hi," she said. "Can I come in?

25

"Sure," he said to Nelda Jo. "Would you like a drink?"

"You got bourbon, honey?"

"You bet. George Dickel and I have gotten real close. It's upstairs. I'll get it."

"No need. I'll go with you."

He led her up to what Selma and Sol called "The Family Room," facing

Prison Alley. They sat on the leather couch in front of the dead TV. The room was dim. "I forgot a glass," he said.

"Where I come from, you share." He poured, handed the glass to her, and she lifted it in a toast. "To your going through a helluva shitty time, Orvy, and to our friendship."

"Friendship," he said, raising the bottle in reply, thinking Why, with Schooners, is it always about friendship? And why the tag team match tonight? The bourbon felt sexy. He followed it with a fresh beer from the sixpack in the cooler at his feet.

"I came over for a coupla reasons," she said. She took his hand. It felt strong, aerobic. "You're a beautiful man, and you surely don't deserve this."

"This?" He glanced at her hand, into her blue eyes, aware of her body.

"Miranda and that darling boy Cray. I worry about them, nobody knowin' what happened. You must be frantic with worry." He nodded. "But you can't isolate yourself from your sources of support, from your family and your friends, from me and from the Good Lord. The first time I saw you I really liked you, Orvy, the gentle way you have, the quiet way, like you're always seeing me like I really am, you know?"

"Thanks. I like you too."

"I can tell." She squeezed his hand. "You and Henry had a rough old time in your youth. I've got no dog in that fight. I'm here for myself." Orville nodded. "You are well aware of how I am my own person, an independent woman—running the health spa 'n' all, running the family. Received my MBA from OU. Not that I use it but still—I write it off as an 'opportunity cost of doing business.' Know somethin'? I think of you a lot. Too much, maybe."

"Why, Nelda Jo, how could that be?"

She laughed, a kind of Southen football hoot, and her breasts shook a little in that tight-fitting pink. He refilled the glass. She drank. "And I pray for you in this time of trial. Even if you don't believe in prayer, I think it could prove right helpful to you. This may sound naive but ever since I was born again, I feel a lot better about my life and life on earth and eternal life, too."

"Good, good. Pray for me. Give it a shot."

"Deal. There's one more thing. A medical thing? Can I ask you to look at something?"

On that body? Have I died and gone to heaven? He said, "Now?"

"I'm so worried! I can't sleep. Dr. Shapiro said it's dangerous, could be a melanoma, and I should get a biopsy but it's in a tender spot. And I don't trust him."

"Join the crowd."

"Really?" He nodded. "Oh, my. Maybe we should all come to you?"

"It'd be my pleasure." Everything she was saying and doing—even praying for him, because someone as fit and sexy and good as she might very well entice God to intervene—was like a sweet dream. He hadn't had any of those kinds of dreams for weeks.

"I'm a little embarrassed," she said.

"Don't be. I've seen everything."

"'Kay." She put down the glass and crossed her hands over her chest and pulled her pink tank top over her head and he was face-to-face with breasts and shoulders and abs as perfect as the woman athletes in Holland. She turned halfway away. "It's this mole. See?"

The mole was on her right side, alongside her breast. His doctor's bag was on the floor, and he reached into it for his high-intensity flashlight. Sure enough, it was a mole, and pitch-black, and he was aware of that awful question floating into the healthy sensual space between them: "Is this death?" Lit up in profile her breast swooped out large, a Mount Rushmore to male fixation, the nipple plumped up. Aroused, he felt like he was again "playing doctor" with Faith as a kid. Diligently he palpated the crown of the mole, ran his finger along the edge, inspected the margins (smooth and regular), asking questions like how long has it been there? ("Years") and has it grown lately ("I don't think so but it's hard to see—my bra irritates it, I've been going without") and have you ever had any others ("Just beauty marks since I was a kid"). Before he clicked off the light he noticed on one arm a nasty fresh bruise, as if she'd fallen or been grabbed, hard.

"Well?" she asked, turning full toward him without bothering to cover up, searching his eyes for the verdict.

"It's just a mole, that's all. It's nothing."

"Jesus!" she said and threw her arms around him, hugging him hard, so that she knocked him over and they wound up with her on top of him on the couch. She pulled away, their eyes met, and she kissed him full on the lips, her tongue an added touch of gratitude for the diagnosis of benign mole. He kissed back.

"Damn but you *are* a beautiful man." She sat back, took a sip from the bottle.

"And you're something else."

"Whew," she whistled, fanning her naked chest with her hand, "hot—and I do not mean the ambient temperachure." They laughed. "I'd better go."

"Yeah. I'll probably get paged soon anyway." He watched her cover those Muscat nipples and gorgeous breasts with stretched pink. *Ah, to be that pink, upon those breasts!*

"Y'know, you shouldn't stand on formality. You oughta just drop in sometime. Nobody up North drops in on anybody. In Oklahoma, people drop in all the time. Don't be no stranger, y'hear? With ole Henry away campaignin' all the time, I get morose."

"Hard to believe, you, morose."

"Wrong word. 'Wantin' company' is better." She stood, smoothed things down, tight, fit, sleek as a swimmer. "Like they say in the South, 'Y'all come see us.'"

He walked her downstairs and waved her along, away. He stood there watching her stroll across the square. In his vulnerable and angry state, he wanted her terrifically. Why had she done that? Was it relief at the diagnosis, or was she really inviting him in? Had Henry sent her? But why? She reminded him of the sex with the athletes in Holland. He wanted her and that, sure, but with Celestina and Miranda he had come to realize he needed something else. Progress had been made. What he needed was what he had lost.

◊ ◊ ◊

For a while Orville resisted the pull toward that glowing golden porch light inviting him into what he nicknamed "Schoonerland."

Sometimes of an evening he'd see the Family Schooner sitting together out on the porch, Henry and Nelda Jo in white wicker rockers, Junior in a colorful Guatemalan hammock, Maxie playing on the steps. They would sit for seeming hours, chatting with neighbors and friends strolling by through the husky summer nights. Orville would watch as these Columbians often would stop, stay—yes, drop in. Before long, snatches of laughter, exclamation and song—even song!—would hurry across the 134 steps of the cement pathway and up the four steps to his front porch, where he sat smoking a cigar, downing boilermakers, feeling left out. Even Selma seemed to pull him toward Schoonerland. From time to time he would have brief glimpses of her heading toward or away from the Victorian, as if she lived there or nested there or had a hangar there, complete with dedicated mechanics for maintenance.

When Orville chanced upon a Schooner—even Maxie or Junior—it was as if it was a great event in their day. They gave normal waves, normal smiles, held normal conversations. Henry and Nelda Jo seemed always to be around, doing normal summertime things, occasionally dropping in together with a homemade pie or a Havana cigar, always with a kind word and an acceptance of his not yet accepting their standing invitation. They never parted without a "God Bless You," and, in Henry's departures, with an added, candidate's "and God Bless America." Whenever Orville encountered the Schooners, even the Columbian weather seemed more normal. The frantic heat lost its edge, the sweating air its humidity. Summer showers were gentle and useful to crops. Thunderstorms brought not just relief but a natural pruning of deadwood and a welcome measure of drama and passed through quickly, doing little damage. Nelda Jo, after that night of the mole, though still flirtatious, never again came alone.

Orville pictured Schoonerland as not just a geography but as a hagiography. It was a suffusion of normal America directly into the Schooners, without harmful additives. It was unfiltered and uncluttered, relentlessly normal, wholeheartedly accepted. Even worshipped, for the Schooners were solid members not only of St. Mark's Episcopal (Henry) and Shiloh Baptist (Nelda Jo), but they made a point of attending various ecumenical services—Jewish, black, Hispanic, Ukrainian, and Dutch Reformed out in Spook Rock. Schooners attended most everything in town and county. Schooners showed up.

Not only was normal America suffusing the Family Schooner, Orville realized, but in a kind of alchemy, normal America, encountering Schooners, was reflected back as an amplified and purified substance, more substantial and crisply defined and even innovated and improved upon. America, through Schooners, made progress, became more perfect. That perfected image radiated back out from each of the smiles of little Maxie, Junior, Nelda Jo, the Filipino servants, and Henry himself, smiles revealing teeth that shone like ice in new Amana refrigerators.

Yes, that perfected image was beamed back out as a happy porch-glow in the July dusk and then, strolling across the putting-green perfect yard and moving lightly past the Courthouse Square with its war memorials to Great Dead Columbians starting with the Revolution and General Worth's War of 1812 and the Spanish-American War whatever that was and the War of the Secession, otherwise known as The Civil, to The Great War, which wasn't all that great if you wound up dead, and then The War To End All Wars, which didn't, and The (strange) Korean War and then, heading toward Vietnam—The War We Lost And Pretended To Win But It Wasn't A Real War Anyway So The Loss Didn't Really Count—the perfected image veered so as not to get too close to *that* war and then, free from the drag of these war memorials, the image gathered itself up in denial and took off through the July dusk and diffused all over Columbia, from swamp to swamp and river to cemetery, and then out through Kinderhook County and America and the world.

America found Schooners, and Schooners illuminated America to the ends of the earth. After all, Orville found himself thinking, what do you hear on top of a Himalayan peak? The Beach Boys. What are they wearing, paddling your canoe up the Amazon? Michael Jackson stuff. What do you drink on the Moroccan edge of the Sahara? Coca-Cola. What's playing in Bangkok? Arnold Schwarzenegger. What's constant in the world? Mickey Mouse. All of it an ad for America the Good—if not the Best.

The Schooners seemed so normal that Orville felt sick.

He had lost his fighting edge. His spirit had sunk, broken not so much by the bullying of his mother telling him he was abnormal but more by the queasy feeling that she was dead right. Given the evidence of his failures to be normal with Miranda and Cray and Amy and the dread Penny and the concrete Milt and the poor ethereal Celestina and the psychoanalyzed Lily and yes, even the Schooners—well, he was finally cowed into thinking she was right.

Your mother is right. You are so abnormal you should be illegal.

From that first afternoon as a child in the field looking up at the clouds passing across when he had discovered the "something else" and when, on bringing it back to his mother he'd been told he was crazy because "there's nothing else but this," Orville had lived with a deep, secret, abiding sense that he was abnormal. His unexplained infertility had sealed it. Abnormal, most definitely. Alternative to the culture, always. Even, years ago in college at Syracuse and medical school in Dublin, alternative to the alternative sixties—talking the talk but not walking the walk.

Now, Orville was more and more fascinated by Henry because the guy seemed to know clearly who he was, what he was placed on earth for, what he was aimed at, and how he would get it. The man was *tenacious.* Orville hated to admit it, but Henry Schooner seemed to know how to live.

◊ ◊ ◊

One lush Saturday evening in the third week of July, Orville found himself immersed in the normal—sitting out on the Schooner screened-in back porch with Henry, Nelda Jo, and Penny. Milt was away in Seattle, pursuing what Penny called "another of his hair-brained computer business schemes, some new company called Microsoft." Orville had managed to get coverage for the practice from noon to ten. The four of them had played golf out at Whale Acres, the Roses against the Schooners.

Early on in the golf match, Orville recalled the observation he'd first made as the manager of the Columbia High School Fish Hawks: you can tell everything about a person by the way they play a sport. Especially with Schooner, seeming so perfect, the way he played golf was revealing.

Although they were all hackers, Henry, under his genial mien and even in a match that meant nothing, was a ferocious competitor. On the last hole, with the match tied, from the opposite side of the fairway Orville saw Henry cheat. He had hit his ball into the rough to the right. A tree blocked his shot to the green. Orville, in the fairway, saw Henry move his ball away from the tree so he'd have a clear shot to paydirt. And then Orville saw Henry see him see. Henry went on nonchalantly, as if what had happened hadn't happened, and hit his shot onto the green, twenty-five feet from the pin. Penny and Nelda Jo were happily thrashing their way down the fairway and out of contention for the hole.

Orville addressed his ball and took a distracted swing that gronkled his ball barely above the fairway surface, a "worm-raper." As he started to curse, he noticed that the ball was heading straight for the pin, slowed down enough by the grass to wind up a perfect shot, two feet away. It seemed that the Roses would win the hole and the match.

On the green, Henry studied his putt. It was a long, tricky, downhill serpentine. He stroked it confidently. It died on the lip, rolling in, for a birdie three.

Now, to tie the hole and the match, Orville had to sink his putt. It was a straight, flat putt, without any break, of a mere two feet. Standing over the ball, he was nervous. He concentrated, trying his hardest. But then a little voice inside whispered *Miss it! Miss it!* He stroked it straight at the hole. The ball rolled up to the edge, and then hesitated. And then, as if controlled by alien forces, or maybe by his mother, it actually rolled back and stayed out. Orville had choked. The Schooners had won.

Henry was gracious in deceit. "Bad luck, but in fiscal terms you're better off, 'cause you only lost a buck and the winners buy the beers."

Nelda Jo took Orville's arm as they marched up the slope to the clubhouse. She was a little taller than him, and he felt her lithe hip a little above his hip and the rolling of her breast a little above his heart and he felt a little less bad about blowing the putt.

In the shower Orville wondered why he hadn't called Schooner for cheating. It was just a friendly match, so what difference did it make? It had been comforting, in a way, to see Henry's flaw so clearly. Like seeing that Henry and Ollie North and Beef, despite their "Secret Ops" with Central American sleuths and U.S. Marines with computers in the White House basement, had failed to locate Miranda and Cray—Orville stopped, stock-still, realizing that during the round he hadn't felt a single wave of grief. Golf had been a four-hour anesthetic. Maybe that's the secret of life: Play More Golf. Could the Milton Plotkins and Solomon Roses of the world be right after all?

They'd all hung out at the clubhouse for a while eating peanuts and pretzels and drinking cold beer in sweating mugs. Henry, a candidate for Congress and a TV personality, was constantly interrupted by his fans. He handled each graciously, in a way that never really took him out of touch with his home foursome.

Then they segued into an impromptu dinner at the Schooners. The Filipino man grilled steaks and the woman served potato salad and corn on the cob from out in the county and a robust Burgundy and generous slices of homemade and still-warm apple pie à la mode with Stewart's vanilla ice cream melting around it, served on the porch. Soon they were sailing, high on alcohol and sugar and screened from the Columbian mosquitoes and frantic cloudy moths and listening to the chirp of crickets in the cooling summer night.

"Gettin' shot off the deck of an aircraft carrier," Henry said, with a twinkly smile, "is the greatest thing you can do in your life—with your clothes on!" He winked at Orville and laughed. Camel in mouth, Heineken in fist, Orville laughed too.

"Can we quote you on that, Your Grossness?" Nelda Jo asked.

"If you do, honeybunch, I'll deny it."

"I'm going out, Mom," said Junior, coming onto the screened porch.

"Dressed like that?" Nelda Jo asked. Junior's cuboid body was in ragged jean shorts and a T-shirt boasting DRUNK GIRLS THINK I'M CUTE, and his blond-white hair was cut boot-camp short, showing an astonishing field of zits on his forehead. His right hand was bandaged, crudely, from knuckles to wrist.

"Yeah. See you later." He was halfway gone when a high-pitched whistle cut the air. He turned. "Yeah, Dad?"

"You be home before midnight, y'hear?"

"Da-aad!"

"It's a curfew, son. Use it or lose it."

"You never had one."

"I'd be a lot better man if I had," Henry said. "Just ask Dr. Rose."

"This is true."

"It's 'cause we love you, Juney," said Nelda Jo. "Church tomorrow too."

"Shit," he said and ran out.

"Get ready for it, Penny dear," Nelda Jo said, "it's comin' to your home right soon."

"You kiddin'? Amy's a terror already. Thank God for all-girls' overnight camp."

Orville was surprised. Amy a terror? Has Penny gone totally psychotic?

"Tomcattin' around with that Scomparza girl," Henry said, "Americo's daughter. Need I say more? When I'm elected I'm introducin' a bill that would make it okay for parents to kill and eat their teenagers."

"Aw, c'mon, Great One," said Nelda Jo. "He's in love."

"He ain't in love," Henry said. "He's in heat. I'm worried about that one. He's turning into a hellion and—hey, look!" They followed his index finger to the TV. "I've been waitin' to see this! Check it out."

The TV had been rolling away on mute while they sat there. Henry flicked up the volume. On the screen now, as opposed to the frenetic sitcoms and shoot-em-ups and harsh bright commercials, was a scene of a peaceful countryside dotted with bright yellow flowers and a cozy white farmhouse in the background. The camera panned to an aerial view of the majestic Grand Canyon, and then to gorgeous children dressed not like Junior but like gorgeous children frolicking in flowery fields, and then to old folks still in love walking hand in hand, and then to strong young black folks all neat and clean and muscular and smiley playing basketball, and then to grimy but proud factory hands at work, and then to a man in a space vehicle. And as these scenes unfolded against a background of music that effortlessly combined hymns and marches and lullabies and waltzes and gospels and symphonies and all somehow blending to a stirring rendition of *America the Beautiful,* the narrator, with a voice of your Grandpa Ed or your dad on a good day or, Orville thought, of an old-time wise and Reassuring Physician, said, soothingly:

It's morning in America. This is America, spring of '84 . . . And this is America . . . And this is America . . . And this . . . And this . . . And this, too, is America. There's a new man for America. A veteran. A patriot. His name is Henry Schooner. VOTE AMERICA. VOTE SCHOONER.

And there he was. Henry and his family right out there on the front lawn throwing a bright white baseball back and forth.

The four of them sat speechless, awed at the video perfection, the way it tugged on your heartstrings with just the right tension. To vote against Schooner was to vote against not only America but against Morning in America, maybe even against Morning itself, and against all those nice people and songs and Grandpa Ed.

"Great ad!" Penny said. "Perfect!"

"Amazing, Henry," Orville seconded, wondering where the hell he'd gotten the money.

"Thank you. Doesn't my wife look incredible?"

"Henry, honey—" Nelda Jo said.

"And I don't just mean in the ad. Lookit her. Is this is one beautiful woman, eh?"

Penny said yes she was and that she'd give anything to have that body, and Orville said he would, too—everybody laughed at this—but what Orville was thinking was something he'd learned as a doctor: when someone calls attention in public to how beautiful their wife is, the marriage is in trouble, especially in the sexual arena. Henry wasn't getting any. Neither was Nelda Jo. Maybe he should "drop in."

"Cost an arm and a leg," Henry went on.

"Nelda Jo?" Orville asked, realizing he must be more drunk than normal.

"What a wit the guy's got! Haha!" Henry seemed to think this was one of the funniest things he'd ever heard and had to wipe tears away from his eyes to go on. "They tol' me in Washington that I gotta go hard now for name refugnition. Name refuni . . . refu-fuckin'nition am I wrong?"

Everyone agreed that this was a fine strategy since name recognition was important. Just look at General Motors, General Electric, General Foods, General Worth.

For some reason he found himself following Henry out of the den. On the way out Orville lost his balance and bumped into the massive old wooden breakfront. It wobbled ominously. As a doctor he was attuned to accidents waiting to happen and made a note to tell Henry again to get it trued up, but then he was going down into the basement, thinking, What's with America now—with all these *Generals*? Whatever happened to *Specifics*? Besides Bill and me, aren't there any *Specifics* anymore?

The basement was the neatest, cleanest basement Orville had ever seen. No clutter, no dirt. On a workbench under a fluorescent light were dozens of small boxes and plastic bottles of black stuff and a serious and severe chrome machine with a hand-pull lever with a Day-Glo orange handle for a real man's fist, a machine that looked like what a wine aficionado would use to uncork his treasured bottles. The boxes contained shell casings, all shiny brass. The plastic bottles held gunpowder. The wine press was a way to tamp the gunpowder into the shells in the comfort and privacy of your home. Henry made his own bullets.

"Hit a squirrel with that mother," Henry said, "all you see is a puff of fur. Hit a deer, motherfucker's done for."

He showed Orville how to make good bullets. Orville said they looked like good nice bullets. Then he showed Orville his guns. They were locked in a freestanding safe like you'd see in a small bank, which Henry said could withstand anything but "nucular attack." Orville said they were nice guns and a nice safe but he was all of a sudden trapped in a déjà vu. Being in a basement with Schooner, no matter how neat and clean, brought back a memory of being in another basement somewhere else a long time ago, maybe the Lutheran Church basement for Boy Scouts with Henry and the nascent pedophile Len Date. The basement where Len and Henry demanded that Orville pull down his pants so they could "see what a Jew-dick looks like."

Now, listening to Henry go on about guns and how you can, with the right equipment, hit a man a mile away but you have to take into account the lift and fall of the speeding bullet due to gravity, Orville recalled the terror. How he would sit in class trying to figure a route home to avoid Henry's chasings and beatings. How his childhood, aside from the concrete boredom, was a childhood of terror. Boredom and terror.

"You terrorized me, Henry," Orville said now. Henry stared at him, puzzled. "When we were kids. You terrorized me and I'll never forget it."

"Me?" His astonishment flew out on a strong scent of toasted oats.

"Don't deny it."

"Gimmee some specid . . . specid . . . specidics."

They were both loaded, talking through ether. Wobbly of stance and glance, they stared at each other, trying to get a bead on each other. Orville had the fantasy that Schooner was about to stuff him into the safe and lock it. And then another fantasy that he and Henry were about to cha-cha.

"Besides, ole buddy, your mom never told me any of that."

"You think I'd tell her? You said you'd kill me if I ever told anyone. I'll never forget it. Never."

"'Course not, old sport. Y'never forget what you *imagine,* nopenope. But to *forgive!* There's the rub! Christian charity—hell Jewish charity, too. Judeo-Christian, it's the greatest! Our damn ticket to *Gott im Himmel,* baby! Ordnance! People change. We both believe in human betterment. We're buddies, now, am I wrong?"

"Just 'cause I'm . . . I'm . . . despert."

"Miranda's great and that kid, too, but tellya something—once you get hooked, even to a gal like Nelda Jo, you're dead. It *does* cost an arm'n a leg am I wrong?"

"No, you're not exactly wrong, Henry, but—"

"Am I wrong?"

"No, you're—"

"You're free, I'm not. Get out of this shithole town while you can. Go fuck your damn way across Italy, Sicily even, the world. Like I did in the navy. Take the cash, hop a jet, and make something bigger out of your life. Look. You got talent I don't, smarts I don't, and freedom I don't. You'll have almost a million for Chrissakes! Go live well. Hell, go out there and do some good!"

Orville was astonished at this hint of nobility from Henry. But there was a double meaning to "do some good"—it could mean public service, but as a boy in Columbia is was slang for "getting laid." His beeper went off. Ten past ten on a Saturday night. Columbians were mutilating each other and he was responsible. He turned to leave.

"Hey," Henry said, stopping him. "I never said any of this."

"Any of what?" Henry's dark eyes seemed shallow, brackish.

"Any of what I said. If it leaks, I deny. I never said what I said."

"Not even that?" Henry looked stupefied. "And you never did what you did?" Orville asked. Henry still looked stupefied. Orville left for the hospital.

◊ ◊ ◊

Later that night, at home again, he discovered another postcard, with a photo of some kind of savage—an aborigine.

Howdy, Doc,
Thanks for the cash. Trip not fun but great. Food terrible, Aussies

worse. Babs bowels bad. Wolfy and Kenni stole her ruby too. Starbusol not working too good in Outback. Headed for the Amazon and points south. Say hi to Our Little Miracle Amy.

Yr frnd, Bill

No word of his coming back, Orville thought, going up to bed. In the bathroom he stared at himself naked in the mirror and was appalled. His hair seemed thinner, his face fatter. He was wearing thick glasses because the contacts hurt his eyes. But for his sunburnt arms, head, and neck, he was a fish-belly white. Because of his lack of exercise, and his compulsive eating and drinking like a native Columbian, he was fattening. Yes, there's a definite beer belly down there, if not a paunch. This, despite his upping his smoking. Camels, like Bill.

With alarm he realized that in eleven months he had gone a significant way down the road to looking Starbuckian—somewhere in the two-ten range already and unfit.

Staring at his image he tried to conjure up a vision of himself finally free of Columbia. *Yes, make a mental picture, a life raft to get you through the next five weeks.*

Nothing came.

Even more alarmed, he realized he had no vision of the future. Just this fat guy, almost forty, in the mirror. That's all.

Shouts outside. He went to the window. The shouts were coming from the Schooners'. The porch light and the lamp in the study were still on. A fierce argument filled with curses. One voice was Henry's, the other was younger. Neither was giving in. Orville glanced at his watch. Almost two. Junior must have come home way past his curfew. He and Henry were really going at it, screaming at each other. And then, as if a knife blade had severed the rage between the fighters, there was silence.

The front door slammed shut and the lights went out. Whatever had been happening was back in the realm of never having happened once again. Schoonerland.

26

"Buon compleanno!"

"Celestina?"

"Orvillo!"

"Orvillo?"

"Celestina! *Buon compleanno e tanti auguri!* Happy birthday and best wishes!"

"Grazie," he said, trying to wake up, checking the clock. 5:10 A.M. *"Grazie,* but it's not my birthday."

"July 24 is your birthday. We celebrated it last year, remember?"

"How could I forget. I mean, the toes."

"I am fainting with the memory."

He yawned. "It's not my birthday. She lied to me, my mother. Had the birth certificate changed. I was born thirteen days later, on August the 6th. Exactly a year before they dropped the atom bomb on Hiroshima, she dropped me."

Silence.

"Don't hang up, please!"

"No, no," she said. "No. And is she still flying around?"

"More than ever. Big, fat, and floaty—like an overfed hummingbird."

"Magnifico! And you have benefited by this gift now for sure, *caro?"*

"'*Caro*'?" He was stunned.

"Si, si. You are my love. I love you crazy!"

"Well . . . um . . . what about the Swiss banker with the elephant?"

"Half the elephant. It was a tax thing. *Non sincero.* Swiss cheese." She fell silent. He heard her breathing. Somehow it was sexy. "Orvillo, I am sorry." Her voice was sad, calm. "So sorry for what I did to you."

"You hurt me terribly."

"I know. I was a fool. I did not realize what I had until I destroyed it." He heard her get choked up. Tearfully, she went on, "I hate myself for what I did."

He was touched. She seemed sincere. "You sound different."

"I am, *caro.* I am changed by my mistakes. In this year I have grown up. Jesus, what I have done?" She broke down, crying into the phone.

"Wait, hold on," he said, amazed at all this. Had she really changed?

"Can you ever forgive me?"

He hesitated. "If you're for real, maybe. *Barely* maybe."

"I am, I am, but it will take time to heal the past, no?"

Again he considered this. Finally he said, "If at all, a *lot* of time."

"*Bene.* And for now, we have only the now. There is only the present moment. Like with your dead and flying mother. Are you healing with her in the now? Is she turning out to be your greatest gift?"

"Gift? It's been hell. A horrible year. A lot of pain."

"I am so sorry for the part of the pain I caused, my love."

This is astonishing, he thought. She sounds for real. Grown-up, almost. "You really have changed."

"*Si, si.* No longer the New Age lightweight, searching for a spiritual shortcut. Now I am focused, on rock-solid Buddhism. This—your pain, our pain—this is The First Noble Truth."

"Yeah, but it hurts! What do I do?"

"Do nothing."

"Nothing?"

"As much nothing as possible, dear one. Sit in silence and follow your breath and when the pain comes? Do not lift a finger—not even the pinkie finger. Do so much nothing that the pain shifts to sorrow."

"You don't understand—I *am* in sorrow and I can't stand it."

"You are in pain. Psychological suffering. Sit there in silence, *caro,* and breathe. Sit there in the present, sit there in a ruthless encounter with the self, the past, the facts."

"And then?"

"And then the pain and suffering will turn to sorrow."

"And?"

"The sorrow moves. Sorrow always moves."

"And what happens when the sorrow moves?"

"Healing. The healing *essenza* of the movement of sorrow. You find what you have never lost."

She said this all quite matter-of-factly, as something she merely understood, without any of the flightiness he'd heard from her before. It now sounded grounded, truth lived. Almost despite himself he found himself focusing intensely on her, on it, tightening his grip on the phone, like a man going under tightens his grip on a lifeline. Whether she was still wacky or not, here was information that might help.

"But what if I can't face it," he said, "and the healing *essenza* doesn't happen?"

"I will love you no matter what."

He was startled to find that for the first time in weeks he felt calm. The sunlight streaming in through his turret window seemed both still and moving—moving faster than any other thing, moving so fast it seemed static. Light is matter, matter is energy. It was, again, a touch of her maybe magic. He thought back to her predicting the two bad things that had happened the last day they'd been together on Lake Orta and he'd gotten the telegram of his mother's death. He asked, "Where are you?"

"Roma. Like always. Your photo by my bed. I am now a banker."

"A banker!"

"Chase Manhattan, Rome office. I teach courses part-time—Yoga For Bankers. The very payment of the rent. So much has happened. I missed you so!"

"And I you," he said cautiously, trying it out, surprised at how much he meant it.

"When are you coming?" she asked.

"Who said I was coming?"

"You did. In one year and thirteen days."

"Yeah, but a lot has happened. A lot of water under the bridge. And anyway I can't leave for four weeks. I get the money on August 27th."

"*Eccolo!*"

"*Eccolo?*"

"'There it is.'"

"Wait."

"I am waiting with my very heart in my throat. Breathing in, breathing out. Speak."

He did not. He was thinking of her and the money.

"*Pronto, pronto.* I am listening," she said, "but you are not speaking."

"You assume that after all this, I'll just forget how you treated me and come to you as if nothing has happened?"

"No, no, as if everything has happened and we have learned. We are more sensible now, both of us. Ready to really love each other, sensibly, walking down the street arm in the very arm. We have our whole future together."

"I thought you said there is only the present."

"Not for lovers like us."

"I've got to think about this."

"Think?" She sighed. "Each day we think maybe 60,000 thoughts. Maybe 59,995 are about what happened in the past or what will happen in the future. Memory or imagination. We fear being in the now. Now, *caro,* come!"

Orville was silent.

"You have someone else?" she asked.

"I had, but no, not now."

"And I do not either. Come. I expect you on the 27th. We will holiday again on Lago del Orta."

"I don't know what to say."

"No, but I can feel your heart saying *si, si*. Wait, I am thinking."

Orville thought to say, But what did you just say about thinking?

"*Si,*" she went on, "I am getting it. We must not talk again until we see each other face-to-face and quickly then toe-to-toe. I will not call you again. Send a telegram with the details."

"But you *have* to . . . we have to work this out!"

"Too much thinking, *caro*, thinking and talking. No more phone calls."

"I'll call you."

"I am screening the calls and not answering you though my heart is breaking at your very voice. No more talk. Telegram me your flight number. Until the 27th in Roma!"

"The plane won't get into Da Vinci until the morning of the 28th."

"Until then, *mio grandioso amore*. I will never leave you again. *Ciao!*"

"Wait!"

Click.

Weird, Orville thought, several times throughout the day as he prodded and patched and cut and sewed and listened to and berated and held back his contempt for and tried to reach out to the sick and wounded Columbians or at least act human toward them. Deliciously weird. As abnormal as the Buddha, as Jesus. She *did* seem different. More sensible, yes. Wanting me. Italy. How can I refuse her? How can I trust her? But Italy! I was happy with her in Italy! Maybe it was good that she never came here. Hard to imagine her and me happy, here.

Like booze and cigarettes and Fritos and golf, this contact with Celestina Polo eased his pain for a while. Now he had an option. He still felt like a total failure as a son, a lover, a stand-in father, an uncle, a brother, a brother-in-law, a bird keeper, a friend, and a Columbian, but now these failures were playing out on a backdrop of the affliction of possibility, once again in Europe.

You know something, Mom, he thought, you're right. I'm wrong and sick and abnormal. So abnormal I can't even make it in Columbia, not to mention America. The hell with it. I'm history. The only thing I'm fit for in this world is to love a strange maybe enlightened Italian Boddhisatva who at least can intertwine her toes with prehensile diligence, and who, at best, is made up wholly of non-Columbian elements.

◊ ◊ ◊

Penny was the only person except Miranda to know the truth about July 24th not being Orville's real birthday. She had told no one. She had suggested that it would be "cleaner," especially with his leaving so soon, to just go ahead and celebrate the day that everyone thought his birthday was.

She organized a dinner party for that night, with Milt and Amy and Henry and Nelda Jo. Amy had come in from her all-girls' overnight camp out at Copake Lake for his birthday. To him, she seemed down. She'd taken Miranda and Cray's leaving hard, and was at loose ends at camp, not wanting to turn into a "girly-girl" and "act silly for boys." Penny and Milt again had sent her to him for advice, which he, like Starbuck, hadn't given, but rather had taken her on a few house calls whenever she could get away. She was losing altitude. Something else was on her mind. He needed to talk with her alone.

The birthday dinner was at an Italian place, Rosie Ahern's Restaurant and Taxidermy. A fixture in town ever since Orville could recall, it was now owned by his childhood friend Marco Tarantelli. Marco also ran the Sports Apparel Shop next door. The shop had had the same pair of shorts, shirt, sneakers, and tennis racket in the window for about fifteen years. Not everyone knew what the shop sold, but everyone knew that the one thing it did not sell was sports apparel. Rumors of slots machines, prostitution, drugs, and loan sharking were rife.

Since the New Yorkers had come, the restaurant—with its camp taxidermy—had become one of the "in" places to see and be seen. Here the antiquers could safely mix with the real Columbians. Ahern's signature take-out pizza had been written up in an antique journal not so much for its content as for its delivery: on the back of a Vespa, strapped with bungee cords over the motor so that it arrived piping hot even on the coldest nights. With a distinct bouquet of *benzina.*

At six that night the birthday party sat at the primo table in the front window, sometimes staring up at the stuffed fox and moose and mink with their frightened eyes, sometimes staring at the New Yorkers, who were loud and current and having a frantic, hilarious time, and sometimes staring out across the intersection of Fourth and Washington at the old jail building that was now home to *The Columbia Crier.*

The narcotic of hope and denial from his conversation with Celestina had worn off. He was again down in the dumps. Orville had spent the day before with a young doctor who had answered an ad for the sale of Bill's practice, to take effect when Orville left town. This was the fifth doctor who'd come through in the last two months looking to settle in Columbia. His name was Patrick O'Lima and he was from Dublin. Trinity, not UCD. When he'd opened the IN door, Orville was surprised to find a man with ebony skin. It turned out that O'Lima had been born Olima, a Nigerian who adopted the apostrophe to make it in Ireland. O'Lima spent the day with Orville, looked around Columbia, and, saying "Are you *serious?*" strolled on out the OUT.

They were finishing their birthday cake, and Schooner was ending his short but heartfelt tribute to Selma Rose. "My only wish is that she could have been here, sitting right here under the mink like she did a lot, to see this great moment for her favorite son." Orville heard this as not just saccharine bullshit but as a put-down, for he had come to see that Schooner, not he, was in a lot of ways his mother's favorite son.

But there was something about the way Henry spoke—the Voice again—that made it sound not only sincere but profound. By the time he finished, there was an expectant hush in Ahern's. The tableful of antiquers were listening in rapt attention, as were the dazed Columbian barflies. When Henry stopped and raised his glass for a toast, so did they all.

Milt chimed in, breaking the hush. "It's been great to have you here—sort of great, mostly great—maybe you'll take one whiff of Europe and come back to smell the roses of Columbia. You're always welcome because we love you. And love what you've brought to this town—medicine, a great personality, and hey, even though it's Penny and my and Amy's loss, we admire you for sticking it out the year and thirteen days to get the money. Shows guts, shows fortitude, shows fiscal responsibility. To my favorite brother-in-law, a helluva guy, *L'chaiyim!*" They raised their glasses again and drank.

During dinner Orville had felt out of it, down in the dumps, walking along the edges of the current of conversation. First it had been an inane mix of talk of new machines. Henry had bought a new Harley-Davidson. Milt had come back from Seattle with a new computer so compact that it fit into a small suitcase and ran on something called MS-DOS, which he claimed was going to make a mint. Penny had bought a new golf cart, Nelda Jo a new Stairmaster. They then talked about movies and TV shows. And then the Schooner campaign and then their children, notably Maxie, who was flowering at his Soccer and Firearms Camp out at the Federation of Polish Sportsmen.

He drank another beer, feeling the buzz. He found himself staring out the front window of Ahern's at the slight dip in Washington as it crossed Fourth, and he was hit by that hard fist of grief. Miranda Braak. She had told him that when the town was created, there had been a deep gully at Fourth Street and that the Quakers, in marching their utopia from the port at Parade Hill up to Cemetery Hill, had built a massive stone bridge to cross the gully. It had been a marvelous construction, a long stone arch in the Roman style, and had become something of a wonder of the time. Later they'd buried the stone bridge under tons of fill.

Eerie, he thought now, to realize that a bridge lies there, buried. Looking at it now, the intersection seemed less solid, for its secret. Settling had revealed something else there, a significant depression. If the fill shifts, will the bridge hold? Orville stared at the dip as if it were a patch of skin over a torso, secreting away the bones of a corpse below. Miranda understood history with a wordless, nameless sense of the town through time, much like a virtuoso in music or math or chess senses their art. Through her, the town for a time made sense. Even the century made sense, through her.

I miss them so much! Where are they?

But he was being roughly hoisted up out of his seat by Nelda Jo and Henry and ushered on out the door. The party was over.

It was still early in the summer evening. The light had that glossy luminescence of late July and reminded him of being in the red rowboat out on the lake with Celestina, looking back through the haze to the *Sacre Monte* with its twenty chapels and the pilgrims moving, stopping to pray, moving again, as they made their way up.

He was off duty and had nothing to do. Facing an evening alone in the house, he felt a blast of desolation. "Henry, can I ask you a favor?"

It was a rare moment—Henry seemed caught off guard. Orville had never done this before. Before, it was always Henry asking. But Henry's response was quick and tight, "Thought you'd never ask, old buddy. Anything."

"Could I take your Harley out for a birthday ride with Amy?"

"Amy on a *motorcycle?*" Penny said. "Over my dead body." What she was really saying, Orville knew, was that motorcycles were for the *goyim.*

"Can I, Uncle O.?"

"Up to Henry."

"Ever been on one, Doc?" Henry asked, revealing a certain and unusual caution.

"Owned a BMW during my year in Holland."

"Nice bikes, those. Here's the key, and here's the helmet."

"Only one?" Penny asked. "It's illegal." Amy was putting on the helmet.

"Maybe, Pen, but hey—if I go down, you get the money, the house, and the Chrysler." He pecked Penny on the cheek, shook hands with Milt, and was about to clasp hands with Henry but was engulfed in Henry's warm hug. Nelda Jo hugged him too, the aerobic push of her breasts against his chest firing up his engines as always.

"When will you be back?" Penny asked.

"September." Orville got on the gleaming bike, showing Amy how to put her arms around his waist and hold tight. Her hands felt great, there.

"What a wit, eh?" Henry said, shaking his head as if in amazement.

"Let's make sure to get together again sometime soon," Milt said.

"I can't, Milt," Orville replied. "I'm busy that day."

"What?"

He started the bike, revved it. *"Ciao!"*

"Hey, old sport," Henry called, over the roar. "We're goin' to a prayer vigil at the AME Zion Church tonight, for that poor kid shot last night, then we're at a campaign appearance out at Spook Rock, so just leave the key on the kitchen table. Door's open."

"Deal."

They roared off, Amy hanging on tight and screeching with delight.

They idled down Washington to Third and turned left and hit the last light and then accelerated down the hill into the Great South Swamp, the pink foam noodles of Styrocusp Corp. whirling in their wake like confetti. Riding the sticky asphalt through the high cattails and the infestation of imported purple loosestrife, feeling the flecks of bugs on his unhelmetted face, Orville recalled getting off the broken-down train and walking the tracks through the swamp up into town. Hard upon this memory was Miranda's showing Amy and Cray and him the Henry Ary painting of the pre-railroad South Swamp, when it was still a marvelous bay, a deepwater port filled with so many whaling ships that you could walk deck to deck all the way across the bay from Mount Pecora into Columbia.

They went left at the entrance to the Rip Van Winkle Bridge and down 9-G before turning left into the curly road rising up a hill through the woods toward Olana. Orville stopped the bike and parked in the lot. A tour bus was disgorging a procession of blue-haired ladies from Wappingers Falls for the last tour of the house that day.

Amy took off her helmet. Flushed, she yelled, "Fantastic! What is this?"

"Olana. Home of Frederick Church."

"Who?"

"A truly great Columbian. Come on."

A great Persian-tiled turret rose before them. The Moorish doorway and the three stories of echoing windows and flirtatious balconies were a shock of color and shape in the lowering sun. This, he thought, was my first sight from the train. Ages ago.

They signed the guest book and joined the tour. The guide quoted an entry from Church's diary: "I think it better to reside on a mountain which overlooks the world than to be a mere creeping thing trying to see it as a mass of details. From an eminence you take in the beauties only. About thirty miles south of Albany is the center of the world—and I own it."

The house—in Arabic, "Olana, Our Place on High"—was Church's living art, done with the care of his landscapes, which had made him the most famous American artist of the late nineteenth century. Olana was zany, a crazy mix of Italianate and Persian, made of polychrome stonework from local quarries, filled with fanciful Moorish arches framing each landscape like one of his landscapes, symmetrical mirrored chambers, purples leading to golds and golds to reds, and furnished with remarkable objects from all over the world—Arabic brass pots and English suits of armor and Chinese life-sized Ibises riding turtles and massive sideboards from Tuscany—all assiduously preserved from the 1870s.

Amid the famous landscapes of Niagara, the Hudson, the Amazon, the view through the dark cleft of rock to the amber desert light of *Ruins at Petra,* all of which held the artist's signature shafts of angel light of gold, and fluid rock, were smaller, darker, unapplauded paintings. In the sitting room were two small landscapes, *Sunrise* and *Moonrise,* each the birth of dim light over the edge of a lowland, both somber yet lit. These had been painted to get through the deaths of his oldest two children during a diptheria epidemic in 1865. On a living room wall over a grand fireplace hung two portraits: one of a stern older man, his father the Hartford industrialist; the other of a younger man with eyes raised to look away, higher and farther, with and toward imagination—his son the artist.

Orville pointed out the small stage of the living room on a platform leading to the grand staircase. The curtain was a Persian carpet hung on brass rings from a brass rail. The Church family loved putting on amateur theatricals with their guests and had a large wardrobe of costumes of silk and satin for pashas and princesses, kings and queens.

Finally, they stood before a ten-foot-high Moorish arched window of amber-colored glass laced with delicate black paper stencils cut out by Church himself, layered between the two panes of glass. The window threw a gold evening light into the room, so buttery a color they felt they could taste it. The amber reminded Orville of *Le Grand Souk* of Marrakesh. How I miss that world, he thought, the vitality, the expansion. He caught himself. But isn't that world right here, right now, with this dear, hurting girl? She and I, balanced together on an edge of pain maybe even of sorrow, keeping our balance by holding each other up and by the potential solace of this art.

"In the days of oil lamps and gas lamps," the guide was saying, "the amber window was placed there precisely with regard to the changing tilt of the planet, to provide what Church called, in his despair, 'perpetual sunlight.'"

As the tour ended, a man was waiting for them. He introduced himself as Orlando Durney, director of the Olana Historical Site. He said he had seen their names in the guest book and "Simply had to meet you." He was bald and tall and slender and kind of splendid in his enthusiasm and clear diction. He wore a lilac dress shirt and red bow tie, the tie wilting in the heat. His most striking feature was a handlebar moustache waxed so severely that Orville imagined it could poke out an eye.

"Simply had to meet you and thank you."

"For what?" Orville asked.

"For your splendid mother. Selma quite single-handedly piloted the movement to save us. The last remnants of Church's family had let the thing go and it was in rather abysmal shape. They were about to sell it as an ordinary house—imagine! Selma took charge and called me. Together we held bake sales and harassed our fascist congressman. She was tenacious, staying with it during some quite high winds, if not tornados. Yes, yes, we stayed with it together and resurrected it, as almost a postmodern passion play. And now it is a National Historic Site, a treasure for the ages." He sighed, a happy man. "She was a force, a powerful lady. What she set her sights on, she got. One wouldn't dare disagree with her, would one?"

"It's tough to, yes."

"Yes, she was a force of nature. Ironically, she was much like what Church painted. Sorry, but if you'll permit me, your mum was quite the 'Niagara', and . . ." he took out a hankie and blew a surge of emotion from his reddened nose into it, "she not only supported me, she accepted me. When no others did."

Orville could almost see him in a Selma letter: "Nice, but *queer.*"

"You must be very proud," Durney said.

"I must be. Thanks."

Durney stared at him intently and then smiled. "Church was *such* an oddball! The man didn't fit in anywhere, really, except here in Columbia. Here, a lot of oddballs have, and do." He winked—he actually winked! "See you at the unveiling next week. Bye-bye now."

She's everywhere! Orville thought, walking toward the door. He remembered Penny saying something about setting a date for the "unveiling"— the Jewish ceremony to unveil the tombstone on the first anniversary of the death. Gotta ask her when it is.

They walked out the Moorish arch into the soft sunlight. The door squeaked close behind them. The bus had eaten the blue-haired ladies, and was grinding down the hairpin slope toward the lowlands and home. Unwilling to leave just yet, Orville led Amy around the corner of the house.

The sudden panorama stunned them. To their right, to the north, the high waves of the ridgeline of the Catskills against the reddening sunset flowed down from Albany. Shading their eyes they could see, far below, sparkling in the sunlight like a silver nail laid across a glittery ribbon of river, the Rip Van Winkle Bridge. To the south, down past the friendly neon of Mike's Pizza and on toward Red Hook, the Hudson ballooned out, a small inland sea, mimicking several of the paintings they'd just viewed. Turning east, they saw a heart-shaped reflecting pond that Church had designed to balance the shape of the ballooned-out river, the apex of the pond's ventricle leading the eye down through an arbor of a hundred or so of the 40,000 trees he had planted, and then their eyes traveled further east, hopping over the spewing smokestacks of the Universal Atlas Cement to the easy green vista slurred in the fading and damp light of the Taconic Hills and the Berkshires. Breathtaking.

"Holy moley!" Orville said.

"Cool! C'mon!" Amy took off across the lawn, running and then tripping and rolling and lying on her back. Orville strolled over. He took out a Camel, lit it, and lay down on his back beside her.

"You shouldn't smoke."

"Thanks for sharing."

"Can I have one?"

He gave her a look. They put their hands behind their heads. They looked up at the clouds passing across. They said "Mmmm" responsively, in delight.

"You're really leaving?" Amy asked. He nodded. "Can I go with you?"

"What?"

"I need a break from here. When my best friend Eliza moved to New Mexico it was bad enough—without her, I don't know if I can *stand* the boys in my class next year! And since Miranda left, it sucks—I worry about her and Cray a lot!" She leaned up on one elbow, looking intently into his face. "I wanna go with you. You can convince Mom, I know you can, please?"

"I don't even know what I'll be doing yet."

"I'll tell you what we'll do. We'll start in Rome with Celestina. But at first we won't live with her, no. We'll get a nice little apartment near the Spanish Steps—no, wait—on the Piazza Navone, my favorite, favorite place!"

"How do you know so much about Rome?"

"Milt and Mom and I did Rome when I was little. So, then, we're living there, and I'll take Italian lessons and you'll work at a free clinic and at night we'll have dinner really, really late and then maybe—hey, yeah—we'll put on little plays at the Piazza Navone for the tourists!"

He stared at her and laughed.

"I mean it!"

"I know."

"Take me seriously, will you?"

"I will. I am. Sounds great, but I'm not sure it's right for you, Ame."

"But I'm like dying here!"

He saw in her eyes that she, like he, in fact was. "Okay, I'll—"

"Yes!" she said, raising her fist in triumph.

"Wait! I'll ask Penny. But she'll say no, and I can't kidnap you. It's illegal."

"Shit," she said, lying down on her back. "Okay, but can I at least come visit you?"

"Sure. Every vacation."

"And can I stay with you at Grandma Selma's 'til you leave?"

"What about camp?"

"I hate it."

"What about 'Finding Your Voice Without Boys'?"

"The boys come over all the time from the other side of the lake. It's a joke."

"Why are they on the other side of the lake?"

"They go to an all-boys' camp run by the same jerky people, a 'Finding Your Warrior Camp' or some garbage. Can I stay with you?"

"I work all the time."

"Yeah . . . Hey, I got an idea! I'll work in your office—I'll be your receptionist. You don't have one, right?" He said right. "And we'll live in your house and it'll be fun!"

"Yes, it would. Okay. Maybe Penny'll agree to that."

"First ask her if I can leave with you, and when she says no, ask her the other."

"You know, for a kid, you're pretty smart." She beamed. "I'll do my best."

They lay there for a few moments in silence, watching the sky.

"Why're you going?" Amy asked.

"Except for you, there's nothing to keep me here anymore."

"Since Miranda left?"

"And Cray."

"You guys were really, really in love, right?"

"All three of us, yep."

"So what happened?"

Without thinking he said, "Our handicaps didn't match."

"Whoa! That's heavy."

"Yeah. Broke my heart."

"Have you heard anything from them?"

"Nothing."

She laid her head on his chest. They watched the clouds, sailing across like ghosts.

"So you're leaving because of her?"

"Her, yeah, but there's more, Amy."

"Yeah?"

"Yeah. It's about a vision. One day when I was six, I lay on my back like this, alone out in a field, and looked up and saw the clouds like that and I had a vision."

"Cool. What vision?"

"That the world wasn't just about what you see and hear and feel and all of that, but that there was something else."

"What?"

"I don't know what, but the words I heard were, 'something else.'"

"Like God?"

"Maybe. Something else that was whole, of which I was just a part. If I were to try to name it now, I'd say something 'Divine.'"

"Far out."

"Maybe not. I was so excited by this vision, I jumped up and ran home

246

to tell my mother. And I told her and she said, 'Sorry, Orville, but there's nothing else but this.'"

"Selma?"

"Uh-huh."

"Bummer."

"So, anyway, I've been trying to hold onto that vision all my life, Ame, and when I was away, working for Doctors Without Borders and running around the world and falling in love with Celestina in Italy—almost exactly a year ago now—I could hold onto it a little bit. And I felt, I don't know, like I was *worth* something, you know? Because I was part of something else."

"I felt that when I was young, too, yeah."

Orville smiled. "But what I've found, being back here, is that it's really hard to keep holding onto that vision. If I stay here much longer, it'll die. And a long time ago I decided that before I would let *it* die, *I* would die."

They were silent again, and peaceful.

"Do you think, Uncle O., that Grandma Selma's vision died?"

He was taken aback. Not only at the question but at Amy's love—no, not the love, the empathy. Amy's ability to flip over into Selma's world, see Selma's lost dreams, the flip that he simply could not make, even after everything.

"Know what, Ame?"

"Yeah?"

"You're a miracle. Let's roll."

"But you didn't answer me."

"Kid, you picked that right up, didn't you? My answer is I'll do everything I can to convince Penny to let you quit camp and move in with me and be my receptionist. And with Selma's money, when I leave I'll be able to bring you over to Europe anytime, even for a weekend if you need me. Deal?"

"Deal."

"Cool?"

"Way."

"Let's go!"

Orville dropped off Amy at home and idled the bike through the twilight back down to the Schooners. He parked it and walked up onto the porch under the gold-painted ceiling and then on in through the unlocked front door.

"Hello? Anybody home?" He knew Henry and Nelda Jo weren't, but maybe the kids were. No answer. He left the key on the kitchen table and headed back out.

For some reason he paused in the den, poured himself a bourbon and a beer chaser, and lit a Monte Cristo cigar. He flumphed himself down into Henry's big leather chair facing the wobbly breakfront and the big blank TV. He had dropped in.

He thought, So this is what it's like to be Schooner? Yeah, must be. But what is it, to be Schoonerish?

He sat, looking blankly out for a long while. Finally he said to himself that maybe what it is, after all is said and done, is to be blank. That's it, that's all, just kinda blank. Waiting for Godot or Nelda Jo—whatever.

The blankness was so vivid he soon dozed off, to be awakened minutes later by the ringing phone, ringing and ringing until the answering machine cut in.

"Hi, Eagle, Sancho here."

Orville recognized the voice of Milton Plotkin, brother-in-law.

"All systems go for the demo tomorrow at oh-six-hundred."

The machine clicked off.

For a second Orville was astonished, mesmerized with disbelief. They wouldn't . . .

And then he believed. They were going to blow up the Worth Hotel.

He was furious, enraged at having been duped. He pictured, again, Henry standing before the angry crowd at the public hearing just a few months ago, calming, reassuring, proposing a stay of execution for the grand old hotel until the end of the year, asking that as a community they not do anything rash or in haste, that they all give the Worth Saving folks a decent chance to raise the necessary "monies."

A lie, all a total lie. As soon as the chance had presented itself to them—Miranda gone, Mrs. Tarr deep in mourning over the death of her cat and the disappearance of her friend, and Orville giving up—they arranged to destroy it.

It all rushed in on him—his first sight of the forlorn three-person picket line that first evening he'd walked into town, his meeting Miranda at the schoolhouse with their sweet good-bye of "Worth Saving, yes!", Amy and him joining the cause, the town meeting. Now, gone. All the air went out of him, in one long breath out. He sank, deflated, into the worn leather. His anger turned to defeat. First we lose each other, and now we lose this too.

He felt powerless, sad, thinking of Miranda, knowing what saving the hotel had meant to her. He stared around the Schooner den, at the perfectly decorated walls, at the massive breakfront, the impenetrable TV. He felt the silent desolation of this beautiful old house that had seen an awful lot of ugliness.

Chance, followed back far enough, is fate. Miranda had told him that once, talking about history, her green eyes alight with mischief. *Chance.*

All at once things shifted. He felt a glimmer of hope, a flutter of relief. Rising up out of the clutches of the soft leather, he faced the glass of the breakfront.

"Okay, you assholes. Now it's my turn. Thanks for the chance. I'm gonna make my move!"

27

The dewy red air of dawn. Silence. Orville lit another Camel and sat back in his rocker, staring across Washington Street at the Painted Lady Lounge. For the past few hours, things had been quiet. As town doctor, he'd come to know some measure of truth of the Columbians, maybe even of Columbia itself. He could sense all around him the dream town, the town the Columbians collectively were dreaming. This, he thought, is the only utopia. Timeless, placeless, tethered lightly by the gossamers of REM sleep to the historical place. He imagined most of the dreams—compared to what the dreamer would awaken to—to be sweet. He imagined that the dreaming Columbians were attending civic functions and having things work perfectly, and that they were fit and thin and sober and nonsmokers and well-off and kind and had no need to go to a doctor. These utopian dreams were a bountiful history of good things to come.

Sound. According to Celestina, quoting the *Vedantas,* sound came before anything else in the creation of the world. Sound came first now, in the creation of the day. A car coughing alive, racheting into gear, moving downhill into the South Swamp toward a job while a tanker tooted past the rotting lighthouse in the river alongside the same Middle Ground Flats of the idiotic horse-ferry-to-nowhere fame, two hundred years ago. An alarm clock, a radio, a tune, an argument, a light in a window across the way and a silhouette of a sleepy, stoop-shouldered Columbian.

Orville saw first light on the gold ball atop the flagpole to his left at Parade Hill, reflecting the rays of the sun pulling itself up out of the covers of Masschusetts and walking over the brow of Cemetery Hill.

B-dangg! Bang!

The explosion of heavy machinery starting up, down on North Second. Coming closer. Massive metal. Diesel-powered massive gears, shifting first to second, second to third, groaning along heavily up Washington in the gauzy light. From his days as a toll collector on the Rip Van Winkle, Orville recognized the sound. A heavy flatbed trailer hauling something heavier. Coming closer.

And then there it was, moving in from his left like a wall, the float carrying a big crane with a black wrecking ball tucked under its lowered arm like an elephant tucking a black fruit into its mouth. It stopped directly in front of him. Scomparza Demolition and Upholstery.

"What the fuck?" A man followed these words out of the cab of the flatbed. Orville recognized him as a patient of his, Jeffrey Liebowski, of Ukrainian descent, deep descent. Bill had gotten his little boy to stop pooping in Jeffrey's motorcycle helmet.

"Holy shit!" This voice belonged to Officer Packy Scomparza. "Hey, Doc, whatchu doin' here?"

A flash of light, and another, and another. Packy and Jeffrey turned toward Toby oop den Dyke, who, with one of those sophisticated news cameras, was snapping away, capturing the moment for the afternoon edition of *The Crier.*

"Aw shit, man," Jeffrey said. "Shit."

"Fuckin' A, Orvy," said Packy, "didya *have* to?"

Toby snapped a few more photos. "Thanks for the tip, Orvy," he said. With a cheery wave, whistling "Some Enchanted Evening," he left.

"So what the hell you think you're doon?" Packy asked.

"Meditating."

"In chains?"

"Jesus was, wasn't he?"

Packy thought about this. "No joke."

"What're *you* doing here?" Orville asked.

"Detail. Traffic detail for the demo."

A truck with a few other workers stopped by. A car stopped, then another. A small crowd started to blossom. People stared.

"Hey, Jeffrey," Orville said. "Who told you to demo this?"

"We got orders."

"From who?"

"Look, man," Jeffrey said, "we got orders not to tell who we got orders from, okay? And if we don't demo this baby right now our ass is grassed, you get me?"

"I do, and too bad."

"Yeah, man," Jeffrey said, "and who told *you* about this, man?"

"Milt."

Looks of astonishment from both of them.

"*Milt?*" said Liebowski in surprise. "Fuckin' A!"

"Wait, wait," Packy said. "Wait. Milt *who?*"

"Milt Plotkin, my brother-in-law."

The workers looked at each other.

Liebowski said, "Holy shit."

"You can say that again," said Packy.

"Holy shit."

"Unbelievable, y'get me?" Packy turned back to Orville. "I mean, chains?"

Chains they were, and Orville was locked into them. The biggest chains and most impenetrable padlock he could find. He had taken his grandmother's rocker from the house and popped it into the trunk of the Chrysler and at three in the morning had driven down to the General Worth Hotel.

Chaining himself to the columns of the portico had been difficult and dangerous. The front portico of the hotel, the columns, and the roof, were a honeycomb of decay. He had checked out other parts of the building, but all were rotted. A hard shot anywhere, and it could all come down. He'd fed the heavy links of the chain around the two Doric columns of the rickety portico—it sagging like the bad side of his mother's face—in through one smashed window beside the rotting door and out through the other smashed window, and then around himself and the rocker a couple of times. The padlock arm slithered into its socket and snapped to with a steely, conclusive *clrokk!*

He sat there, dressed in his suit and wearing the tie Cray had given him, elephants grazing on a silk veldt. Orville had spent the dark hours rocking, chained to what the sign now said was the GENE   HOT   . As if the dear old hotel had become a Columbian biotech company. Rocking in the dark, waiting. Given Selma's fashion show triumphs at the hotel when she was still beautiful, he half-expected to see her floating or flying. From time to time he scanned the sky, half-hoping. But no.

"Okay, Doc," Packy was saying now, "youse made your point, okay, so now unlock yourself and go home."

"Not until my demands are met."

"Demands, man?" cried Liebowski.

"Damnit I just *knew* you was gonna say that," said Packy.

"Dee-fuckin'-*mands?*"

"What do you think this is," Packy said, "one of them flower-power protests against 'Nam? They're over, Orvy. The war's over, okay?"

"Maybe not. This is an emergency. Get the mayor."

Packy looked at Jeffrey, Jeffrey at Packy. Their level of discomfort rose.

"Look, Doc," Packy said, "we only get the mayor in an emergency."

"I *know* that," Orville said, "and *that's* why I said to get the mayor. This *is* one."

They thought about this, whispered about this. The bystanders were more numerous now, a real crowd. Someone shouted out, "Save the Worth, yeah!" and another shouted, "Go for it, Doc!"

"Okay, Orvy," Packy said. "We decided."

"Good. I like decisiveness."

"We decided we'll go ahead and like, you know, wreck *around* you, okay?"

"What?" Orville cried, terrified suddenly of what these dopes could do. A shock anywhere could bring the portico down on him. The end. Dead. Here? Like this?

"Jeffrey says he can like just wreck around you a *little,* right, Jeffrey?"

"Yeah, man, I can just wreck a little, yeah. Like you say to your patients, you won't feel a thing." He paused. "Man."

"So just relax, Doc," Packy said. "We'll start over there where the ballroom used to be, remember?"

"No!" he said, thinking *breakage!* "No, you can't do that."

"Why not?"

"You'll kill me. This front part will come down on me."

"No, it won't," said Liebowski. "You don't get me. We're just gonna wreck a *little,* man, a *little* little, the side part, over there."

"The ballroom," said Packy.

"But it's all connected."

"Which is why I'll be extra-careful. No problem. I'll wreck over there."

"Wreck?" Orville asked. "You're not even *in* the wrecking part, Liebowski, are you? You told me in the office that you were in the upholstery division."

"I can see where you might question my competence, man," Liebowski said. "But I assure you, you pick up a lot here and there. The problem is, the real wrecker's in Vegas this week."

"No problem, Doc," Packy said, "you just sit there and relax."

"Yeah, keep meditatin', Doc," Jeffrey said, laughing. "Think like nice peaceful thoughts!" He roared with laughter, shaking his head in disbelief as he went back to the wrecking crane and got into the cab and powered it up. His helpers put down the steel ramps to unload it from the flatbed. As the ramps slid out and clanked down on the pavement, the crane sat there idling, an unruly wooly mammoth, well-rested and ready, warming up.

"You touch this hotel," Orville called out, "my lawyer'll sue for all you're worth!"

At the word "lawyer," everybody froze. Packy went over to Jeffrey in the cab of the crane. He shouted up at him, and Jeffrey shouted down. Orville couldn't hear over the muttering of the crane's diesel engine. Then Packy got out his walkie-talkie and clicked it on and put it to his ear and talked a little and then he screamed in pain and pulled it back away from his ear and clicked it off and sat down on the edge of the flatbed and lit a cigarette. The diesel wrecking crane, perched on the start of the downslope of the two ramps, kept idling—*ka ba doommmm, ka ba doommmm, ka ba doommmm.* To Orville the sound was a comfort, a throaty, oiled steel mantra on internal combustion.

Nothing happened, except the crowd grew bigger. They were mostly passive, but a New Yorker put a flower in front of Orville. Then other people went to get flowers and put them in front of Orville, too.

By the time the diminuitive mayor's big pink Cadillac El Dorado rolled up, stopped, rocked a little on its shocks, and disgorged Americo, the crowd, by Columbian standards, was huge. Some were chanting "Worth Saving!" and some were chanting "Worth Wrecking!" Americo was up for reelection, and it was the first time anybody had seen his new compaign slogan, on the Caddy's bumper stickers:

PUT A LITTLE ITALIAN IN YOUR LIFE
A. SCOMPARZA FOR MAYOR

Americo headed straight for Orville, looking as if he would kill him and eat him. "What the hell do you think you're doing?"

But then a bright light went on, and Orville and Americo turned toward it. A TV crew had just arrived and were about to capture on videotape whatever happened next to broadcast on the morning news and the noon news and the evening news and the late news and, if it were salacious enough, even on the national networks and in print—*Time, Newsweek,* and *People.* Maybe even into the two opinion leaders, *The National Enquirer* and *The New Yorker.*

Caught in the spotlight, Americo shifted direction. He gathered himself, and walked deliberately toward the portico where Orville and his cousin Packy were. To the TV camera Americo said, "As mayor of this fine town, I am outraged. Outraged!"

He turned to face Orville and Packy, maintaining his good angle to the camera.

"Yes, I am outraged by this!"

His eyes went from Packy to Orville, Orville to Packy. It wasn't clear which "this" of the two of them he meant.

"Outraged at *you,* Officer Scomparza, to think that a public employee would aid and abet the demolition of this sacred old historical landmark hotel. Outraged that someone—some disgruntled citizen of our town—would even *think* to knock down this fine hotel. And though I disagree with your action, Dr. Rose, I fought in a war to protect your right to act like an—like a patriot. Free speech. I'm ashamed, Officer Scomparza and Mr. Liebowski, ashamed that you'd even of thought of knockin' off this fine old historical hotel." He considered, and, seeming to realize he had been too wordy for the TV camera, moved closer to it and said, "Freedom is due process for all Columbians!"

The TV light went out. The crew started packing up.

Americo turned to Packy and Jeffrey and shouted, "Why are you doin' this?"

"We was just followin' orders, Mr. Mayor," said Packy.

"And who gave you your orders, Officer?"

A pause. "Am I under oath?"

"Not unless you wanna be."

"Nope. Okay." He considered, brow furrowed in thought. "I forget who."

Americo shook his head and spat on the pavement. He looked up into the cab of the crane and shouted. "Liebowski?"

"Yer 'oner?"

"Come here. On the double!"

Jeffrey did so. He and the mayor and Packy conferred. The shouts of the crowd rose, but the officials ignored them until the shouts turned to screams as the wrecking crane without Liebowski in it began to move down the two steel ramps toward the street and the vehicles parked there, including the TV crew's minivan and the mayor's pink Cadillac.

People scattered. It looked for a second as if the wobbly crane would topple over off the ramps toward the Worth and demolish it, and Orville thought he would die, but then it tilted back the other way toward a meticulously restored eighteenth-century whaling house with a widow's walk, the bottom floor of which was now the high-end store called Misery Antiques.

In a fit of bravery, Liebowski leapt onto the flatbed, mounted the crane like a cowboy a runaway horse, and managed to keep it on the ramps until, going too fast, it hit the street with a terrible *mmMRONKCH!* which shook the old hotel ominously and set the columns creaking over Orville's head, the dust raining down so thickly he feared the whole thing would collapse and that in fact he would end up dying there and then.

It didn't, but the impact with Washington popped a manhole cover and busted a pipe, which sent a geyser of suspiciously brown water up, and then down, spreading messily across and down the street. All cleared out except Packy, Americo, and Orville.

The TV cameras gone, Americo said, "Unreal. So what the fuck you want, Orvy?"

"That you keep the agreement we made at the hearing, where you don't knock the hotel down for six months—and that you add another six months to it because of this."

"Done."

"And that you yourself sign a note to guarantee that personally."

"*Personally?* You want me to assume that kind of liability?"

"Yes."

"Go fuck yourself."

"Kinda hard to do, chained up like this. I'm staying. Staying right here." He looked around happily. "It's nice here."

"Tell you what I'm gonna do. I'll guarantee it *politically*, okay?"

"What does that mean?" Orville asked.

"Executive privilege. We'll get the town lawyer to draft it, okay? Len Date?"

"Isn't he still suspended? Awaiting trial for what he did with that little—"

"No, no, the little boy's parents are settlin' with 'im. For a bundle he'll beat it."

255

"Looks bad for Columbia, though, if he stays on, doesn't it?"

"What *doesn't* look bad for this place these days! I can't argue with you there, but he's blackmailin' us to the tune that he'll sue for some kind of bullshit federal workplace discrimination bullshit if we fire him. He's one sick fuck, ya get me?"

"Okay, as long as I get my own lawyer in on it too. Happy Thorne."

"Whoa!" Americo waved his hand up and down in front of his belly, palm up, in a gesture of admiration. "Them WASP lawyers out in Spook Rock are balls-out!"

"That's why I got him."

"Okay. So c'mon. Unlock yourself now, okay?"

"Don't have a key."

"He doesn't have a key?" Americo asked Packy. "Did you know this all along?"

"We didn't get that far."

"He doesn't have a fuckin' key. So what—we're supposed to find a blow torch?"

"But I know where you can *get* a key," Orville said.

"Where's at?"

"First we sign the document. *Then* we get the key."

"What the hell, Orvy—you've known me all your life—don't you trust me?"

"Americo, I've known you all my life—of course I don't."

"Aw c'mon, don't be a fuckin' hardass. Think of the town, your town, my town, our town—this is an embarrassment, okay?"

"Then you better hurry up. I'm happy. You can be happy too. I'll wait."

It took a while to draw up the document and sign it, but it got done.

"So where's the key, Doc?" Packy asked.

"In my office, on a table below the twelve-point buck, under the big bottle of Starbusol."

As he sat and rocked and waited, the saying that came to mind was, "Beware the weak, the strong have no defense against them."

◊ ◊ ◊

That afternoon, *The Crier* ran the photo on the front page, it taking up much of the space above the fold. Amy rushed the paper into Orville's office. He stared at the massive crane facing the frail old hotel, at Officer Packy Scomparza and Mr. Jeffrey Leibowski, wide-eyed and open-mouthed, facing the smiling Dr. Orville Rose, in a suit and tie, in a rocker,

256

in chains. One link of the spanking new steel chain was caught catching a ray of dawn sunlight and reflecting it back into the imperfect lens in a big dazzling X of light which, Orville mused, a postmodernist antiquer would falsify to the level of art. The caption read:

TOWN DOCTOR SAVES HISTORIC HOTEL
RISKS LIFE, LIMB, JAIL FOR CAUSE

All that day as he doctored Columbians as usual, fielding their more intense interest now that he was a celebrity and answering their arguments pro and con about saving the Worth, and as he worried whether he could find someone to buy the practice because he didn't want Bill to return to find it dead, a strange word kept floating through his head: *ahimsa.*

It was Ghandi's word, meaning "nonviolence." He had heard it from time to time in disparate corners of the world when he worked for *Médecins Sans Frontières.* He had a vague recollection that the word didn't really mean what everyone thought it meant, didn't really mean "nonviolence." But all day long he couldn't recall what it did mean. He'd walk along and his feet would tap the pavement *ahimsa, ahimsa.* He'd eat lunch at the Hendrick Hudson Diner and chew his French fries *ahimsa ahimsa.*

Finally, late in the day, it popped into his mind.

Last July at Lago del Orta, perhaps even to the day, Celestina Polo had told him that the Sanscrit *ahimsa* is wrongly translated into English as "nonviolence."

"The true meaning, *caro,* is 'creative love.'"

28

Howdy, Doc,
Cold and wet. Ugly place. Makes you not believe in God. Close as you can get to Antarctica. Babs wants to go there to see Emporer Penguins. Seen one penguin seen 'em all but that's married life. Both bowels blocked bad. Worse than the Army. When you leave, lock office door and throw away key.

Yr frnd, Bill

The front side of the postcard showed a desolate mountain range, all ridges and hollows and no trees, overlooking a more desolate rocky beach. In the foreground was a single, piercing, scarlet and gold wild-flower. Tierra del Fuego, the southernmost tip of South America. So far south it's always cold.

Orville read the postcard while sitting in Bill's chair. He realized that the ridges and hollows in the seat of the chair that had fit Bill's big butt beautifully now fit his own fairly well. His very own Tierra del Fuego.

It was late afternoon of August 6th, his real birthday.

Weird, he thought, for the first time in my life after forty years, to celebrate my real birthday. Some celebration. No one except Penny and Miranda and Celestina knows. Celestina and Miranda are unreachable, and Penny is enraged and no longer speaking to me. Some celebration.

In the almost two weeks since he'd chained himself to the Worth, things had gotten a bit better, and then a whole lot worse. Better because he had a brief high when he knew for sure he'd be leaving. He'd bought a ticket to Rome for August 27th and sent a telegram to Celestina with the details. Everything else was worse. No good deed goes unpunished, he'd say to himself as he walked from one disaster to another with his patients and his family.

Word had gotten out that Milt was the culprit. Totally pissed at Orville, he denied being the one—maybe with Henry Schooner—who'd ordered the demolition. *Maybe* Schooner, yes. Orville realized that while he assumed from Milt's message that Schooner was part of it, he couldn't be sure. As usual, to the naked eye everything about Schooner seemed obvious and clear, but when you looked deeper you realized that you knew nothing for sure. Henry hadn't been in town the day of the chaining and hadn't been back since.

Orville had phoned the house and got Nelda Jo. She said he was on a fund-raising trip to Washington and then on to the Deep South and the Sunbelt. "He's followin' the money—that's where the deep pockets are. My daddy has clout with the oilmen of Tulsa, and Henry's buddies in the navy all seem to have settled in around golf courses in the desert, makin' it hand over fist. He'll be back on the tenth. Honey, I think what you did was great, brave and great. If we don't save that dump, what won't we save? Makes good business sense, an opportunity cost for tourist return. How 'bout droppin' in? Or comin' over for a barbecue on Sunday?"

"Sorry, can't." He didn't inquire about the fate of the mole.

"Next time. I'll tell the Great One you called."

That very night Henry called Orville back. Out of the phone came puzzled concern.

"I'm shocked, shocked, at what Milt did," he said, "and saddened, too. What is our great little town without due process. I swear on the Bible, Orvy, that I had nothing to do with it, and thank God you stepped in and saved that dear old lady. Your mother would be proud. God Bless you."

Orville waited for "—and God Bless America," but it didn't come.

Amy was thrilled at what Orville had done, and Penny, trying to find a way into Amy's life, had praised his public-spirited action. She allowed Amy to move in with him for the few weeks until he left. Amy was helping out at the office, functioning as receptionist, scheduling appointments, and helping with the billing. This made everything in the office run a lot better, and Columbians resented it greatly. In particular, they didn't like having a set appointment time, a time when they could be seen without waiting.

"*Bill* never saw us without waiting! When's he comin' back anyways?"

Penny had good reason to be enraged. Not only had Orville provoked her husband's public humiliation, but he had missed the unveiling of their mother's tombstone

"You did it on purpose!" Penny said, eyes full of venom, when Orville arrived after everyone else had left.

"No," he said, "I swear not. I'd been up for two days straight and was finishing up another all-nighter doing a delivery way out in Red Rock and I got into the Chrysler and was going as fast as I could down 66 to get there and nodded off once, and woke up, but then the line down the middle of the road started wobbling again and I nodded off again and only woke up when I felt the car shudder off the road—I pulled out of it just in time. I was too tired to see straight, to drive. I fell asleep—it was a deep sleep and I missed everything and I'm sincerely sorry, Pen. I overslept, okay?"

"No. Your oversleeping is your unconscious hatred for your mother."

"Hey, I love my mother. Selma's a great Columbian."

"Do not mock me, okay? I mean, even after a whole year when you're supposed to be mourning her you hate her more. You should go under psychoanalysis—fast!"

"I was nodding off in the car! People die that way! You'd rather have me dead?"

"Don't tempt me but I've had it with you and when are you leaving?"

"The 27th. I get the check that day, and I'm gone."

"For sure?"

"Got my ticket."

"One way?"

"That's sweet."

"No, it isn't. Your leaving Columbia, leaving us with one less doctor, is one of those good news/bad news situations."

"Is that right?"

"Yes, but not the way you think. You think it's bad for Columbia and good for you, but I've got news for you—it's the opposite. You've done a lot of harm here this year and we'll all be better off without you."

"Thanks, Sis."

"You're welcome. The problem was that you got our expectations up—me, Amy, even, would you believe it, Milt. Over the years we'd gotten used to expecting nothing from you, so your staying for a while was more than we bargained for. But now, hell, it's clear that you were just doing it for the money. I wouldn't like to live in your head for a day, even for a million! Thank God you're going. When you're gone we'll be all set. We can all get back to normal."

Her viciousness rocked him. He still felt shaky three days later.

And so it was August 6th, his first real birthday. That morning he'd gone up to the attic of his mother's house to the Scomparza Moving and Funeral box. He found the pile of Selma's letters and took the top one off the pile. It was marked "Number 15, To Be Mailed On the Eleventh Month and First Week He Is Back." He opened it and read:

Dear son,

    Maybe writing these letters to you is having an effect on me.

    I had a strange thought today. It brought tears to my good eye.

    Maybe you weren't running from me, you were running for me.

    I can't write anymore now, dear, I'm crying too hard to see.

Til next time,

Love, Mom

Orville was surprised, touched. He remembered as a boy lying next to her on the couch, his head on her breast, his grandmother Molly sitting in her rocker, all of them watching what his grandmother always referred to as "The Ed Solomon Show"—mistakenly thinking Ed was Jewish. Lying there, feeling his mother's breathing. Soft rise, soft fall. Feeling her laugh at the jokes on the show.

He looked at the letter again, turned it over, searching for the dagger, the way that, whenever she opened him up, she would plunge the knife in.

No dagger.

He reached into the box and picked up the next letter, "Number 16, To Be Mailed on the Eleventh Month and Second Week That He Is Back." It felt light. The flap was unsealed. He looked inside. It was empty.

He looked back down into the box again, and took the next one off the pile. "Number 17, To Be Mailed On the Eleventh Month and Third Week That He Is Back." This one, too, was unsealed and empty. And so it was with all the rest of the letters. They were marked to be mailed at closer and closer intervals until the year and thirteen days was up, two a week for a couple of weeks and then one a day for the last seven days. All of them were empty. Stamped, but empty.

Sometime between Letter Number 15 and Letter Number 16 his mother had died. He flashed on her complaining in previous letters about her indigestion, brought on by exertion, and not helped by Maalox. Bill had blown the diagnosis. It wasn't indigestion, it was angina, her heart.

Orville felt light-headed, and slumped down onto the rough dusty planks of the attic floor. She's dead. This meant she really *was* dead. No more letters. She was out of touch for good. He felt sick to his stomach.

"Running *for* her?"

◊ ◊ ◊

It was a long lonely day doctoring. Longer and lonelier for it being his fortieth birthday and no one else knowing it. No "Happy Birthdays!" to carry him through the day and no one to welcome him home. That evening as he trudged through the sluggish damp night from Bill's office to Selma's house, his heart was heavy and his spirit sunken. His feet hit the warm pavement softly, sadly. At the entrance to the Courthouse Square he had a sense of being watched and raised his eyes.

There she was! Not flying, hovering only a few feet above him, at the level of a first branch of an oak. He felt a strange relief—glad to see her now that she was somehow more dead. Her head was turned away from him. She was not wearing the cobalt-blue satin gown but something white—maybe a housedress? And she had something on her head, also white—a white hat?

"Selma?"

She did not respond.

"Your indigestion? Remember your indigestion?"

Still she floated there, at the level of the oak branch, facing away, and silent.

"Bill blew it. It wasn't acid reflux, it was your heart."

Nothing.

"Mom?"

On this she turned toward him. He reeled back, in shock. Her face was hideous, one facial nerve cut by the surgeons so that half of her face was fallen, as if in sorrow, and one eye was sewn shut with black sutures, to protect the cornea because she could no longer blink. The white house-dress was a hospital gown and the white hat was a turban to wrap her head and cover the hairless flap of skin over the hole drilled in her skull. He lost his breath and stumbled back. It was how she had looked when she'd come home that morning from the hospital, when he, taking one look at this woman he'd always seen as beautiful and being totally unprepared for anything being wrong with her, anything at all, had run out of the house across the Square and down into the woods. In that first moment he hadn't stayed with her, and he hadn't stayed with her all summer.

"Mom? Are you okay?"

Instead of an answer, a look of inconsolable sadness passed over her mutilated face. She floated away.

Shaken, he groped for a park bench and sat down. Trying to catch his breath, he stared at her house. It was dark, forboding. How can I go in there?

Sounds from Schoonerland came from behind him. Rock music. Must be Junior. Was Henry back? He turned to look, thinking he might go over. But the oversized sign on the front lawn—VOTE AMERICA VOTE SCHOO-NER—was a deterrent. Breathing more easily, he took out a Parodi cigar and lit it. The sharp taste stimulated a craving for bourbon and a cold beer, which lived in the house. He got up and walked slowly, shakily, toward Selma's house, thinking, Now I've even been rejected by the dead.

The front door was unlocked. Strange. He'd been locking the door ever since a break-in last month, a "Below Fourth Streeter" looking for drugs in his doctor's bag. Had he forgotten to lock it this morning? Not like me. Is Amy home? Hayley? But there were no lights on. He went in cautiously.

"Amy?" No answer. "Hayley?" None. He tried again, louder. Nothing. A touch of fear. He shivered. Hayley always waited around if she knew he was coming home, and she knew tonight. They would talk and watch TV while he ate. A comfort. He thought he remembered Amy saying that they would all have dinner together tonight. Something was wrong. And then he realized that Starlight wasn't shrieking. The bird always shrieked when he came in. Better than a watchdog. Something was definitely wrong.

He picked up an umbrella from the stand in the hall. Scared, he tip-toed down the dark hallway to the kitchen door, raised his umbrella, and opened the door and felt something roar and come crashing down on him and saw a flash of light. As he reflexively slashed out with the umbrella, he realized that the crash was a hand slapping his back and thrusting him further into the room and that the light was from flashbulbs and the roar was Columbians shouting "Surprise! Surprise!" A banner read: "HAPPY FORTY-ETH AND FAIRWELL!"

Like a rowboat on a friendly lake, Orville floated among friends and dear nurses and hospital workers and patients and enemies. Someone took the blanket off Starlight's cage and the bird began to shriek. Going person to person and then blowing out the candles and cutting the cake, Orville was touched. As he stood between the small squat Hayley and the taller, thinner Amy, Orville, feeling appreciated, felt appreciative. At one point, looking into Hayley's eyes—noticing behind the thick glasses the gathering clouds of cataracts and thinking she should have those done, but not here, up in Albany—he said, "This is great! Thanks!"

"So, O.," Hayley said, "you finally believe people care?"

"Everybody but you, maybe."

"Gimmee a break!" she said, punching him on the arm.

"'I see,' said the blind man, and he picked up his hammer and saw." It was Hayley's favorite proverb and he'd heard it ever since he was a kid. She smiled.

Milt was thrust forward by Penny. Milton Plotkin the Patriarch held a plaque. Under duress, sweat pouring down off his forehead onto his chins, his eyes twitching as if, Orville thought, in a nascent case of Tourette's. "You and me have had our differences, Orvy, like in hotel management."

No one laughed.

"Just read the plaque, Milt," Penny said tightly.

"But, in fact," Milt went on, trying to recover, "it hasn't been all that bad having you here." This, too, went over like a lead balloon.

"Daddy, stop!" Amy said. "Just read it?"

Milt held up the plaque, one of those blue historic markers they put on buildings.

HERE LIVED THE TOWN DOCTOR

ORVILLE ABRAHAM ROSE

AUGUST 14, 1983–AUGUST 27, 1984

"Jesus, Milt," Orville said, "you make it sound like I've died."

"Maybe you have," Milt said, "and this, with me, is Heaven!" Finally, a laugh.

Henry Schooner, exuding the wholesome scent of toasted oats, rode the laughter to the front of the crowd. The marvelous public Voice made some brief remarks, ending with, "I knew Orvy as a boy, I knew his mother as a great lady when I, too, was a boy, and a great mother, and now I can say from the bottom of my heart that Orvy the boy has grown up to be Orville Abraham Rose the man—a fine man, our very own, however brief, 'Dear and Glorious Physician.' He's cared for us for richer for poorer, in sickness and in health—"

"What're you gonna do, honey," Nelda Jo called out, "marry him?"

"We can all dream, Mother," Henry replied, "can't we?"

Everybody thought this was about the funniest thing going.

"And Dr. Orville Rose," Henry went on, "has shown us something incredibly important: that despite our differences we can all work together for the good of Columbia, the good of America, and the good of the world. It's like what a friend of mine who lives in New York City told me the other day, when I asked how he could possibly stand to live there. 'It sucks,' he said, 'but we're all in it together.'" He paused. "Well, friends, we're one up on New York City, as our dear friends the New Yorkers who have come to Columbia to live and make their fortunes can attest to—in our town it doesn't suck, it *shines!*" As he said it, his face, too, seemed to shine. "Yes, friends, it shines, and it shined brighter this whole year with our dear town doctor here, the *good* doctor Rose. Yes, it shines, and we're all in it together. God bless you, Orville, and—"

Many in the crowd shouted out with him, "and God bless America!"

"And vote Schooner!" someone cried out. "Vote early and often in the Republican primary on September the 15th."

Henry smiled, and said, "Thank you. One more thing. In Orvy's name, Nelda Jo and Junior and Maxie and I are donating the use of Schooner's Spa three hours per week for disabled boys and girls of Columbia. The Orville Rose Memorial Hours will start next month. Thank you, friends, and, again, may the Good Lord bless you and keep you."

Pure *kitsch,* Orville thought, but he's right. A town this size, you have to get along. People who hate each other for a time are nice to each other for another time—like tonight with Milt, Americo, Packy, and others. One minute they're screwing you, the next they're friends with you, and there's no connection in between. What's real? What's fake? Who cares? Maybe Selma was right in her rules—so WHAT? and WHAT'S NEXT?

Looking around, he realized that over the year he'd doctored just about everybody in the room, except the Schooners and Penny and Milt. I know all their secrets, he said to himself, have kept their secrets, and when I see them out in the world I hear all their lies—and they see me hearing their lies. As Bill had said, "In this office, you lift up the lid and look at the truth." Corny as it sounds, he thought, the right word is "privilege." Yeah, it has been a kind of privilege. And the most corny thing is that they seem sad to see me go.

Penny, too, showed no sign of her prior viciousness. She handed him a present from her and Amy. A black sweatshirt, on the front of which, spelled out in glittering sequins, was:

ROME

PARIS

LONDON

COLUMBIA

Toby oop den Dyke gave him a framed blowup of the photo of Orville chained to the GENE   HOT   —which got a lot of laughs, even from Packy and Americo and Milt—and Tommy Kline and Whiz, cocaptains of the Fish Hawk basketball team, gave him an old framed black-and-white photo of the three of them holding aloft a trophy with the caption FISHHAWKS IN ROMP TO CLASS B TITLE, 1962. Johnny Holsapple, a smart classmate turned into dairy farmer, presented him with a brass cow engraved with BOTHWAYS FARM, WEST GHENT. Orlando Durney gave him a framed photo of himself and Selma in front of a dilapidated Olana, clearly before the start of Selma's campaign. Americo's two gifts to him were a key to the city and no official remarks. Mrs. Tarr, pigeon free, had done a pen-and-ink sketch of the one-room Ichabod Crane Schoolhouse where he'd first met Miranda—which tipped his heart over and sent it plunging weightlessly down into nowhere.

"Speech, Orvy, speech!"

Shyly, Orville rose to speak. Someone called out, "Look out for breakage!" People elbowed each other, laughing, but glanced around furtively, some in fact positioning themselves along the sightlines and pathways for safe exit from the house.

"When I came here a year ago," he began, "I thought it would be, well . . . a kind of hell. But now, while I can't exactly call it a kind of heaven, it's been a year filled with . . ." He stopped. *They're gone! Miranda and Cray, gone!* He stopped, unable to shake it. He tried to breath. For a few seconds he was silent. Finally, fighting tears, and with his voice trembling, he said, "with love for those who are no longer with us. Thanks."

Silence, broken by sniffles and coughs. Stillness.

Many times in his travels Orville had experienced moments like this, when a gathering of people falls silent, and then still, at about eleven at night. All over the world, he found, people would give the same explanation for the stillness: it was a sign of angels passing overhead.

Could it be? he asked himself now. Here in Columbia? In the ongoing stillness, he considered it. Maybe it could. I mean, how could you ever prove that it wasn't?

And then, like Fish Hawk hoopsters after a moment of prayer in the locker room before the big game with the dread Niskayuna, the crowd broke. Talk and laughter and shouts and cries and party tricks like picking up a chair by one leg with one hand resumed and carried the Columbians along. The group split into smaller and smaller ones and then the niggle of babysitters and the next day's work and dyspepsia and sciatica and rheumatica saw most of them take their leave.

Just after midnight, as Hayley and Amy and Orville were cleaning up the plates, glasses, and cigarette and cigar butts, the front doorbell rang. Orville went to answer it.

Miranda Braak. Before he could say anything he heard a cry and felt something hit him in the stomach, almost bringing him down, and he knew it was Cray.

"Hi, Orvy—" the boy started to say but then he was overwhelmed with joy and started bawling like a baby. Orville started to cry too. The boy wanted to hide his tears, and so Orville pulled him up into the crook of his neck, the boy's hair against his cheek, both of them crying. Orville recalled for the first time in his life how, when he was Cray's age and had been taken by Selma for a month-long trip to California to see Selma's crippled Aunt Anna and hadn't really thought of Sol at all the whole time, when the old propeller plane had touched down back at La Guardia and he had seen his father, he had felt a breakout of love and had found himself crying crazily and doing just what Cray was doing now, burying his face in his dad's neck. And then he had started talking, talking wildly about California and the paddle boats at Catalina Island and Disneyland and the tar pits and the farmer's market—and that's what Cray started doing now, only it was about North Dakota and the seas of wheat and Auntie Heyward's farm and the horses and the pigs.

The boy in his arms, he turned to Miranda across the threshold. As gently as one would brush aside a stray tear, they each took the one step to each other, he sensing that she was stepping with her good leg, she realizing how substantial he was in real life and how he'd lost matter in her memory during the months apart, and then there they were, Cray and Miranda and Orville all in each other's arms, crying like crazy.

"Happy Birthday, Doc," she said, wiping away tears. "Sorry we're late. We just drove in from North Dakota."

"Unbelievable! But why?"

She ignored the question. "We saw the photo in *The Crier.* That was great!" She was beaming. "Simply great!"

"What the hell happened to you?"

Her eyes told him it was too much to tell right then, in the whirlwind of Cray and the re-meeting. "Give me a little time."

"Orvy, listen! I learned how to milk a cow and milk a goat and drive a combine, wanna hear?"

"Totally!" Cray started to tell him, but then Amy was there and started crying and that set everybody off again.

Soon the hour caught up with the boy. Orville carried him up to Selma and Sol's big bed. Then he and Miranda unloaded essential items from the car. The Ford Country Squire looked battered and worn but triumphant for making it back from North Dakota. He carried their suitcases and the birdcage with the zebra finches. The finches sang and Starlight shrieked. For anyone to sleep, the birds had to be separated and so they were. Miranda carried in a big typing paper box containing her thesis.

All, exhausted and high, went to bed—Hayley in the guest room, Amy in Penny's old room, Miranda and Cray in Selma and Sol's, and he in his turret.

At two in the morning Orville was still awake, staring out his window onto the square. He was too wired to sleep, sensing for the first time since he'd been back that the house was *full.* It was a home to real live sleeping people with lives all the subtle colors of rainbows and all the power of diesel combines harvesting those seas of wheat, machines that were the whales of the plains. *As if a family, yes.* He could almost hear the breathing of each of them—Amy, Hayley, Miranda, Cray, the finches, Starlight who still believed it could fly but could still only fly down and always slept facing the water dish. He sensed so much life in the house, the place suddenly so full of hope, that he was sure that in this love nest there was no way that his dead mother would dare appear.

A knock on his bedroom door. Miranda stood there in one of Sol's bathrobes, one with the logo of a Spanish conqueror's helmet and the name of their golf course in Florida, *El Conquistador*.

"Hi," she said. "Can we talk?"

"Sure. I have a special place. Can you climb the ladder to the roof?"

"With help."

"Let's go."

He helped her up to his boyhood sanctuary, the flat tin roof. He brought up a folding chair for her to sit on and sat beside her on the warm tin. This, he told her, was the only place in the house where he'd found any peace or privacy or fullness, the only place for him in the Family Rose. He pointed out his old pals the copper beech, the larch, the giant maple, and the summer constellations of the tilting stars, the shy sliver of moon. They fell silent, comforted.

"I left for a lot of reasons," she said, in answer to his unasked question. "I probably know only about 60 percent of them, even now. I was hurt—but that wasn't the main thing." She hesitated. "I just couldn't bear to watch what we had together fall any lower, not with the savageness we both showed, the last time, on the bench under the catalpa, by the stream."

"Horrible, yes. I'm so sorry."

"Me too." Tears rushed to her eyes, and she blurted out, "It's incredible to see you again. I . . ." she paused, swallowed hard. "I haven't stopped loving you, you know."

He was startled, affirmed. "And I you. You and Cray were with me every day."

"But I shouldn't say that. You're leaving, right?"

"Right. I've got my ticket out."

"Where to?"

"Rome."

The word sank in. "Ah." She tried to breathe. "Maybe we shouldn't even talk," she said. "Just forget it?"

"Can't. Just seeing you and Cray again, it's hard to imagine that there's not still a sliver of hope for us, isn't it?"

"Yes." She wanted desperately to say more but could not.

Crickets did their thing with their hind legs for a while.

"Tell me everything," he said at last, "from the time you left."

She told him about packing up everything and then slipping away at night, dropping off the Scomparza box on his porch on the way out of

268

town. Mrs. Tarr was the only one who knew where she was going, but not why, and was sworn to secrecy—she would be her lifeline to Columbia. They drove west across the grand, seemingly optimistic sections of America and in a few days reached her Auntie Heyward's farm, an island in the archipelago of farms in the ocean of wheat, hundreds of miles west of Grand Forks. She told Cray nothing except that she and Orville had had a falling out—as he had noticed—and had broken up and that they were taking a geographical cure for the summer. Cray would be the man of the house and the farm and he would love it.

"Which he did," she said, "though he missed you terribly. Nightmares, tears, moping around—the works." She choked up, but then gathered herself. "It was hard to tell him not to write you, call you, but he's a good kid. He picked up right away that I needed him to be big and to help take care of things, of himself, and me. So he helped—he grew up so much this summer! Grew closer to me again, too, like when he was a child. He told me on the drive back that he wasn't a child now, he was a kid."

"Yeah, I noticed."

"And then there was my thesis." She glanced at him with a furtive smile.

"You finished it?" She nodded. "Yes! Good for you! 'The Columbian Spirit!'" He reached up to hug her, but it was too intimate—like when they first met—and he held back.

"Funny," she said, "but looking back on the history of my working on it here in town, I realized that I was becoming the latest victim of the odd spell Columbia casts. I'd always been facile at writing history, in my pre-Columbian days, but here I just couldn't do it. I was in a weird kind of limbo, like my brain had turned to lard and my fingers were heavy with weird breakage. Only when I got away did I get any perspective on things, catch fire again, and I just raced through it all, and it's . . . well, it's all right."

"I'm sure it's brilliant. I can't wait to read it."

"I have to revise and do the bibliography. I'm really going to dive into it the next two weeks, night and day. I have to finish it before Cray goes back to school."

"Will you make me a copy? Signed by the author?"

"Sure."

Their eyes met and held for just an instant—as if there was too much gravity in the glance to keep afloat—and then fell. They stared straight ahead into the night at nothing visible, except maybe a glint of moonlight off the gold cross on the top of St. Mary's steeple. With what seemed enormous effort he put his hand on hers, his palm over the back of her hand. She raised her hand and turned it over so that they were at least palm to palm. Their fingers intertwined, feeling *known,* alive with their shared history.

Orville felt himself losing substance, starting to fade, as if part of him was already gone.

Miranda felt displaced, knowing now that it was truly over and that all she had left to do was ride out the couple of weeks before he went back to his life with his Italian lover, no kids and no family, and that would be that.

It was the best they could do, and the worst—sitting together staring into the night, being somewhere else. He in his somewhere else, she in hers.

29

Dear Orvy,

By now it is two months since you left, and I hear from Amy that you are happily settled in Rome with Celestina. What I am about to tell you will unsettle you emotionally, but I sincerely hope it will not change your relationship with her. It is over between us and, I feel, over in a good way. With one caveat, from our history.

I am now five months pregnant. Yes, it is yours, ours. Given what you told me, it is a miracle, but I guess miracles happen. Yes, I thought to tell you, many times before I left for North Dakota. I found out soon after our disastrous day of the benefit for the Worth. The first time I sensed I might be pregnant was just before I came outside with the punch bowl and cups. You were waiting for me at the car, we were late, and you were angry. The reason that I was late coming out of the house was that I was in the bathroom being sick. I put that together with the way I had been feeling ("the flu that was going around") and the fact that my period was late, and despite the impossibility of it being real, I decided to go for a pregnancy test the next day. I almost told you then, but it was such a jagged, terrible time. I held back, thinking that if it were positive, I could tell you. The next time I saw you was when we had that talk out at the bench by the stream under the catalpa tree, when we saw, I think, the worst of each other and had a terrible fight—the worst fight I have ever had with anyone. We could not accept what we saw in each other. It was over.

There was no way that I could tell you, then, and there was no way I could stay. I would never want you to stay in Columbia under that kind

270

of duress. You chose not to be with me, and I you, and that was that. When I came back, we had reached some level of . . . well, yes, a level of love that was based on your leaving, and it was hard, but it was—in your mind anyway—a clean break. When we were up on the roof at your house that first night back I thought to tell you, wanted to tell you, but I didn't want you to stay simply because you felt you had to. Clearly you needed to—to use your mother's word—"fly." And that, of course, is one of the things I loved about you.

This will upset you greatly, and I am sorry. I am profoundly sorry.

But I want you to know, from the depth of my soul and my love for you, which right now feels like a sun-warmed metal charm deep inside me, that whatever part you want to play in the child's life is fine with me.

I have confidence that we will move through our unspooling history around our child in a way that will bring out, in both of us, our very best—which, I believe, is remarkable.

Love,
Miranda

She sealed the letter, wrote her address where it should be, wrote his name where it should be "c/o Celestina Polo," and, skipping the street address—she would have to make sure to get it before he left—wrote "Rome, Italy."

The next day she went to the post office and bought the correct postage and the Air Mail stickers and affixed them carefully.

She put the letter in the top drawer of her dresser, which Cray would never open. She would mail it two months after Orville had left.

30

A week before Orville was due to leave, he sat in the kitchen staring at one of the framed photos he'd dug out of the bottom of the Scomparza box. It was his bar mitzvah picture—*before* he performed. Sol, Selma, Penny, and he were dressed up. Sol in his suit looked schlumpy, Penny in her neck-revealing beige suit looked aristocratic, and Selma, her face whole, wore the cobalt number she'd flown around in, which made her look pretty gorgeous. Orville was in an ill-fitting brown suit. He'd been dragged down to the garment district in New York to get it wholesale from a second cousin's brother-in-law in the business. He recalled watching a cutter sail a power knife smoothly through foot-high piles of material as if it were so much butter. He was measured up precisely. The suit would be custom-made to fit. When it arrived in Columbia, it didn't.

Selma was the tallest, Penny next, then Sol, then Orville. Sol looked like he was in significant hemorrhoidal pain, Penny looked noble, and Selma triumphant and maybe a bit flirtatious—definitely flying high. Orville looked like he was about to fall off a cliff.

In many ways it would have been a lovely photo. The problem was that the photographer was a Columbian. The camera was tilted, off-kilter, and a touch out of focus. All members of the Family Rose, like four stick figures, were leaning to the left, as if on an ocean liner and caught precisely at the instant of impact, the crashing into the iceberg.

Orville noticed a scrap of paper tucked into the back of the frame. In Selma's handwriting: "Interviewed new cleaning girl. Darling, but *Ethiopian*." Doorbell. Telegram.

BEEL NOT FEEL WELL

RETURN HOME MONDAY AUGUSTO 20

ON SLEEPY HOLLOW 16:39 IMEEG LOVE BABS

"IMEEG"? What the hell was that?

◊ ◊ ◊

Two days later Orville stood at the train station watching the Sleepy Hollow tilt scarily as it rounded the sharp bend into Columbia. His heart was beating fast—he realized how much he'd missed Bill and was looking forward to seeing him again.

During the week or so since Miranda and he talked, they had not seen each other much, and when they did it was always in the presence of Cray and Amy. Miranda was totally preoccupied with her thesis, and the kids had renewed the best of their big sister/little brother thing. They joined forces to try to convince Orville to stay. When that failed, they made him promise that they could all visit him in Italy. Miranda and Orville were treating each other gingerly, like a man and a woman who have survived the crash of a small plane and don't want to risk air travel again anytime soon.

With Orville leaving, Penny had attacked his mother's house with a neat-freak vengeance and a goal of obliterating every micron of dirt and every trace of his year living there. An army of cleaners scoured and scrubbed.

Most of the furniture was covered with sheets. Every time Orville came back to the house to sleep, he had the impression of its being, if not a house of the dead, a house of the dead furniture. These sheet-covered chairs, tables, and sofas reminded him of draped corpses in morgues wherever he'd gone as an itinerant doctor, some with pennies over their eyes to bribe the guards of heaven. Corpses are a kind of furniture, he mused as he waited for the train, are they not? After arriving home he would snatch the covers up and off, relieved that beneath were not bodies but couches and ottomans, bureaus and lamps. The next day they would be shrouded again.

As the train pulled in, Orville saw that something was wrong. The conductor was leaning out from between two cars, waving frantically, shouting something. Finally, he was close enough to hear.

"A doctor! Get a doctor!"

"Call an ambulance!" Orville shouted reflexively back at the stationmaster, as he started running toward the train. The train slowed, shuddered. Orville ran at an angle to it, trying to gauge where it would stop, overshooting, then jumping up on the lowered metal steps.

"I'm a doctor."

"C'mon." The conductor disappeared into the car, Orville following.

The dear old man lay slumped over onto his wife, drool coming out of a flattened corner of his mouth.

"Orvy! Thank God!" Babette cried out.

"What happened?" he asked, automatically doing all the emergency things—airway, cardiac, breathing.

"He wasn't feeling well, you know, high up in Peru, but was not bad all the way here until . . . suddenly he just keeled over."

"How long ago?"

"Just after we rounded the bend around Mount Pecora and started across the swamp and he saw Columbia again. He was so . . . so happy!" She wept.

By the time he heard the crescendo cry of the approaching ambulance, Orville knew the diagnosis. After his triumphant trip around the world, upon entering the outskirts of Columbia, Bill had suffered a massive stroke.

◊ ◊ ◊

Bill's fall from health had been severe enough to kill him. And yet he lived—sort of. He was comatose, gravely ill. Orville had considered sending him up to Albany Medical, but Babette told him that she and Bill had discussed things and he'd said that if anything happened he wanted to be taken care of in Kinderhook Memorial and taken care of by Orville. That first night Orville stayed up all night with him doing what he could, making sure that his cardiac medications were on board and putting in a pacemaker and starting him on steroids to reduce brain swelling. He called the best neurologists and neurosurgeons in Albany. Many of them knew Bill, and one made the trip down to examine him. All agreed that he had suffered an occlusion of a major vessel; the prognosis was grim. All of Bill's risk factors—obesity, smoking, sedentary lifestyle, heart disease, family history of cardiovascular accident, bad lipid and cholesterol pro-file—made the prognosis even worse.

Orville knew that the critical period for strokes was the first twenty-four to thirty-six hours. During that time he rarely was far from Bill's bedside. Babette stayed at the hospital much of the time, too. Bill had been taken up to the top floor, the Schooner Suite in the Wing of Selma Rose. Orville hadn't been up in the suite for a while, and his first look out the west-fac-ing windows was startling. The hospital was high up on Cemetery Hill, the view unparalleled: straight down Washington to Parade Hill, up over the pathetic pink-and-blue ski chalets of Plotkin Village, skimming out onto the broad river and skipping up off it, climbing the Catskills speckled with the first fall colors and, on the peaks, a hint of the first snows. It was ach-ingly beautiful, all the more so for Bill, in coma, being unable to see it.

A bed was brought in for Babette. Everybody knew everybody, of course, and everybody was upset. Bill had been their doctor, and much more. He had become the true icon of Columbia. Forget the phony whale icon in-vented by Milt and Schooner and SPOUT. This man was the heart of the town. After all, Orville thought, wasn't Starbuck linked to the forgotten utopia of its Nantucket founders by his name, and linked tightly to the century by his eighty-odd years? Bill's stroke was the town's stroke. Orville saw, in his patients, a shadow cast.

He had seen a lot of strokes, coming to understand that strokes have their own way with brains and souls, and the best that could be done was to prevent complications and to rely on the tincture of time. Bill had not been lucid since the train. There was still light in him, but it was flicker-ing. After a week he was stable but still in a coma. With the pacemaker beating his heart, with excellent nursing care and the attention of Babette and friends and patients, he seemed at peace.

Orville began each day by checking in on Bill and ended each night with him, too. Babette would sit on the other side of Bill's bed as Orville examined him. He came so early in the morning and so late at night that often Babette was in her flannel nightgown and her ram's horns of curlers.

Over the years, he had seen a few patients who had come up out of coma, and he had learned that sometimes they could dimly hear and sense what was going on around them. He was careful what he said in Bill's presence and asked others to be careful too. Babette, with Orville's encouragement, would talk to Bill, tell him the news, the weather, the gossip, and replay the status of the grudges. Bill himself had once told him that coma is a balance of the soul between the living and the dead, a kind of tug-of-war between powerful adversaries so equally matched that the little flag tied to the midpoint of the rope trembles constantly with the effort, even if it does not perceptibly move. Those of us who are braced solidly in life can be of great help, for the dying sometimes sense that we are reaching out, pulling hard, back. The rope, stretched taut between life and death, is not like other ropes—there's always room on it for more hands. For Bill there were hands aplenty. Four generations of Columbians came by.

Orville repeatedly did a checklist of his treatment of Bill, always coming to the dead end of medical knowledge. He had fitted his mentor into the tight boxes of diagnosis (occlusion of the middle cerebral artery resulting in contralateral hemiplegia, hemianaesthesia, and homonymous hemianopsia), of treatment (none, really), and prognosis (despite Bill's being left-handed and thus having more bilateralization of brain function, poor). One side of Bill's face and one side of his body were paralyzed. Every time Orville saw Bill's face he could not help but see the half-fallen face of his mother.

The end of Bill's first week back, the 27th of August, would be the day that Orville fulfilled his mother's will and the day that he had arranged to fly to Rome. As it approached, he realized that there was no way he was going to leave Bill in such dire shape.

On the 26th he called Celestina at her apartment in Rome. No answer and no answering machine. He tried several times, all day long, into her night. Nothing. So he sent a telegram.

MY FRIEND DR. STARBUCK IN COMA
CANNOT LEAVE HIM YET
CALL ME ALL MY LOVE ORVILLE

A few hours later she called, waking him. It was two in the morning on August 27th.

"*Allora,* you are not coming?"

Orville heard the tension in her voice. She seemed on the edge of significant anger. "I am coming, baby, but I can't leave yet."

"This Dr. Starbuck, he is your guru?"

He was surprised at the word, but then not, and said, "Yes." He explained what had happened.

"Ah . . . *Si, si.* I get it." She said this in a somber, thoughtful tone.

Most of the time as they were falling in love, Celestina had been light-hearted, funny, and outrageous. But once in a while a dead serious look would come over her face, and they would have remarkable, revealing conversations about things he'd come to imagine as impenetrable—life, death, love, the soul, transformation, forgiveness, compassion, loving-kindness. By that time he'd mostly given up on these themes. Her Buddhism had given him a whole new way of understanding them, and he loved her for this.

Now as she went on, her tone was steady and sure, like the day on Lago del Orta. Hearing her this way again now made him yearn to be with her. She *has* changed, he thought, she's onto something. There's a whole world of possibility now with her.

"*Transizione dell'anima,*" she said, somberly. "The transit of the soul." A sigh. "I regret to say, *caro,* it is for you another gift."

"I think so, babe, yes," he said, smiling. How he had missed this, her!

"And have you seen the first gift, your mother flying around?"

He realized that he had not seen Selma airborn since the night of his surprise birthday party, the night Miranda and Cray had come back. She'd flown a lot when they'd been away, but not since they'd been back. Like Selma, he was superstitious, and now asked himself: Is there a link? The dead don't fly in the face of love?

"No," he said, hiding these thoughts from her. "Not since my real birthday."

"Ah. Then it is now safe to leave."

"Yes."

"So then, *caro,* when?"

"I'm not sure, sweetheart. With Bill it's day by day."

"Okay. *Eccolo.* We stay in the most intimate touch. Stay in the 'now.' If we touch the ground of the present moment, we touch the peace and joy. Full of peace and joy, when we do come together toe and toe again we will see each other as if for the first time, and the very sensuality will blossom off the charts. *Conclusione? Uno:* stay in the present. *Due:* we talk every day, okay?"

"Okay."

"And I will wait for you."

"Promise?"

"Promise."

There was silence on the line.

"Hello? Hello?" He was afraid that she would turn back into her old self, turn flighty, and slip away.

"*Si, si,* I was just thinking."

"What?"

"How you and I, such passionate lovers, are *sciocco.*"

"*Sciocco?*"

"Silly. *Comico.* Like everybody." She seemed sad. "We are all ridiculous, but created by God."

"God?"

"Who else?"

"Not the Buddha?"

"The Jesus and the Buddha, *si, si.* I have read recently *La Vangeli Gnostica—The Gnostic Gospels.* From age sixteen to thirty, Jesus travels in India and walks with the disciples of the Buddha. It is all the Divinity, so why split the hairs?" She yawned. "I have not had my *espresso.* I called you at once. So now I go to work."

"Where?"

"Chase Manhattan. Teaching the greedy to let go. Today I teach the story of the Buddha and his monks meeting a cow farmer. The cow farmer is frantic. He says, 'I lost my cows! They are valuable and they are gone! I have to find my precious cows—have you seen them?' The Buddha says, 'No, we have not seen your cows.' The farmer runs off, crazy. The Buddha turns to his monks and says, 'Aren't you glad you don't have cows?'"

Orville laughed with her. "It's a wonderful story, baby."

"I love when you call me 'baby.' *Allora,* dear heart, this year has brought us closer. We have each changed in the same way, do you feel it?"

"I do, yeah."

"It will be the dynamite. But be aware, *Orvillo,* we cannot go back."

"What do you mean?" He felt himself tense up, on guard.

"We can't go back to what we had, to what was. We have to find out what is."

"Hold it. You always said that what was, is, and what is, will be—"

"—will be, *si, si.* But with us it has to be new, or nothing."

"I can't take another 'nothing'! What do you think? You think it'll work?"

"With what we had—and with no more worry about money? Of course, *caro*, of course. *Certo! Ciao, ciao!"*

"Ciao." As he hung up, he felt a hit of apprehension. Something rankled. And why at the end had she again brought up money? But as he thought about it, he realized how right she was. They couldn't go back. It had to be new. Scary, but true.

Later that day Orville fulfilled the terms of his mother's will and was given something shy of a million dollars and the deed to his mother's house and the title to the Chrysler and the trunk space. He felt a flicker of relief that money would no longer be an issue for him, but only a flicker. He was surprised at how little it seemed to matter.

"Now *you* have to make out a will," Penny said that afternoon.

He realized that he was now the guy with the cows.

"Fine," he answered. "I'll pull a Selma. Leave it all to you if and only if you shave your head and wear sackcloth continually for a year and thirteen days. Or to Milt if he pierces his ears and nose and penis and attends the Baptist Church religiously for the same 378 days. Deal?"

"Sadist."

"Exactly," he said, feeling afresh the enormity of what his mother had done. From the grave, to actually do that to someone? To not let go? What gall, to treat someone you say you love, like that. He felt a surge of anger and looked up, hoping to see her, to yell at her or try somehow to bring her down—to do *something*. No luck.

He phoned Celestina, venting his spite.

"Momento," she said, and the phone flew down, *clonkk*. He waited. She came back and read him a verse from something called *The Upakkilesa Sutra.*

> In this world
> Hate has never yet dispelled hate
> Only love dispels hate.
> This is the law,
> Ancient and inexhaustible

"I agree," he said, "but I'm not there."

"Not even in being the good doctor to your Columbians?"

He was taken aback. At first he had resented the Columbians, had contempt for them. Now he realized that somewhere in the arc of the year things had changed. Now, mostly, he didn't.

"Hello?" She was calling into the receiver. "Hello?"

"Maybe," he said. "But I'm still living with a lot of bitterness inside. I'm no saint. You know that."

"None of us down here are saints."

"'Down here'? You mean 'up there' there are?"

"Of course. But let me be *essenziale,* simple, and Christian—in your case, 'do unto others as has *not* been done unto you by your mother'—this is the very Selma gift!"

The money part of his will turned out to be simple: half to Amy, half to Cray.

The house and car were harder. He toyed with the idea of giving both to Miranda but knew she wouldn't take them. He thought of donating the house to Columbia for some kind of institution, say a Sanctuary for Songless Lovebirds or a state-of-the-art Plotkin Whorehouse or a Home for Abnormal Idealists. Or, all in a single breakage-proof structure built like a nuclear bombproof bunker, a combination Home for Songless Idealists and Plotkin Whorehouse for Abnormal Lovebirds.

He asked Milt to put the house on the market, take his commission, and wire him the cash.

And the Chrysler? He decided to give it to Amy. He would have it stored and serviced until she was able to drive in five years. If the windows were tightly closed, it might even still smell of Selma, which she would like.

The trunk space he kept for himself.

31

About a month later, at the end of September, Orville sat in the kitchen facing the strangely early fall. High above Columbia, there had been a breakage in the weather pattern. Up north, something had fractured. A slippage of frigid air down from Hudson Bay brought a premature cold snap. Chlorophyll drained from the veins of the leaves, revealing their true colors—scarlet, yellow, gold, purple, brown. The joints where the stems met the twigs weakened, trapped by the fatal genetics of autumn. The leaves needed only a rainy wind to let go and carry them fluttering down.

A mass of warm spongy air sailed innocently up from the Gulf of Mexico. Encountering the higher cold, the wet sponge was wrung out and its contents fell on Columbia, bringing two days of snippity wind and insistent rain, ripping the stems from the twigs, laying a rainbow of dead leaves all over the backyard.

Orville sat with the bird at the kitchen table of what was now his house, staring out the window at the flurried descent of the leaves. His big old friends the beech, the maple, and the larch were letting go in true copper and scarlet and needles of gold. He was stalling, surprised to find himself reluctant to go spend Saturday afternoon with Miranda and Cray and Amy out at Miranda's house. He felt torn apart—lonely, but being with them might make him feel more lonely. Loneliness when you're alone is hard, but loneliness when you're with people you love is hell. The problem, he realized, was that with the coming of fall, with the real start of the year, based on the harvest not on the calendar, everyone but him had started a new cycle.

Cray and Amy were back at school, so he didn't see them nearly as much. Miranda was diligently finishing up the final details of her thesis, "The Columbian Spirit: Breakage and Resilience." Mrs. Tarr was ecstatic about it and had shown it to a few of her antiquer friends who "loved it!" and passed it on to a New York agent who had unwittingly bought a grand house in the bad part of town and who said it had "great commercial potential—it's so funny, this place!—there's already a buzz!" The agent wanted her to revise it with an eye for publication, emphasizing the irony, the humor. Miranda was scared, excited, and hard at work. She had a chance to connect her work to the larger world—and she could use the cash. A big chance, yes. He had not seen much of her. When he did, it was hard to get a fix on her. She seemed preoccupied with her own future—her writing, Cray. He felt even more adrift among the Columbians.

They've all got clear purposes, he said to himself, staring at the captive bird. They're gaining substance, stepping out briskly upon the autumn ground on their way to appointments, someplace else. Me, I've lost substance, purpose. Columbians act as if I've already left, forgotten but not gone. I'm floating—much like Selma!—apart and above the town, unloved and dead.

But, he countered to himself, he was surely loved and alive with Celestina. The two of them had kept in touch pretty well, speaking to each other nearly every day. The amazing thing, to him, was how rich and expansive their conversations were, full of humor, allure, sensuality and the promise of great sex, mixed with the Celestina Polo School of Buddhism, which now seemed more relevant to his pain. It was an alternative view that made sense.

On the phone with her everything was heightened for him, as if without eye contact or the chance to lay hands on her—on her lips, her eyelashes, her breasts, her thighs, and her toes—it was all so much easier. Looking straight into a woman's eyes and at the same time dealing with his or her feelings had never been easy. But he had come to understand over his years with women—his first love Laurice, Lily, Celestina, Miranda—that *not* looking into their eyes was, for women, much harder. Eye contact was a turn-on for them. Somehow his connection with Celestina had deepened, no question. Would it hold up eye to eye? He'd soon see.

Orville got up from the kitchen table and put Starlight back in its cage. He wiped the dollop of lovebird poop off his shoulder and went out the front door.

"Fake! Fake!" A cry came from across the square. Through the leafless trees Orville saw Henry Schooner on his front lawn playing soccer with Maxie. Orville headed over.

Henry had a cigar between his teeth and a beer can in his hand. He suspended the beer from the top rim, between thumb and index finger, with surprising delicacy. Here's a man, Orville thought, who really knows how to hold a can of beer. He had learned something in the navy after all. My tax dollars at work.

Henry's campaign was sailing along. With the Republican incumbent deciding not to run, with the district being overwhelmingly conservative Republican and riding along in the "Morning In America" Reagan theme park, and with a hapless Columbian novelist named Leston Moore as the Democratic nominee—Leston's main support was from the CAVE people of the town, and his campaign slogan was the inane LES IS MORE—Schooner looked like a shoo-in. The Honorable Henry Schooner, my representative in Congress? Unreal.

Henry didn't seem to notice Orville approaching. Unusual, that, Orville thought. He stepped behind a tree, peeked, and listened.

"Damnit! I'm tryin' to teach you to fake. You know what a fake is, doncha?"

"Nope," Maxie said, head down. He seemed cowed, beaten down.

"It's when you act like you're goin' one way and you go the *other* way. You fool 'em. A fake is when you fool 'em, fool 'em all, and then you go by 'em and score! C'mon. Try again to stop me. Be tough, be tough." Henry dribbled the ball toward the kid, juked one way, the kid went for it, and Henry easily jived the other way and booted the ball past him into the goal. "Damnit, Maxie, you went for it too easy. Don't lemmie fool ya. Focus on what the other guy's tryin' to do to you. Get into his head. Be tough be sharp, be tough be sharp. Mentally tough, physically tough. Focus!" He relit his cigar. "This time you try fakin' me out. Be tough be tough!"

Maxie got the ball out of the goal and they reversed positions. Maxie started coming at Henry. Henry seemed to relax, to move slowly to let the boy beat him and win. Maxie made a clumsy, halfhearted attempt at a fake, and Henry couldn't help but take the ball away from him.

"Dammit, Maxie, you weren't tryin'."

"Was too."

"*That* was a try?" The boy nodded. "Bullshit. I told you a hundred times I don't care if you succeed as long as you give it your best shot. And you didn't and it—" he seemed to try to control himself but could not "—it pisses me off!"

"I did."

"That's your best shot? That little girl bullshit move?" Another sullen nod. "If that's true, we got ourselves a big problem." Maxie said nothing. "You're not focusing, son, not really focusing on faking. And not being aggressive. Life's about focusing, faking, and being aggressive, okay?"

"Can I go in now? I'm cold."

Henry stared bullets at him. He seemed on the verge of exploding. Even from a distance, Orville could feel the ice in that stare. It was a glimpse of Schooner he hadn't had over the course of the year, but it was familiar because it was the Schooner he'd known before.

Orville strolled up nonchalantly and said, "Hi, Henry."

"Why, hello there, Dr. Rose!" Henry's tone was the very excellent public one, the musically soothing one, down a few notes to the husky world of buoyant grandfathers. It said that he viewed the good doctor's arrival and greeting as a great honor, maybe even the high point of his day so far. "Nelda Jo's due back today from getting Junior settled in at Valley Forge," he offered, as if Orville had been waiting for this important news bulletin, "and I'm teachin' Maxie a little soccer."

"Valley Forge?"

"Military Institute. Gettin' that boy back on track!"

"You coaching soccer again this year?"

"I wish. I really enjoy coachin', but there's no time this fall, with the campaign."

"Amazing, Henry, how well it's going. They say you're a shoo-in."

"Ain't over 'til it's over. But hey—maybe, given the competition, I might even get your vote? It'd mean a lot to me, Orvy, given our differences, old and new. A real lot. Kinda seal our friendship at the ballot box before you go, know what I mean?"

"If I'm still here, sure."

"Great! Just great! It'd be an honor to get your vote, doctor. And hey—there's always an absentee ballot, of course. You can pick one up before you go. It'd mean a lot to me. Every vote counts, but some votes count more. So when you leavin'?"

"Depends on how Bill does."

"Noble. Damn but that's just so noble. Our noble and glorious physician. You will be *missed*. Let's get together. I'll stop by."

"Yeah. I gotta go now."

"Sure. Thanks for dropping by. Okay, Maxie, let's play. Let's see some happy feet happy feet!"

Maxie's feet at the moment were a little way away, plonked down onto the top step of the porch, his rear end on the porch itself. The feet had taken him there in relief, as Orville and Henry had talked, but had not taken him inside. To Henry's "happy feet happy feet" command, the feet didn't move. Orville noticed that his lips were blue, his teeth chattering. The kid did not look well. Henry put a few fingers in his mouth and gave a high-pitched whistle. The feet started to move down off the steps, but they didn't look happy, not happy feet happy feet definitely not. There was no bounce, no twinkly toes, no anticipatory dance that Cray often did when he was about to play something he liked. In fact, Maxie fell. As he came down the steps into the yard he tripped over a fallen branch and wound up sprawled among the leaves.

Orville walked away and, looking up at his mother's house, offered a silent prayer: Please God Moses Jesus and Buddha or Whoever, please let Bill improve by the November election so that I don't have to make good on my promise to vote for Henry.

32

Later that afternoon, rake in hand, Miranda surveyed her yard, covered with the truth of fallen leaves—red swamp maple, yellow sugar maple, scarlet sumac, and the latest to turn, deep purple sycamore. The seasons had come round, to a time you'd be crazy not to think of as foreboding, given the Columbian winter.

Orville was raking by himself, on the crest of the slope.

She stared across the sluggish river at the indolent rolls of hay with their elongating shadows on the foothills, the pink glow of the sun falling toward the peaks of the mountains. Straight overhead a series of lumpy gray clouds were spread far apart, but as they neared the lowering sun they packed more tightly into formation, turning pink. A wedge of pink-tinted geese flew west, homing to all that red, that heat.

She planted her good leg firmly and reached down with the rake. Using it as a support, she pulled the leaves slowly into her pile.

Scritch . . . scritch. Move your feet, plant your leg, reach out, pull. *Scritch . . . scritch.*

She had worked down the slope of the backyard from the two pines. Her pile was in the corner where the raccoons attacked the garbage, on the edge of the dirt road heading toward the turnaround at the railroad tracks and the river. The afternoon was clear and cool; as the sun fell it would be cold. The raking was warming her, as did her sense that Cray and Amy were having fun doing something with water, somewhere upstream, maybe even up at the ruins of the old Wild Brothers Mill, built in 1824 as the English tied up the textile trade in the valley, up at Stuyvesant Falls.

One of the good changes, she thought, was how close Amy and Cray had gotten. And the buzz about her thesis among the New Yorkers was a strange new affirmation of her perspective and skill as a writer. The agent had helped her emphasize the irony of the text and had gotten her an assignment for a small piece in the Travel section of the *Times*. The idea of suddenly having some paying writing assignments both terrified and thrilled her. She and Cray might just be okay. As she worked to bring out the humor, she could hear again Orville's big laugh, how he enjoyed learning of the folly of the Columbians. The memory, now, brought on a certain sadness. She blinked, back in the reality of the raking, the leaves, him. She was constantly worried that she might start to be showing—at just over three months now. Her body was feeling full and warm, breasts and tummy stretched, nipples tender. To her surprise, her body felt whole, even healthy. Sensual. It reminded her of the first time she'd been pregnant, with Cray, with Joe. A happy, expectant time. Not like this.

Scritch . . . scritch. Trying to fathom it all. *Scritch . . . scritch.*

As of a month ago, he was free to leave. He'd gotten the money and the house. Bill was in a coma but stable. He and I, she said to herself, have leveled off. We don't see each other much, and when we do, it's more like good friends, or a sister and a brother. And yet beloved sister and brother

412 207 8148

Regency Gold
169-609

818-284 3100

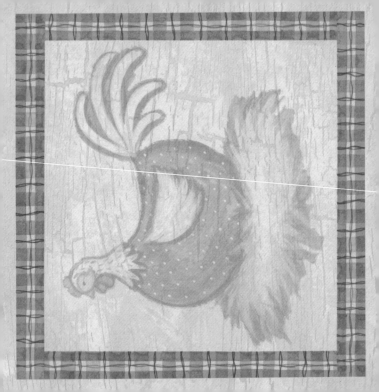

who know it's fruitless to talk about the trauma of the past in the family. We find ourselves sitting together and talking, side-by-side rather than face-to-face. I love that, having him as a good brother right now—and it'll help in the future. The past is too big for the present. We're out of our depth. And his going back to his Italian? Sometimes it bothers me, sometimes not. We've settled into finding a distance at which we can be kind. Wary, but kind. Except for one thing: he's still *here!* Right over there! If he stays much longer, I won't be able to hide the pregnancy from him, not even with these bulky clothes. I'll have to tell him face-to-face.

A week ago, more out of frustration than bravery, she'd asked him, "What are you waiting for? Why aren't you leaving?"

"I can't yet."

"Why not?"

"I'm waiting for Bill to live or die."

She leaned on the rake and looked up the slope at him.

Scritch scritch . . . scritch scritch . . . Orville looked down the slope at Miranda. She was wearing the same bulky white fisherman's sweater and cute sailor's cap that she had last autumn when they'd fallen in love, on that first picket line at the Worth, just after the schoolhouse meeting. His breath caught, more in his gut than his chest. Trying to steady himself, he looked up at the two pines soaring high over her house, but they only brought him back to that day coming out of the schoolhouse and catching the scent of cedar and staring up at the spruces and seeing the hawk in the rain.

Again he looked back down at her as she leaned on the rake, looking at him. A flame of red hair peeked out under the knobbly white of the cap. A glint of green eye under dark lashes, the creamy white cheek, rouged a little from the effort and the chill. Her face lately had looked beautiful, all aglow. She was so happy at the stir her thesis was making. Strong shoulders, strong chest, white wool rounded over her breasts, which moved like live animals, say whales, why not, underneath as she raked. Sexy. Bad leg, good leg. Worn jeans, solid boots. *Grounded.* He felt a jolt of the old excitement for her, for all she was. His passion sailed up, leveled off. Before it could fall he started raking intensely down the slope, to bring his pile of leaves into hers. *Scritch scritch . . . scritchscritchscritch . . .*

She heard his insistent *scritching,* saw him working fervently at the pile, pulling the lumpy center along down toward her, leaves tumbling over each other like loose fur on a big, rainbow-colored dog. And then she watched him charge back up the slope to herd in the stragglers and entice them into the edges, *flumphphing* them up onto the heap and then tumbling them all down toward her. He did this with happy abandon, a big kid at play. She laughed.

He heard her laughter and renewed his effort. Soon the front edge of his pile was near her pile. He got down on his knees and pushed his into hers, onto hers, over her rake, over her boots, and then just lay there, to her mind like a big puppy, looking up at her.

"A big pile!" he cried out happily. "A humongous pile! Gargantuan, man!"

"Nice raking."

"I was lonely up there."

"And now?"

"Not lonely at all. Come on down in here with me." He patted the enormous pile. "Soft and scratchy and sexy and fun." He smiled. "And sexy."

"In a second," she said. "There's something I want to talk about."

"Oh, God!" he cried, clutching his chest in feigned horror. "Get ready for World War Three."

"*You* don't have to talk if you don't want to, but it's something *I* want to say. As a way of . . . how to put it, a historical explanation."

"Sounds okay. Will it hurt?"

"Don't think so. All you have to do is listen."

"What's it about."

"Selma."

"Yeoww!" he screamed, jumping up, holding his belly where the rake/ sword had gone in, struggled to pull it out to no avail, and, whimpering and staggering, fell on his back into the huge pile, sinking down, feet up, rake like a lily, playing dead.

She laughed hard. It was the first time in a while that she'd let go, let him break through the muted, hold-your-breath portent of whatever it was they still had together.

"You big jerk."

"Okay. Ready." He leaned on an elbow. "Selma."

She leaned on her rake looking down at him. How cute he is today. Sexy, yes. Ever since she'd been back she'd been surprised at how big he was, heavier and more solid than she recalled. His short chestnut hair with its bald spot, his large forehead and blue eyes and hawk's nose and delicate lips, his surprising reddish beard—the year had given him more substance, made him more substantial. His leaving made him less so.

"In particular," she said, "Selma's lie to me about your staying with her."

"Go for it,"he said, with trepidation.

"When you told me it was a lie, I was shocked, angry. She had duped me totally."

"Classic Selma. So far so good."

"But then—"

"I knew it. A Selma-justifying 'but.'" She stopped, gave him a look. "Okay, okay. Sorry. Fire away."

"But then I started thinking. Maybe what she was doing was imagining you as better, or imagining the better part of you, something like that. Imagining . . . putting what she held as the best of you out into the world."

"Keeping the worst of me for herself and me?"

"Maybe," Miranda said, a thoughtful look on her face.

"Like she did with herself. Showed the public a saintlike Selma, and inside the house, at least to me, she was ferocious."

"But which one was real?"

"Selma at home was dead real. I knew who she was, believe me."

"But people in town would say the same thing—that they knew who she was—and they'd say she was terrific. She did accomplish things here, which we know isn't easy! The Library, Olana, the Hospital Auxiliary. And she stepped in and helped a lot of people directly, too. I watched her. She was amazing. People loved her."

"Did you?"

"I want to say no, and that's mostly true—she was hard to love—but when I think back to the only heart-to-heart we had after a committee meeting at the Library, well, right then I did. The story she told me that evening was loveable, and she was loveable telling it. Screwy, but loveable. After all that had happened to her, her surgery, her losses, she still had a vision. I had a sense that as a girl and young woman in New York that vision had been bright, but that when she came here she had to put it aside. She put her head down and took care of Sol and raised her kids, figuring that after things calmed down a bit she could get back to her vision again. And then, years later, she looked up and it was gone. She was left with, well, 'the Columbians' and with the two adults who'd been her children. And Sol's model airplanes. So, I guess she was a woman with a lost vision, lost out there or up there somewhere. A woman forced into a lesser life, historically a fifties life, down on the ground. And she went after that life with passion." She paused, considering this. "Almost as if it were the other one, the old one."

"Like a Sherman tank."

"In a way. Driven—or trapped—by her time and her history."

"Well good for her, and hurrah for Columbia. But it's just a lit-tle bit difficult—even if she is a public saint—to have her beat down your spirit in the comfort and privacy of her home. But, hey—don't listen to me, I'm selfishness incarnate. I care more about myself than about the welfare of the Columbians, imagine?"

"I can't." She smiled. He did too.

"She's like Schooner that way. In public a winner, in private . . ."

"What?"

"God knows. They were friends, Henry and she. I never knew that. He hung around the house when he first came back. Now I see why. To her he was the good son, I the bad. I never told her about his beating the shit out of me when I was a kid."

"Why not?"

"He said he'd kill me if I did, and because whenever I did tell her anything she always managed to make it worse. The woman had the empathic skills of a rhino." Orville felt his spirit fading, just talking about her. He didn't like the way this was going. "Look. It's simple. She told me that I was, at heart, one of the most ungrateful, selfish wretches who ever walked the face of the earth and then, when she talked about me to you and others, said I was a combination of Moses, Sandy Koufax, and Dr. Kildare."

"That's how I saw you too, of course."

"Not still?"

"Could be," she said, and immediately regretted it. It was going too far, toward hope. "The only way to justify it, I guess, is that that's what mothers do. I do it myself when I talk about Cray out in the world. I try to show him at his best out there—and it's not a lie. Mothers tend to imagine the better parts of their children to others. Not unusual."

"No, it isn't. What gets me is the extremes of her two Orvys and that she never put the two together." Heat was rising around his collar. "One minute she's accusing me of being the greatest narcissist who ever lived, the next she's saying I'm the greatest humanitarian. It's called 'delusion.'"

"Or hope."

This surprised him. He stared up at the fall sky, the light flying fast from it, west. "Thanks, but that's all I can take today."

"Me too."

They stared at each other.

"Come on down in here with me," Orville said, "just for a second."

288

"No."

"Why not?"

"Has to be longer."

"Deal."

She lowered herself carefully, using the rake as a support. The tines bent, but held. The leaves felt soft and scratchy through her sweater. She lay her head on his shoulder, sharing his view of the sky. Their bodies fell slowly down further into the pile, like one of those soft dream-fallings. They could see the low light hitting the tops of the pines.

They lay together, acclimating to the touch of each other's bodies. Since she'd come back, they'd touched each other only as friends do, slight kisses and hugs at hello and good-bye. Now something else was going on. The sensual, even at their worst times together, had been a refuge, and it started to happen again.

They kissed, first softly and then more. They hugged each other, their motion sinking them deeper so that the leaves mostly covered them, the light coming through all scarlet and gold and purple. It was so deliciously secret. They fluffed the coverlet of leaves up over them thickly, so the filter of leaves against the sun was too fine to let in much light. The earthy scent reminded Orville of lake water, and Miranda of childhood before the polio, playing in the Gulf of Mexico on the swampy shoreline of "the walking trees," the banyans.

"Feels like we're under water," she said. "Like big sea creatures. Without gravity."

"Sounds good to me," he responded happily, "to have a little less gravity."

His fingers were feathery on her cheeks and her lips, and hers caressed his neck. With care he moved his touch up under her sweater, stroking her breasts through her bra so that the nipples rose, as he did too. The leaves prickled their patches of naked skin like lovebites.

She felt his hand move down toward her belly—she grabbed it, stopped him.

"What's wrong?" Orville asked, jolted by the suddenness, the roughness of it.

For a second she rethought it—but just for a second. "I can't do this."

"Why not?"

She said nothing. It was too dangerous.

"Why not?" he asked again.

"I . . . I'm not sure we can talk about it right now."

289

"Now or never."

"That's not helpful."

"And your stopping this is?" he asked. No answer. "You did come down in here with me. I didn't force you."

"I just wanted a cuddle."

"We cuddled."

"And it was nice. Great, even."

"And then?"

"It turned into more, and I can't do more now."

"If I were staying?"

"No, no," she said, drawing away. "No. I will not get into the 'if' part again."

"Not into the possible?"

"Not much is possible, Orvy, with you going back to her."

"You're the one who left!" he said, angrily.

"And I came back. I'm *here*. I'm staying; you're not!"

"You just can't seem to imagine that *you* can hurt somebody, that *you* have power! Jesus!" With an exasperated sigh, he fell back down into the pile. She, too, lay back down. They lay there on the cooling earth, still mostly covered up by the leaves, the lowering sun drawing away the warmth.

"Hey, guys what's going on?"

Voices, from above. The leaves parted. Cray's face was expectant. Amy's too.

"It's all right, Cray," Miranda said, "we're just in a little leaf hollow, here."

"Can we make hot chocolate?" Amy asked. "The first cold day and all?"

"Sure," Miranda said. "You go start it.We'll be right there."

"Race you into the house!" Cray shouted and took off, Amy following.

Orville got up first, reached back for her, helped her to her feet, to solid footing on the sloped lawn.

In a stretch of low sunlight, two fatally tardy monarch butterflies fluttered in, played around flashing their orange and black, and fluttered out. Someone once, somewhere in the world, had told Orville that butterflies are trapped souls. Should he share it with her? He looked at her. In that lovely face her eyes had a look of yearning, a wistful look. He did tell her, an offering. She took his hand tenderly, and they walked slowly around the house toward the kitchen, the hot chocolate, and the kids.

◊ ◊ ◊

A few hours later Orville was sitting with the lovebird, morosely wondering to whom to will it, when he heard horrific screams outside. Schooner-land.

He grabbed his bag and ran out across the square to the house. The Filipino woman was standing on the porch, hopping up and down crying and shrieking, holding her arms out to him. As he approached, his pager went off and he heard the first wail of the ambulance. He ran into the foyer and then turned left into the family room.

Henry and the Filipino man were grunting and cursing, hoisting the old wooden breakfront up from where it had fallen. Nelda Jo was kneeling, eyes wide with shock, ashen faced, above little Maxie. He was lying amid the broken glass and smashed crockery, face down, crumpled up. The breakfront had fallen on him.

Orville's focus went laser onto the boy. He knelt down next to Nelda Jo and pushed her aside, and, pushing Henry's hand away, shouted, "Don't move him!" He put his cheek down on the carpet to check the boy's face. Breathing. Eyes open. Stunned, in pain.

"Wiggle your toes," Orville said to the boy as he took his pulse, praying he hadn't broken his neck. His toes didn't wiggle. "Maxie. This is *important*. Wiggle your toes." Maxie wiggled his toes. Thank God, the spine is intact. The ambulance arrived. He and the EMTs carefully turned the boy over on his back. A shaft of bone protruded through the bloodied dungarees—a spiral fracture—the worst kind. "Call the medicopter," Orville said. "We've got to get him up to the orthopedic surgeons at Albany Med. I know the best guy there." He looked at Henry and Nelda Jo. "Okay?" Nelda Jo was too shocked to speak.

"Absolutely, Doc," Henry said. "Call in the 'copter. I'll ride shotgun."

It wasn't the moment to ask how it had happened. With disgust, Orville realized he didn't have to.

33

"Aww crap! Aww crap! Aww crap!"

Bill Starbuck had been crying out intermittently for almost a week. Occasionally he would sob.

Before the crying and sobs had started, Bill had been deteriorating rapidly. At first Orville and Babette and the nurses thought that these words were signs he might be coming out of his coma. But as the minutes and then hours and days wore on, there was no other sign that he was improving. His vital signs, in fact, were heading in the other direction, showing a deterioration of all organ systems. Orville's only conclusion was that somehow Bill, the savvy doctor until the last, was sensing his imminent death and was feeling a lot of pain, in body and soul.

For a while everybody tried harder. Orville increased his attentiveness. Babette intensified her vigil. The nurses worked around the clock to make Bill comfortable. They even tried squirting hefty doses of Starbusol down the feeding tube and, at Babette's suggestion, puree of scallions. Nothing made Bill better. He continued his decline.

By now, the ninth of October, the curses and sobs had become fairly continuous. People were avoiding going into his room. Bill was getting more isolated. Even Orville began dreading his nightly checkup.

Tonight Orville stared at Bill, sunk down on the pillow, burrowed under the covers as if wanting to go to ground. Only his Humpty Dumpty face was visible. No longer jowly and without those thick glasses, he seemed younger. His head had edged closer to being a skull. The skin seemed to have thinned. Veiny and translucent like a baby's, each hill and valley of the bony terrain beneath seemed to shine through as if lit dimly from within. His thin black hair was mussed, falling forward across his bald top, reminding Orville of the comic actor Zero Mostel. His lips were still purled in that girlish way, but more cyanotic. A sign that his heart was less a beat than a whisk, a riff around death.

"Aww crap! Aww crap!"

Bill's eyes were shut. One lowered lid glistened with tears, the other, on the paralyzed side of his face, was dry. Orville heard his mother's voice—"I hate crying out of only one eye."

He noticed that Bill needed a shave. The nurses had been too broken up lately to do it. When Orville sat down on the bed, Bill started sobbing again. As Orville searched out his carotid for a pulse, Bill barked out:

"Aww crap! Aww crap! Aww—"

"Stop it, Bill, damnit!" Orville shot back.

Immediately ashamed, he rose and walked to the west-facing window. Terrific. Is that what you've learned this year? To yell at people in pain?

He stared out the window. It was dusk. The sun was just down behind the mountains, leaving a fiery red afterglow, cut sharply by the rise and fall of the frozen pulse of the rock. The river reflected the red as purple, and the purple of the bare-branched orchards and forests as black, and the scattered lights of the hamlet of Athens across Middle Ground Flats as yellow and red flickers, more like in oil than in water. Closer below him, Columbia was lighting up against the early autumn night. Its checkerboard—the five long straight streets from the river to the cemetery and the eight cross streets from swamp to swamp, all rotated forty-five degrees off sensible— was pegged by those bold argon streetlamps, as if in declaration that any down-and-dirty nightlife would be under the strict illumination of the most high-minded utopians. A wedge of geese flew past, right to left, heading downriver toward Rhinecliff, Poughkeepsie, West Point, honking through Yonkers to Manhattan and Staten Island, to winter maybe at Kill Devil Hill or even, like other snowbirds, in Boca Raton.

When Orville turned back to Bill, there was a strong sense that something had changed. It was not definite and not spooky, yet it called to him clearly. What was it? For some reason he thought of Mrs. Tarr.

Several months ago, after Mrs. Tarr had kicked out the magician and recovered from the pigeons, her dry cough worsened. Orville found lung cancer. She'd never smoked, but sitting in the smoke of the Columbians for forty years in the DAR Library had finally gotten her. Since diagnosis and treatment, she had gotten rapidly worse. Lately, to him, she became an example of the classic Columbian whose blood values and physical state were pretty much incompatible with life. Yet there she was, walking around alive. Bald from the chemotherapy, sporting a red turban, toting her mobile oxygen tank to and fro on a leash, much as she had toted her cat Randolph, sitting in her seat at the borrowing desk at the DAR under the arch of the whale jawbone, checking books in, checking books out. Sometimes, even, with Miranda and Amy and Cray and her tank on Sundays, she still walked the walk in front of the Worth.

What surprised Orville was the generosity of the Columbians toward Mrs. Tarr. People mostly had been kind. In tough times, Columbians mostly tried. Helping each other through to the desk at the Library, to the checkout counter at the supermarket, to the parking lot and even beyond. Walking the walk, with each other and some oxygen. Coming in the IN, going out the OUT.

At that moment, turning back to Bill, he saw that his old mentor, here in the best private room in the hospital, had gotten pushed aside, isolated. No one was really with him. He understood, then, what Bill had shown him all those years ago when Orville had come to him as a bewildered, Selma-and-Sol'd adolescent, looking for somebody with some sense—no, more—with some *expanse*. Bill hadn't told him, no—he'd shown him. Through his being with patients and laying a hand on a shoulder and saying "Heh heh" and taking a crate of scallions for a tonsillectomy or a chicken for colitis, Bill had shown him that what healed people had less to do with diagnosing and treating and more to do with connecting.

For the first time Orville understood the force of isolation. Even in the face of cancer or coma. Understood, too, that the moments of healing had been when he, often inadvertently, had been present with people. Bill had shown him that, that this is what good doctors do. We're present at the crucial moments, and at the ordinary moments. We bring someone who is out on the edge of the so-called sick into the current of the human. We take what seems foreign in a person, and see it as native. This is healing. This is what good doctors do. Isolation is deadly. Connection heals. Even in dying.

What Orville then understood was that if he were to stay in this room with this dear old doctor, he had to be *with* him.

Yeah, Mr. Bigshot Doctor, he said to himself, and how do you do that, eh?

Mundanely. Down to earth. Nothing heroic. Do something small.

So Dr. Rose decided to give Dr. Starbuck a shave. After all, the first doctors, the surgeons, had evolved from barbers, had they not?

Orville's constant transitions from finishing his day or night as a doctor and starting his night or day as a person had taught him to carry, in his black bag, a shaving kit. He took out his wooden shaving mug and a safety razor and screwed together the chrome-plated Crabtree and Evelyn Genuine Badger Bristle shaving brush. He wet the brush with steaming hot water and worked it into a lather. As he propped Bill up higher, the slippage of the sheets down from his neck was like an exhumation. The scent was that terrible mix of stale sweat and residual excrement and urine and baby powder—all too familiar to doctors and nurses, signifying bodily decay and hospital neglect.

He began to lather Bill's face. It wasn't easy to shave someone else. The brush felt awkward on Bill's skin. Try to feel his face from *his* side, Orville thought. What if you could do that anytime you chose? Shift from "I" to "you," take on the other as yourself. Better yet, take on all of it—"I" and "you" and "we." What if you could go through a whole day without using the word "I"?

As he worked the brush, trying to feel it working from Bill's side, chin-to-sideburn, cheek-to-fallen-lip-corner, it started to feel different, as if he were working it on his own face, in that unconscious way you get into, so habitually that—like tying a necktie—if you *try* to do it you can't do it at all. Bill continued to curse and weep. When Orville started moving the razor through the lather, he had to time his strokes carefully. He set to work.

"Oh, you shouldn't have to do that, Dr. Rose," said a nurse from the doorway.

"No, that's okay," he said, "I'll finish him up."

"But it's not your job. I'll call a candy striper."

"I want to do it."

"Doctor," she said firmly, with a hint of anger, "it is against hospital policy." They looked at each other. "There's a candy striper at the nursing station."

Orville started to see red. All of his frustration seemed to gather just behind his eyes, and he felt his face get hard—he felt himself about to lash out at her.

But then he saw her not only as she was just then, but as her story, her life. He knew it well, for she had been a classmate of his in high school and a patient of Bill's and his. He saw her, then, as the dairy farmer's daughter who'd gotten involved with one of the high school brutes who'd impregnated her in her junior year. She dropped out in disgrace and married him and had twin girls, and the brute, when the twins were about a year old, finished bathing one girl and came out of the bathroom with her while the other girl fell into the diaper pail and drowned. Things went to hell. The brute left. Single motherhood. Somehow she pulled herself up and became a nurse known in the hospital as a stickler for protocol and for her insane dedication—it had become her life, now that the surviving daughter was out of the house and living in Tucson—but she was a good nurse. You don't recover from that, Orville said to himself now, from that baby head-down in the diaper pail, you don't recover, you change. And she had.

"I'm sorry, Cindy," he said softly, meaning he was sorry for her suffering and appreciating her making it back, to here with him and Bill, to now.

"You see, I feel so bad for Bill and I want to do something for him, some last thing, before he dies."

His softening softened her. Tears came to her eyes. "Sorry, Orvy," she said. "You go ahead. Call when . . . if you need us."

"Thanks, Cindy. I will."

She left. He resumed shaving.

With Bill's sobbing and cursing it wasn't a neat job. Nicks oozed poorly-oxygenated blood the color of a sluggish stream reflecting a dark red sunset. He stopped the oozing with a styptic pencil. As Orville got into it, feeling, as a guide through the lather under his fingertips, Bill's bristly skin, it was as if he were feeling his own stubble and the razor cutting through his own lather. And then, under his attention it transformed again, so it wasn't even that he was shaving Bill or shaving himself but that shaving was happening. So, he thought, either there is attention, or there is "me"—take your pick. The shaving became a suturing up, across a mirror, across a fleshy gap.

He wiped the last flecks of lather away and took out his bottle of Aloe Vera With Swiss Herbs handcreme he used to keep the skin of his too-often-washed hands from cracking and splitting. He massaged it into Bill's papery skin, softening it.

"Okay, Bill," he said, "now you get the extra-special super-duper treatment, for only our best customers. Miranda gave me this." He took out a spritzer of Caswell-Massey Cologne Spray Number 6, which Miranda had told him was the one made by the same firm two hundred years ago for the Father of Our Country, George Washington. It wasn't until he'd George Washington'd Bill up that he realized the old guy had fallen silent.

Something else is happening, he thought. In him, in me, in us, beyond us. I'm his mother now. He's my son. Help him go.

He pumped the bottle of lotion and took Bill's hand and stroked it firmly, drawing the skin over the bones so that he was making deep contact, the knuckles like marbles in a child's velvet bag, the bones like long stones. He bent to Bill's ear.

"You can go now, Bill."

Orville's only clue to his getting through to Bill as he moved on to his chest, the ribbed box above his thrumming bird's heart, was his own feeling inside his own chest, an answering thrum, a chill, a sense of excitement and sadness all at once at a leaving and also an arrival. Bill is leaving and arriving, he thought, and I'm arriving and leaving and it's the same trip, really.

Bill was still. Breathing lightly but still. Announcing that he was now dying.

His dying is forcing me to announce that I'm still living, Orville thought, right here, right now with this old man. It isn't his heart or my heart, it's the human heart, the human journey, common and ordinary and a big deal and a small deal both and the only deal really and available to us all at no extra cost if we can face it, bear it, share it.

The moment wasn't mystical or sad or scary or corny, it was just a moment. It shone.

Having forgotten to spray Bill's thorax with cologne, he went back and did it, whispering in Bill's ear, "Hey old friend, you can go now, y'see?"

And so on down his body, patting his still-fat tummy, this little boy's universal tummy that a mother had once patted with such delight, playfully, patty-cake, patty-cake.

"You're going out a little under your fighting weight, Bill, but it's okay."

And even Bill's groin, the purple-crowned penis that had had its share of adventures in repayment for his tending the whores on Diamond Street.

"Two dollars a house call, Bill, and you never came away empty-handed."

He took out his comb and combed Bill's thin hair, gray lines on a shiny dome.

"You can go now, Bill."

Orville arranged Bill's flaccid gleaming limbs in as dignified a position as possible and drew the sheet back up, leaving the arms and hands outside, palms up. Sitting there still for a moment, in silence, Orville knew that he was talking not just to Bill, but to his own mother as well. She was still dead and had stopped flying. He felt a rush, a yearning, rocking him back in his chair. He tried to get his arms around what he yearned for. It was the same heartrending yearning he'd felt for the woman he loved when he lost her, and for the boy. Maybe the yearning is feeling seen by death, a boy gone.

He rose and walked to the door and gestured down the hallway for the nurse. He asked her to tell Babette to come in.

Babette came quickly. She had changed into a billowing muumuu with hibisci in bloom and a panther about to pounce, and a straw hat sporting guavas. Earrings featuring plastic bananas hung down. She saw in Orville's glance what was what.

"No, not yet!" she cried out. "Please, no!"

Orville brought her to Bill's bedside. She sat on the bed and removed her hat.

"He looks so sweet," she blurted out. Tears were running through her makeup like rain through dust. "So young. He's like a little baby! Sweet. And he smells so nice."

Orville took her hand and showed her how to massage his hand, his cheek, with him. Soon her hand relaxed. He felt her feeling what he had felt: her husband's torment lessened, lightened, as if the light from the room had been drawn into him. Within that body lying there, almost a glow. Lambent.

She started sobbing. Orville sat beside her and put his arm around her broad back. She cried into his neck. The spasm left. She pulled away.

"Babette," he said, "listen." He took her hand. He turned to Bill and put her hand upon Bill's open palm and said firmly, "You can go now, Bill."

"No! No you can't!" She tugged Orville's hand away and held it up above the sheets.

"Go on." He put her hand once again on Bill's open palm. "You tell him."

They sat motionless, and silent, for what seemed a long time.

Babette moved Bill's hand, in hers, to her lap. Looking down at it shyly like a little girl who is talking to an imaginary friend so important that she's more real than a live one, she said, "Scally?"

Embarrassed, she looked up at Orville and said, "That's what I called him, y'know, all these years, our secret name. 'Scally' for the scallions he loved so much. He called me that name too, 'Scally.' We never told anybody, it was so silly—'Dr. and Mrs. Scally' we called ourselves at home and we laughed—oh, we laughed! It was silly but it was ours, our whole lives . . ."

She broke down again. Then, lifting her head to look at Bill squarely, and with each word more sure, she became the wife, the woman who had stayed right there with him just like this all these years no matter what. The woman who had, in a pinch, shown up with him and helped him as a good mother might. Through the early death of their handicapped only child and the trials of doctoring Columbians and all the secrets and lies and truths of the life of the town that they shared, because the only person he could tell them to was her.

"Scally, can you hear me? It's all right. You . . . you. . . ." She turned to Orville. "I can't."

He smiled at her. Put a hand on her shoulder.

"You . . . you can go now, my . . . my dearest love."

They both felt a wave of sorrow. Tears came to Orville's eyes, eased down his cheeks. Babette sobbed hard. Her whole body shook. The plastic banana earrings swung wildly against her neck, trees in a hurricane.

They sat together on Bill's bed. Everything was still.

As they calmed they became aware that the light had gone out of Bill. Orville leaned over and felt for a carotid pulse. Still there, some. His body was not dead, but his spirit was somewhere else. You could never have measured it, yet for the past hour Orville had felt it had been there, as the pilot flame of a furnace in an old house is there—and now it was not. There, not. The old house, floor by floor, cools.

Babette wept more gently now, tears of release washing out the fear.

"He'll be all right now, dear," Orville said, rising. His hand still rested on her shoulder, much as Bill's, at the right times, had rested on his. "He'll be fine."

A few nurses were in the doorway.

"He'll be going now," he said to them. "Soon."

They began to cry. He started to make his way out, past them, feeling really old. Old age spread its wings in him, and he felt the creaking of betrayal.

"Are you leaving?" Babette cried out, again fearful.

"No, dear. I'll just be down the hall."

Bill's body kept on for a few more hours of its eighty-third year in the world and then stopped. By that time their tears had softened, washed of fear. What was there to be afraid of anymore? The softened tears were those of surrender to Bill's life, to the way his life had been aligned with all of theirs for both a long time and a brief time and a final time. The surrender was to being part of something greater, which can't help but bring a sense of awe.

Like, Orville thought, when you stand in a redwood grove and look up or stand on a canyon rim and look down or you hold your baby in your arms who one day if you're lucky will be holding you in his or her arms, and you realize that your life is a speck in the time of that redwood or in the stone of that canyon or the revolution of that baby and that man. The awe of being a part of a whole, even for a moment of your life.

Out of nowhere came a crush of despair, knocking him down mercilessly, a hellbent descent. I'm alone. Alone! Who can I call? Miranda? No. Who?

He looked at the clock. Past midnight. Morning in Rome. He picked up the phone.

34

Two days later, on the morning of the Columbus Day and Bill Starbuck Funeral Parade, Columbians awoke to find their town prematurely glazed with ice. During the night a freak ice storm had hit. Worse, it had hit on one of those "bad cement days," when the dust spewing from the Universal Atlas and the Lone Star was fierce and the wind was wrong.

Everything was coated in ice. Thick ice. Concretized ice. Over and over, Columbians, walking out their front doors, looked with wonder at the fairyland of glazed trees and bushes and houses and cars and were startled to find their legs going out from under them and the porch or steps or walk coming up to meet them. For a sickening instant they were suspended above the world. Then came a sickening *thwaPP!* Down, they tried gingerly to move things like elbows and knees and backs and butts to see if anything was broken. It did not bode well for the combined holiday and funeral parade.

Cray and Amy had stayed over at Orville's house. Orville would be leaving the following day, and Cray had come up with the idea that he and Amy, together, should have a sleepover with Uncle O. After all, there was no school on Columbus Day. They could all go to the parade together. Miranda and Penny could meet them there.

The sleepover had been wild and fun—they stayed up until two in the morning. Cray had lost a tooth, and they'd put it under the pillow for the tooth fairy. Cray wondered how she'd know that he wasn't at home. Amy assured him that she had her ways.

Both kids slept late, so late that Orville had to wake them both and rush to get the finicky Cray his ritual breakfast. The tooth fairy left a five-dollar bill. Cray was high as a kite.

"When I put my tongue where my tooth was," Cray said, "it feels all like soft butter."

Finally they were done and dressed warmly and out the front door. They stood for a second staring at the crystalline world. The Courthouse Square was glistening in the bright sunlight. All the trees, every single one and every single inch of each one, were coated in ice. The pricker bushes just off the porch steps were bent over by the concretized ice, as if in pain. Orville stared at the black twigs at the core of the icy fingers. Further off, the black skeleton of each bush and tree diminished into a hazy dendritic array much like, he thought, the nerve cells in our brains haze off to connect with other hazed-out dendrites, making the connections that allow us to build bridges and go to the moon and tell stories and get lost and find each other again and see the pattern in the ice storm and the connections with the pattern in the brain and be in the mysteries of flight and of the divine. From a distance, all that was left of trees were vaguely treelike clouds of sparkling ice, delicate as water or rain, transformed to huge glittering lollipops, enticing in the angled light of the autumn sun. The ice gave off a bluish hue—a shade of portent. He breathed deeply, trying to take in the moment forever.

Cray took a running start, skidded down the steps and then, waving his arms to balance on the walk, fell into a pricker bush, grabbing at it to break his fall. Twigs snapped off.

"Look," Cray said, holding up a bunch and looking at the core of black in the white-blue ice, "like the legs of insects, or crabs."

"Or of elephants," said Orville.

"Elephants? Are you crazy?"

"Yes, I am."

"He told me once," Amy said to Cray, "that his mind is so crazy it should be *illegal.*"

"And it is, you know," Orville said. "Americo issued a proclamation the other day saying that it's illegal in Columbia to have a mind like mine. But in Italy it's not."

"It's not illegal in Italy?"

"Illegal?" he said in mock amazement. "In Italy it's not only legal, it's a religion. They've built a fountain to it called the Orvy's Mind Fountain. Tourists throw pennies into it, and—"

"Really, Orvy?" Cray asked, wide-eyed.

"Don't believe anything he says, Cray."

"Exactly," Orville said. "You'd be crazy to. Come on, my little miracles, let's rock and *roll!*"

They did, slipping and sliding and sprinting and sailing along the iced pavement, around the edge of the square to Fourth, and down Washington to the Episcopal Church for Bill's memorial service.

Because of the weather the church was not full. Driving was impossible, walking a risk. Fewer than a hundred hardy souls had come out to say goodbye to Bill. In the front row was Babette, all in black with a pillbox hat and veil almost covering her silver hair. Something on her lapel glittered green and white—a small jade scallion? Beside her was a man in deepest black with a large head of shocking white hair.

Henry Schooner. Alone. Orville hadn't seen him since the night the breakfront had fallen on Maxie. At Albany Medical, they'd set the leg but the prognosis for full recovery of the leg was not good. They'd flown him down to Texas Children's Hospital in Houston. Nelda Jo's father, a rich oil and gas man from Bartlesville, Oklahoma, had contacts there. Henry had been in Houston for the past ten days. He'd issued a statement about the tragedy and was suspending his campaign until further notice. Someone had taken a photo of them leaving Albany Medical for the airport. Henry and Nelda Jo, in perfect black, on either side of Maxie on a stretcher, a desolate look in the boy's eyes.

Good for him, Orville thought now, to come for Bill. And yet, and yet. No one had talked much about *how* the breakfront had come to fall on the boy. Just a tragic accident, that's all. But Orville knew it would have taken something much more for it to fall, not just a boy bumping into it or even running into it. Not even an "accident-prone" boy, no.

Orville consciously lifted his gaze up over Henry's head to the altar, to Bill.

His casket lay in the front of the soaring nave, a relic of times without breakage in Columbia, when soarings were possible. Orville was surprised to find himself so aware of the history of the town and of how Bill fit into it. Everything he saw and heard reminded him of Miranda showing him things in their "historical outings" when they first fell in love. Like her pointing out to him the name "Starbuck" on the original "List of the Proprietors of Columbia," the 1783 parchment brought out by Mrs. Tarr in the DAR Library after they—with Amy—had picketed for the Worth. Like why he and Cray and Amy and the other mourners were sitting in an Episcopal church rather than a Quaker one—because the discovery of oil had led to the victory of the whores and gamblers, depleting the Nantucket Quaker stock until all that was left of their grand utopian endeavor was that one-room Meeting House down on Coffin.

That day with her at the Meeting House, he recalled now, I had let go. Told her of my dismay at being the doctor for the Columbians. She laughed, said "Yes!" and took me to the Library and showed me the documents, the Town Seal, told me the story. For the first time, *my* history linked arms with *history.* She understood what I'd gone through, made me feel I was okay. That day, in the cold outside the Library, we fell in love.

Miranda was supposed to have met them at the church. He figured the weather had prevented her from getting out of the house—the walk was too icy to risk it alone, and scraping her car off and getting it out would have been too much. Or maybe she'd tried and had fallen down and couldn't get up? He felt a touch of cold sweat. Should he go back to the house and call her? No, calm down. She's resourceful, sensible. She'd never put herself in danger that way. Probably waiting for the salt she threw down to work. Or was she reluctant to see him again after the argument in the leaf pile?

The eulogy was going on. Toby oop den Dyke, editor of *The Crier,* was telling Bill's story. With muffled coughs and nose blowings, Columbians started to weep.

The day before, Orville had closed down Bill's office. He went in the IN, sat in Bill's chair, feeling how the seat now had a year's worth of his own butt indented in its leather—a small refinement of Bill's big butt sitting there for a half-century, but still a kind of signature. He stared up at the twelve-point buck with the glazed eyes, at the photo of the early Columbian town doctor with his gun and jaunty cowboy hat and tragic end, at the chrome stirrups, at the big ornamental bottle of Starbusol, more bottles of the stuff stashed all around the place. Saw himself as a boy being understood—no, loved, for it *was* love between Bill and him, wise love—being started on his journey of trying to care, trying to help.

Leaning back in the leather chair, staring up at the stamped-tin ceiling, a thought came to him: *What if I stayed?*

Suddenly it was as if he were seeing himself floating up there, looking down on himself ten years on. There he was down there—older, fatter, balder—sitting with a patient, half-listening to her, someone he couldn't identify. Ten years on, sitting there doing his thing as Bill had always done his thing and as had all the other doctors all the way back to the days of the Wild West.

Great, just great, he'd said to himself, getting up to go, you're starting to see *yourself* flying around! Time to hightail it outta town, partner.

Leaving, he'd taken two souvenirs: a small bottle of Starbusol and a prescription pad reading *Willam Starbuck, M.D.* He'd failed to find a successor. This was the end of the line. Even if a new doctor came to Columbia, he or she would never want this little old house in the bad part of town as an office. He went out the OUT and locked the door behind him. The circle of doctoring here had gone flatline. He felt shaken.

"In 1830," Toby oop den Dyke was saying now, "when the Columbian economy died and the other Quaker merchants left, Bill's great-grandfather, Caleb Starbuck, stayed. A hundred years later, Starbucks were still here. Bill

303

opened his practice in 1929. He left just once, to serve in World War II in England. Thus, today, our military parade. He came back and practiced until 1984. Fifty-five years. And for all those years, if we called, Bill came. In tough times, he always would tell me, 'Y'know, I think I've had enough of this work. I'm gonna leave, day after tomorrow. Heh heh.'"

Everybody laughed—they'd all heard Bill say it.

Orville found himself wishing that he had been asked to speak, that he could have publicly shared his love of Bill with everyone. But you haven't earned it, he said to himself. You're nothing to this town, to these people. In their minds, you're history.

"Many of you were brought into the world by Bill," Toby was saying. "Many more of you were cared for by him, and the cemetery where we'll lay him to rest in a few minutes is filled with those he helped on their last . journey out. What better tribute could there be to a man's life than to know that if you go anywhere in Columbia, or even anywhere in Kinderhook County, if you mention the name 'Bill' in a certain way, people know who you mean. More than that, people *understand.* We all love you, Bill, and we'll miss you." Toby stopped. Even he, the epitome of journalistic deflection and Yankee control, choked up. Columbians broke down and wept with him. The coughing and nose blowing and little cries signified the softening contagion of grief. "Bill," Toby finished, "go in peace."

The casket was carried out by the men and placed in an old open farm wagon made of wood and iron, with iron-rimmed spoked wheels, a relic from a farmer whose life Bill had saved three times in three different ways. It was driven by the farmer and pulled by a team of two matched roan mares. Ahead, a saddled but riderless black gelding at the end of a long lead line pranced on the icy roadbed, startled by the crowd, its hooves going *Clack, tee-clack! Clackettee clack!* like gunshots off the concrete ice. Its breath made tailed cylinders of clouds in the clear air of the strangely cold October morning. The image of the horse-drawn carriage and riderless black horse called back to those old enough the funeral procession of John F. Kennedy, that bitterly cold and shiny day—much like his Inaugural Day when Robert Frost couldn't see to read his poem because of the glare and recited it by heart—that bitter day that broke America's spirit.

Bill's war marched first. Following the color guard and veterans of Bill's war came the Fish Hawk Marching Band and the riderless horse and the wagon with the casket and the veterans of other wars. The sole remaining Spanish-American War veteran had been carted in from his nursing home and bundled up and wedged upright in between Babette and Americo in the mayor's pink Caddy convertible. Americo waved politically, Babette nodded uncomfortably, and the vet wobbled to and fro with each grand arc of the mayor's arm. Just behind them walked the dignitaries of Columbia, and in that line was Henry Schooner. He wore a smart full-length black cashmere coat and a serene black homburg hat. His hair was a white ring under the black rim—the very picture of mourning. Mostly he walked with his head bowed. Occasionally he would lift his chin as if bravely confronting some inevitable horror that lay ahead for him and for America.

Every war after was represented nicely, even Vietnam. The Vietnam vets, Hayley's son Whiz and Tommy Kline of Whale Oil and Gas among them, were classmates of Orville. They wore combat pajamas and floppy jungle hats in contrast to the snappy regimentals and dress hats or movie helmets of all the other wars. Greenie Sellers, in what Orville recognized as an Italian traffic cop's uniform and hat, marched hand in hand with Blinky the Clown, who carried a flag with a flower that read, I LOVE BEGONIAS.

Orville walked with the regular Columbians, Amy holding one hand and Cray the other. Penny joined them. Her colorfully feathered black hat was enormous. Good for her, he thought, adding a *zetz* to the parade.

Columbus Day itself was the minor motif this year. The Knights of Columbus carried fake blunderbusses as they walked alongside a float in which three little girls in cutout ships labeled the *Nina,* the *Pinta,* and the *Santa Maria* walked around among a passel of lolling, pipe-smoking Indians.

Public Works had sanded and salted Washington, sort of. It worked okay from Second to Fourth, where the grade was a little downhill, but after the parade crossed the dip at Fourth where the bones of the old stone bridge lay buried, the path was uphill, and there was much slipping and sliding. The horses had the hardest time, their iron shoes uneasy on the ice. The wagon slid here and there, the flower-strewn casket sliding too, bouncing against the wooden slats on either side of the wagon bed with an ominous *Thunk! Thunk! Thunk!* so that everyone began to fear that sooner or later they would get to see dear old Bill one more time, popping out of the smashed coffin and sliding back down the middle of Washington Street toward the river, as if he wanted to put in one final morning at the office.

But no. The parade made it up Washington and went left on Cemetery past the hospital, the ranks of nurses, orderlies, and candy stripers, in white and green and peppermint uniforms, crisp and bright in the glancing sunlight, standing tall, many of them weeping. They would miss this roly-poly man who always seemed to be present, chuckling to himself at the latest folly of human beings—and somehow turning that chuckle into compassion. Something, Orville thought, seeing it all, that I've failed to do this year.

Finally they turned into the Fish and Game Club Road and then into the cemetery bordered by what Orville had always known as "The Artificial"—an artificial small pond. They walked up to the highest hill. Soon, everyone was gathered around a hole in the ground in the shadow of a granite obelisk featuring what else but a whale in relief and the chiseled name STARBUCK. Sure enough, here were however many generations of Starbucks it had taken to get from 1783 to 1984. The plot faced east toward Nantucket, a long way away even as the crow flies across the rolling, stream-stitched land tended by the farmers Bill had tended, land that bunched up into the Taconics before they themselves bunched up into the Berkshires. The air was so cold you could see a long time.

The burial ceremony was brief. Prayers were said. The Quaker hymn that ended with "turning, turning, we come down right" was sung. Tears were shed as Bill was lowered into the ground. Orville was dry-eyed, feeling more somber than sad. He had already said good-bye. Dirt was thrown. Pebbles danced on the coffin lid. Flowers were strewn. Guns were fired into the air at an acute angle. The sun went behind a cloud, the wind whipped up. As "Taps" was played, Cray tugged on Orville's jacket.

"I gotta poop."

"Really?"

"Bad."

"Okay." He whispered to Amy, "Cray's gotta poop. Back in a few minutes."

But it was hard to find a place, and it took a long time. When they walked back up the path to the cemetery everyone was gone, including Amy. Where was she? Should they leave and walk back downtown? Wait for her here?

Cray was impatient. Orville scanned the cemetery, from the rippling pond cradled by the yellowing willows around to the newer part. Nothing. He started walking back down the hill, and soon got a little lost, except for knowing most of the names on the headstones.

I've treated a lot of these families this year, he thought. I know who they came from, who they've left behind. Nowhere else in my life and my travels have I felt that kind of depth. No, not depth exactly, more a longitude and latitude, a people's history of this place.

He thought he heard something and cocked his head toward the sound. There, on top of a hill, in silhouette against the low sun, were two figures, one small, one large. They were gesturing and shouting, but they were downwind and their words were carried away from him. The small shape started sliding on the ice down the hill toward him and Cray, whirling on its butt, throwing its arms around. Amy! She was red-cheeked and screaming happily and plowed into Cray, knocking him down, to his great delight, so that the two of them spun on the ice together a few yards until they stopped.

"Who's up there?" Orville asked Amy.

"Mom. She wants us to follow her."

"Why?"

"Got a present for you, a like going-away thingee. C'mon." She held out her hand.

"Is her car over there?"

"Yeah, she's got her car."

He saw that Penny was gesturing them vigorously to meet her around the other side of the hill, to the left. He took Cray's hand. It was bare. "Hey, where are your gloves?"

"Lost 'em," he screamed proudly. "You'n me are in double trouble with Mom now!"

The kids didn't want to go on the road around the hill but straight up it. The three of them started up the slope toward where Penny had been. Slipping and sliding, sometimes Amy or Cray holding Orville up, sometimes Orville, standing, lifting them up, all the time falling, rolling back, laughing. Only by falling and getting up and leaning on each other at the right time and even on their bellies for a while with shared clawing fingerholds, did they make it to the top. All the way up they were laughing 'til the tears came at who fell how and who dragged who down and who picked who up. Orville took a few hard falls. As they neared the top he was sore and cold and breathing hard. Kids have a lower center of gravity, he thought, less far to fall. With us grownups, so much always seems to hang on so little.

Penny was no longer at the crest of the hill but way down below. The feathers of her hat were a lone spot of color in all the blueish white.

"Let's slide!" Amy cried, sitting down and pulling Cray down with her. Orville lost his footing and went down too. The kids pushed off. He followed, whirling around, losing his bearings, loving the losing. They tried to steer toward Penny and her hat. In a sweet instant the three of them were lying there looking up at her, laughing hard.

"Hi, Pen!" Orville cried excitedly. "What's up?"

"Look." She pointed to a tombstone into which was chiseled SELMA ARIEL FLEISHER ROSE. Beside it was a stone for SOLOMON ROSE.

"I come here every time I'm at the cemetery," she said. "I talk to her. Amy does, too. I don't talk to Dad. I mean, I never really could. You've never been here, have you?"

"Not since Dad." He got up, first knees, then one foot, then feet.

They stood side by side staring at the matching stones, each a polished pink granite. Hebrew letters straggled across. Orville looked down at the red-haired little boy beside him, focusing in on how all this death would affect Cray.

His father is lying dead somewhere, below ground. And I'm about to disappear too. Take care. For the boy's sake.

"Okay, everybody," Penny said with high purpose. "Now we take a stone and put it on top of whichever tombstone we want. Then we say something to that person."

"Why can't we do both people?" Amy asked. "Both Grandma and Poppa?"

"Fine," Penny said tersely. "You can do both."

"But where are the stones?" Cray asked, looking around the ice field. "They're all under the ice."

"I brought stones," said Penny reaching into her purse. She took out a plastic bag in which there were smooth round stones, which she placed in their open palms. "Four stones. One for each of us."

Penny and Cray tried to place their stones on the top ridges of the tombstones—Penny on Selma, Cray on Sol—but the ice-film wouldn't let them stay. They kept slipping off, dropping down onto the icy ground, popping up and skittering away like live beings.

"They won't stay!" cried Cray.

"We'll chisel little hollows for them," Orville said, "little homes." He took out his Swiss Army knife, chose the chiseling blade, and started hacking away at ice coating the top of the tombstones, carving out four neat resting places for the stones—three for Selma, one for Sol.

They all placed their stones. The stones stayed.

"Now," Penny said, "we talk to them."

"Penny, I'm not sure that's such a good idea—" Orville began, trying to indicate the presence of Cray.

"Me first!" cried Amy.

"No, me, me!" cried Cray, louder.

"Okay, Cray," Amy said, "go ahead."

Cray just stood there, not knowing what to say. "I don't wanna any-more." He slid behind Orville's back, holding onto the man's pant legs.

"Penny, I really mean it, that's enough. Cray doesn't want to."

"Okay, then," Amy said, "I'll go next."

"Wait." Orville bent down and whispered in Cray's ear. "You wanna leave? You and me can go if you want. Really. We don't have to stay."

Cray looked down at his feet, then up at Orville, then at Amy. "I wanna stay."

"Okay. But anytime you want to leave, you tell me and we're outta here."

"'Kay," said Amy. "My turn." She closed her eyes and considered.

The wind whipped them savagely.

"Darling," Penny said, "it's really cold, and if you could hurry up a lit—"

"Grandma Selma, I love you and miss you. I'm doing good in school and theater. I'm gonna miss Orvy. He leaves tomorrow morning. See you soon." She paused. "Not *soon* soon, I hope, not in Heaven, but see you in my mind's eye, like you really are. Wait, no—not *are*, but like you really *were!* I want to end with a quote from *The Merchant of Venice*. I played Portia—'a wonderful, pint-sized Portia' *The Crier* said." She looked up and spoke to the sky—making Orville wonder if she, too, had been secretly seeing Selma up there. "'That light we see is burning in my hall. How far that little candle throws its beams! So shines a good deed in a naughty world.' I will always love you, Grandma. Forever."

Penny looked to Orville. He gestured to her to go ahead.

"Mom," she said, "it's good to be here again. Amy, as you heard, is do-ing great. Milt's doing, well . . . Milt's doing Milt. He just came back from Hong Kong this morning, imagine? Something to do with what he calls PCs, personal computers. Milton Plotkin, Hong Kong? Me? I could lose a few pounds but. . . . We're happy Orvy's finally made up his mind to go—I mean, he's better off in Italy, and our stress level will fall with him gone. Um, I mean, we'll miss him terribly, but *bon voyage!* Now. Going through my stuff I found this letter you wrote. When you were at home recovering from your brain surgery. Orvy's never seen it."

Inwardly Orville groaned. Another letter? He looked up, thinking he'd see her. Nope. He got more concerned for Cray. The boy was standing in front of him, and Orville put both arms around him. Selma might say *any-thing.*

Penny dug into her purse but didn't come up with the letter. She dug and dug, and finally bent down and emptied her purse out on the ground where Sol lay, so that the lipstick tubes and BMW keys as big as mice and wallets and sugar-free candies and Mars Bars and pill bottles spilled out onto the ice covering him. No letter.

"Try your pocket, Mom."

Penny tried. "Found it!"

"I'm freezing!" Amy said. "Hurry up. I'll pick up your things while you read."

Penny read.

Dear children,

When I was in the hospital after my surgery I wasn't sure I wanted to live. When your father brought me home, as Hayley and he helped me upstairs into the house, my hair gone and me wearing a turban and veil covering the dead half of my face, that first day, Penny, you saw me and I saw the shock in your eyes, and that was hard, but the hardest was when Orvy saw me—I could only make him out dimly through the veil and my one good eye—I saw his horror, as if instead of seeing his mom who had left as a beautiful woman many weeks before he saw a monster and he took one look and ran out of the house and didn't come home 'til after dark. Do you know what it's like to see your child be disgusted and terrified by your *looks?* I could have given up then and not ever gone out again. I could have just been a cripple. I sat in the bathroom in front of the mirror and asked, "Why God, why should I live, after what they did to me, after my looks have been destroyed?" I cried and cried. And then God said to me, "Selma, you have to live for the children, and for their children." So, I lived for you. I sat in the bathroom day after day moving my shoulder so my face would move a little—they transplanted a nerve they said might take, grow a millimeter a month, and I'd be able to blink my eye, and smile my smile, half a smile, anyway. (Good surgeons, *bad* men.) And I turned my attention to trying to do good for others, and for our poor neglected little town Sol brought me to against my will for the toy store. I lived for you two.

I hope now you live for me. I was about love. I never was all that good at it, I mean love, but I tried my best. Maybe love is just not giving up on people?

All my love my dears,
Your mother

Penny's voice shook. Tears ran down her cheeks. She folded the letter and held onto it.

Orville was moved by Penny's sorrow. But his focus was on Cray, on what the boy would make of all this. He felt sad at what Selma had gone through, sure, but his heart was closed.

The irony, he thought, is that her convincing me that I'm selfish and coldhearted forced me to be that to her. With her, I acted like the most selfish person in the world. But not with others, no. I wasn't as bad with them. Not a monster, no. Selma's contempt produced the very thing she was contemptuous of. She blasted me with the worst of herself and got the worst of me back. Maybe I can't be open to this letter of hers because of all her other letters?

But seeing his sister in pain, knowing that she was stuck for the rest of her life with a real *schlemozzle* of a husband in this neglected backwater, got to him. He put his arm around her shoulders. To his surprise, she stopped crying and pulled away.

Looking at him expectantly, she said, "So?"

He felt a sense of dread, rising.

"*So?*" she said again, more insistently.

"The lady sure writes a mean letter."

She gave him a look. "Please, do not joke. Your turn to talk to her." She waited.

He faced the stone. Faced it more. Finally he said, "Mom, I'm sorry."

Silence. He turned away to leave.

"That's *it?*" Penny cried. "After all this, and your leaving again tomorrow, and *that's it?*"

"Seemed like a lot, to me."

"But Mom," Amy said, "he *said* he was sorry."

"It was nothing," Penny said coldly. "Virtually, I mean."

"I thought it had a lot of good qualities," he said.

"After all *this,*" Penny went on, "just *that?*"

"Mom, I don't believe you! He meant it! It's what he wants to say to his mom! To Grandma! I think it was neat!"

"Fine," Penny said, her tone making it clear that it might have been a lot of things but one thing it was not was fine. She took out her plastic bag. "Let's put the stones back in the baggie and we're done." She picked one off Sol and moved on to pick off the three others sitting on Selma.

"No!" Amy said. "You can't take 'em back, Mom. They have to stay.

Sometimes I think you *dream* of plastic baggies! Like you'd put me and dad in 'em if you could only find ones big enough!" Amy started to cry.

"I . . . I'm sorry, honey," Penny said in a shocked voice. "You're right, I mean, they should stay." Penny was losing it, looking around distractedly as if, Orville thought, she was expecting to be rescued by a flying Selma. "They stay. What a mess I've made. Don't worry, I . . . you . . ." Penny started to cry, too, really hard.

Amy stared at her, amazed.

"I'm sorry, sorry sorry, honey, okay?" She paused. "Okay?"

Amy did not say okay.

"Oh!" Penny cried. "I always do everything wroooonnng!"

"It's okay, Sis," Orville said, putting his arms out to her. She fell heavily against his chest so that he started to slide and had to do some fancy footwork to stay up. She was sobbing, really hard. "Now, now . . ."

Penny blew her nose. "Okay. See those three markers, Orvy?" She pointed to three small marker stones, lying flat under the ice. "The two together on mom's side are for Milt and me. The other, Orvy, next to Sol? It's for you. If you'll, you know, well . . . accept it?"

He was startled. To be brought back from wherever he died to lie *here?*

He stared up at the clouds and again it was as if he were seeing himself up above the scene, looking down at his own funeral a few decades ahead. People were laying him to rest. A surprisingly large crowd of Columbians had gathered, as if appreciative that he had stayed on as their doctor for all those years.

"I'd be honored, Pen," he said.

"You would? *Honestly?*"

"Don't push it."

"Right. Now. Let's all go home and have a nice hot cup of . . . of hot nice chocolate." She turned to go back to the car.

"My turn." It was Cray. He went to Sol's grave. "That's your dad, Orvy?"

"That's right."

"He died. My dad died. I'm sorry you died. But you were old. My dad's plane crashed and he was young." He turned to Orville. "And you're going on a plane tomorrow, a long way away and *you* can die." The boy was looking up at him, his eyes pleading.

"Those big jet planes are really safe now, Cray."

"But you can die, right?" Orville nodded. "And Mom and I'll be left?"

"Yeah."

"Maybe Mom and I can go with you, so if you die, we die too?"

"Your mom and you can't go with me."

"Why not?"

"Well, because you've got school and she's got her work and—"

"I hate school."

"Yeah, I know, everybody does, but she can't come with me."

"Well, why you goin' then?"

Cray's green eyes were asking him for the truth, but the only truth Orville could tell him was a lie. It was like Bill showing him that the truth for some patients is a lie, a lie against the life force because if you tell them they're going to die, you'll hasten their death. And besides, you never know anyway, because even if everything points to their dying soon, well, they're Columbians and sometimes it's as if they've aquired a measure of immunity to the final breakage, and they can go on and on. Just look at Mrs. Tarr who yesterday with her oxygen tank went *bowling* for Chrissakes! It's not about their bodies, it's about something else. The truth Cray needed then was a lie.

"I've got a job there. You'll come visit, you and Amy."

"But if me'n Mom went with you and the plane crashed, we'd *all* die, so me'n Mom won't be left alone standin' here cryin'." He walked away.

Orville hurried to catch up with him and put a hand on his shoulder. Cray looked up, his face somber, older, sadder. Orville took the little boy's hand, and that was when he started to cry.

35

Is this crazy? Miranda was asking herself later that evening, as she walked carefully around the icy puddles and up the steps and onto the porch of Orville's house. Yes, this is crazy. Especially after the disaster in the leaf pile. Be brave.

By noon that day the wind and weather had done one of those Columbian inversions. The sun came out and the temperature rose, so that the ice was melting rapidly, flushing the cement dust into puddles and pools of gray ice water. The twigs and branches and limbs, liberated from the weight of concretized ice, were springing up higher, resuming their shapes, seeking out just that little extra sunshine to turn into nutrients that would carry them through what promised to be another severe winter.

She had waited until late afternoon, when the footing was solid down her flagstone path to her car. The Ford Country Squire sailed easily over the ruts and rolls of the dirt road out to Route 9 and then south into Columbia. After the parade, Cray had called and asked if he could stay with Amy and Orville the rest of the day and for dinner. Fine by her. She needed the time to finish up some work on her magazine piece, run some errands, and come to final terms with Orville's leaving, not to mention saying goodbye. In her mind all day long was the death of her husband and the effect of Orville's leaving on her son. After dinner she drove over to his house.

It was a bright twilight. In the Courthouse Square the warm air falling down onto the icy ground was combusting to mist, rising in spirals and floating in whorls under the argon streetlamps. Bravely she rang his doorbell. Bravely she was greeted by Orville, Cray, and Amy.

"Can I have another sleepover with Orvy tonight, Mom, please?"

"No," Miranda said.

"Aww, Mom, c'mon!" Miranda said nothing. "Why not?"

"Because tonight it's my turn." She watched Orville's jaw drop. Watched Amy and Cray take it in—at first puzzled, then glad.

"Yeah, but what about me?" Cray asked.

"I checked with Penny. You can sleep over at Amy's tonight, and Penny can drive you all down to pick up Orville and me in the morning so we can take him to his train. If it's okay by Amy." Cray looked at Amy.

"Hey," Amy said nonchalantly, "works for me. Okay, little brother?"

"Yes!" Cray said, fist punching the air.

"Cool," said Amy. "When do we leave?"

"Now. I'll drive you over." She had barely glanced at Orville during this, and now did. "Okay by you?"

He felt a rush of trepidation but then, admiring her gutsiness, said, "Better than okay. Much."

Left alone in the house again after so much kid activity, still raw from walking away from the grave with Cray, he felt lonely and a little frantic. Might as well finish packing. He poured himself a bourbon and relit a Parodi and went up to his bedroom in the turret. He worked for a while, recalling how he'd come into town with only a backpack and an Italian Women's Swim Team sweatshirt. Now he could fill three suitcases. But he was determined to take only the backpack and one suitcase. Starting to travel light again. What do I take with me? What do I do with all the stuff I leave behind? Storage? Trash? What about Starlight? Cray, for some reason, didn't want it; nor did Amy. And the birthday presents? The plaque

314

saying what a great doctor he'd been, the framed blowup of him chained to the Worth, the brass cow from BOTHWAYS FARM, WEST GHENT, the photo of Selma and Durney at Olana, the pen-and-ink sketch of the one-room Ichabod Crane Schoolhouse where he'd met Miranda, the ROME PARIS LONDON COLUMBIA sweatshirt? All these and more he packed in a box for Penny to keep in her basement. Let go, he said to himself. Go lightly.

But then he took back out of the box the photo of the Worth and the sketch of the schoolhouse. These—and a small brass whale and the *Guide to Good Morals* Miranda had given him—he would take with him back to Europe. He turned to the last box, Scomparza Moving and Funeral.

Selma's letters would stay. The bar mitzvah photo of the Family Rose tilted to the left would stay, as would all the other stuff Selma had left him. As he got ready to put the things back in the box and seal it, he found something else that he hadn't noticed before, jammed flat on the bottom of the box. He pried it out. A large wrapped framed something or other. He took a deep breath. She can't hurt me now. He started to rip the brown paper wrapping off one corner, and then heard the front door slam and Miranda call his name.

"Up here," he said. He heard her uneven steps on the stairs.

She came into the turret and saw him sitting on the polished oak floor in the curve formed by the five windows, caught in a shaft of final sunlight. He was still in the white shirt and dark slacks he'd worn to the funeral. The sleeves were rolled up, and he was leaning back on his hands looking up at her and his eyes seemed different—more open, more open *to* something. She had always loved his hands, his doctor's hands, with their fingers more long and delicate than his bulky arms would suggest and, she knew from his touch, more gentle. With his fingers splayed on the floorboards, now, his hands, too, seemed somehow more open. They weren't tight with doctoring. His doctoring here, now, is history. Eyes and hands. Vulnerabilities and innocences. Kindnesses. These were what she loved in him.

All this came to her in a moment, the moment of his smiling at her.

"I didn't think you should be alone tonight," she said. "No one should be alone, their last night anywhere. In front of the kids you said it was okay, but maybe . . . if you don't want me to stay—"

"I do," he said, surprised at what rolled into his head, a line from a Shakespeare sonnet, "My mistress when she walks treads on the ground." "I really appreciate it." How lovely she looked just then to him, standing

315

in the doorway, the last light of the day playing on her red hair, her reassuring green eyes in which he for the longest time had seen not just her but Cray, her lips, strong shoulders, breasts under her baggy lilac sweater, her rumpled jeans with their asymmetric legs. Pain nested in his heart and spread out its wings, much as it had done that moment he'd left Bill's deathbed and had the sudden sense of being old, too old.

He struggled to rise and said, "Let me get you a chair."

"It's okay. I'll sit here on the bed." She did. "There's something I want to tell you," she said.

"Yes?"

"I keep thinking back to our, you know, our horrible argument in the pile of leaves, a few weeks ago, the last time we . . . well, you know."

"Me too."

"Yeah, and I have to clear the air about one thing. It came to me early this morning, as I lay there listening to the sleet come down . . ." She took a deep breath. It all seemed too formal, too wrong—as it always seemed lately with him. "What you said to me, that I didn't know how much power I had, how much I can hurt another person?" Orville nodded. "You were right. I *don't* know that. I can't see that. And this morning, you know, lying there like you do at times like that, I . . . well, what I thought was that maybe it had to do with my own history."

"In what way?"

She knew, but could not say the word. "I'm not sure."

"Polio?"

The word, said out loud, had always filled her with revulsion. She herself would never volunteer it. But now, hearing it from him, she was surprised to find that it was okay. She understood that he understood. She got teary and looked down into her lap.

"Hearing you say that right now, seeing you look so—forgive me, Orvy, but so, so damn handsome and caught in that beautiful light, hearing you, it's strange. I mean, that such a horrible thing could have such a . . . a cheery, musical name."

"I know."

"Even if it does sound Italian." She smiled through her tears.

"I can't win."

"You are," she said kindly. "You're doing fine right now."

"So how does it make sense to you now?"

"Maybe, sometime . . . . But I'm not saying that or doing anything like this just because you're leaving."

"I never would think that you'd—"

"I don't want anything from you tonight. I mean it. But I just had that to say, and didn't want you to be alone."

"I'm glad you're here. Really truly. I'll never forget it. Never."

They sat for a few moments, quietly.

"What's that?" she asked, pointing to the wrapped, framed something.

"Don't know. It was jammed into the bottom of the Selma box. A final blast from the past. Let's see." He ripped the brown paper off. A large, old, black-and-white photograph of hundreds of people in a hazy, gaslit ballroom.

The doorbell. They looked at each other.

"I won't answer," he said.

But right away it rang again, and again. They heard someone try the door, with no luck, and then pound on it.

"I must have locked it when I came in," Miranda said.

"Good. They'll go away. No more patients anymore. None."

"Hey Orvy! Orveee! It's me!" It was a familiar voice, shouting up at them from the square.

"Oh no," he said. "Schooner. I'll get rid of him."

Henry was standing outside at the end of the walk, staring up at the lit-up turret. He saw Orville open the door and started up the pathway, that bulky body rolling smoothly through the mist and the puddles. Orville met him on the porch. For once he was better dressed than Henry, his white shirt and tie and dark slacks and shoes outclassing Henry's jeans, T-shirt, and what looked like a jungle-green flak jacket.

"Everybody's gone!" Henry said, as if this were an important news flash. "My boys are gone. Nelda Jo's gone. Tomorrow you're gone." He sighed. "Can I come in?"

"Not now."

"Aw, c'mon."

"I'm busy."

"Yeah, I know she's here and that's great, just great, but I'm friends with her too. Maxie and Cray, you know, so we can all sit down, have a drink, cup of tea, whatever."

"You been drinking?"

"Not a drop." He crossed himself. "Swear to God. Please?"

"Sorry."

"See that? Y'still don't respect me. Sure, things were rough way back when we were kids, but your mother forgave me, and I've come back and done well." He paused. "Haven't I done well?"

"Depends what that word means."

"I'm gonna be your congressman."

"Not mine, Henry. I'm on a morning train, and I'm not coming back."

"So why don't you respect me?"

"How'd the breakfront come to fall on Maxie?"

He paused, considered. "I don't get your question."

"It didn't just fall. I saw it wobble all year long. In fact, I told you you'd better get it fixed. It wobbled, but it never fell. It would have to be hit hard, real hard, to fall."

"Like from someone bumping into it, sure."

"I bumped into it. It rocked, but it didn't fall."

"What are you implying?"

"That you hit Maxie—or pushed him hard—and he crashed into it. *Hard.*" He paused. "All year long, broken bones, bruises . . . "

Henry stood there in the shadows cast by the porch light, dead still. He didn't look down, or glance away, but kept looking straight at Orville. He just stood there. Bulky, solid, closed.

Strangely, Orville felt himself rooting for Henry right then, rooting for him to tell the truth, whatever it was. Cut the denial bullshit. Ask for help. Redeem yourself.

Finally, taking a step into the porch light, Henry spoke. His voice was the deep, calm, resonant one that was so appealing. "Where to start?" Henry asked, softly, sadly. "I can see, given everything between us, how you would make an insinuendo that I could do something like that. To tell you the truth, my friend, I have done a lot of bad things in my life, things I'm ashamed of, things a man does in war that he can never forget and never tell, things that make what you say I did to you when we were young, well, sort to speak, 'child's play.'" There was a glancing smile, quickly erased.

"But I am a human being," he went on, "with a heart, and with pride, and love. And right now I'm down. But I'm still standing, still trying to answer your . . . accusation. Because I know it comes from your heart. Look at me, Orvy. Look. Am I a man that could even *live* if I'd done something like that to my son, to my little baby boy, my flesh and blood? Could I even *breathe?* No way! I'd have to be some kind of monster. And I'm not. You know I'm not. I swear to God I'm not. And you're right, my friend, you did tell me to get that damn thing fixed, trued up, and I kept saying, 'Tomorrow, I'll do it tomorrow.' And tomorrow was yesterday, now." He fell silent again and just stood there, shoulders hunched, breathing heavily, head fallen on his chest.

A creepy feeling came over Orville. Maybe he's telling the truth? He found himself wavering. The thing *had* wobbled. Maxie *was* a wild kid. Couldn't he have been slamming around the house and crashed into the breakfront and *bam?* But I've believed him before, believed guys like him before and been fooled. With him, you never know. With all these guys, you never know. Maybe they really did kill Kennedy, Martin Luther King, Bobby. Maybe Bush really did go to Paris secretly and bribe the Iranians with money and guns not to release the American hostages until after Reagan won the '80 election. How can you ever know the truth? Years later, maybe. You find a hint of it in the paper ten years later buried on page 17. Discredited by experts. Never happened.

"And so, my friend," Henry was going on, "just for the record—and you can check this out with Nelda Jo or the maid or Maxie himself—I wasn't there when it happened. I was upstairs, getting ready for bed."

Up until that moment, Henry had rocked Orville's certainty, cast doubt. But something about this, a kind of alibi, rocked Orville back. Of course Schooner would lie. Schooners lie. He could not afford to admit it. It might leak, destroy him. Everything he'd fought for since that humiliating day when he'd walked away from me and Tommy and Whiz and the other Fish Hawks and became a soldier and somewhere along the way became A Great American would be lost. At that moment Orville felt that things had become untethered from solid ground. Maybe Henry had done it, maybe not—there was no way to tell. But that's the problem with these guys: not being able to tell, *tells.* We will never know. But we need to know, like a little boy needs to know the truth from his dad or mom. Like Cray needs to know. It *matters.*

Staring into Henry's obscuring ink-black eyes, Orville had a sense of a person to whom it didn't matter, a hollow person, an absent person, creating a hollow world, an absent world. The person as TV, as "president." An impossible world as advertised, taken for normal. It's a world, he thought, that I can't live in.

"Henry," he said bitterly, "as a human being, you're lower than whaleshit."

"Whaleshit?" He thought about this, as if inspecting this with all the presence of mind and objectivity of a marine biologist. "Whaleshit. That's pretty low."

"You bet. You don't even seem that sad about it all."

"I don't?" He was astonished. "I tole' you I was."

"Told me, but you don't really seem it."

319

"I *am* it, pal. I'm pukin' my guts out every single day." He sighed. "But I'm doin' my best to, y'know, be an example. Put a good face on."

Orville had had enough. He started to turn away.

"And what would your dear mother say, hearing you say that to me?"

"What?" He stopped, his hand on the doorknob.

"Your mother. What would she say? She and I were close, you know, after I came back. Told me the truth about you, you know."

"What truth?"

"That you ran. That you ran, pal, that you ran. When she came home, needing someone, all alone with that terrible face, after that terrible surgery, and she asked you, begged you—that was the word she used, *begged*—and what did you do? What the fuck did you do, buddy? You ran. Right?"

"Right," Orville snapped back. "So what?"

"So what goes around comes around, Orvy," Henry said, now with a different voice, a street voice from when they were kids, a bully's voice. "And don't you talk to me about who's low and who's high, who's whaleshit, okay? I have my flaws and I face my flaws every fuckin' day. I've got a son now who can only and *maybe* learn to be a good kid at a military school, and now I've got another son who maybe's never gonna walk right again let alone run, play sports. And I got a wife who, well, never mind—and her *father?* I got shit here, now, in my life, and I got nobody with me in that fuckin' house except those Filipinos and I come over here wantin' to be a friend and only really wantin' to wish you safe journey and what happens? You call me low? *You* call *me* low?" He raised his hands as if to God. "Well, I'll tell you somethin'. I've got shit, and am *I* runnin' away? Is Henry Schooner runnin' away? Am I goin' off to a guru in Europe? Eatin' pasta and drinkin' wine in a place where what happened 300 years ago is more important than what's happenin' now? Am *I* runnin' away?"

"Go to hell!"

"I'm stayin', old sport. I'm a stayer. My life is for shit—thanks to those fuckers out there who are trying to pin every last damn thing on me— thanks to people like you, to the ones who never take a step to try to make things better. For *shit,* now, and am I runnin' away? Am I droppin' out? Think I don't want to? I want to, but I don't."

"You yourself told me to get out, that day in your basement. Told me that if you could, you would too, remember?"

"I want to, but I don't. You want to, and you do. Call *me* whaleshit? God!"

They stood in the gathering night, the night now strangely warm, the drip of the last melting ice the only sound. Rage in both sets of eyes. Orville was trembling.

Henry reached inside his jacket.

Orville flashed on their trip down to Henry's basement, the bullets, the guns. He braced himself, thinking, This is how people get killed. I've seen it over and over again this year in emergency.

He grabbed Schooner, one hand on each side of the jacket, grabbed him hard, to keep him from pulling out the gun. He squeezed, bracing himself for a lot of tough muscle fighting him off. To his astonishment Henry's body wasn't hard and muscular, but soft and fluid, as if filled with toneless flesh. Air-pocketed. Vacant. Orville felt no gun. He let go and backed off, fingers spread in the air.

"What the fuck?" Henry said, astonished, slowly taking a cigar out of his pocket. And then he got it. "You thought . . ." he blinked. "Me?"

"You bet."

"You crazy mother!" He reached into another pocket, shaking his head in amazement, and took out a silver cigar cutter. "Is that what you think of me?"

"That's what I fear about you."

Meticulously, Henry cut the cigar, lit it, and blew a smoke ring up at the light. "Shit. Runnin' from the woman who loves you—you don't even see it, do you? Runnin' from that sweet boy who loves you like a father? Shit."

"Running from people like you."

"Yeah, well, people like me made this country what it is today."

"Exactly."

"Can't run from a town. Y'find another town just like it down the road."

"What's it to you? What the hell do *you* care that I'm leaving?"

"I care 'cause we're like brothers, and I cared—"

"Oh for Chrissakes! Cut it out!"

"—and I cared about you more'n you cared about me. You'n me are alike, the both of us just tryin' to catch up to where we are in our lives, right? Your mom was like a mom to me. 'Henry,' she said to me, 'you're like a good son. I wish Orvy'd be like you.' I said to her, 'No, dear, he's a good son too, just a little rambunctious.' I stood up for you, respected you, and you spit on me. Everybody always spits on me. Underestimates me. Well, guess what? 'Blessed are those persecuted for righteousness' sake, for they will enter the Kingdom of Heaven.' Matthew 5:10."

"You're crazy, really crazy."

"I always wanted your respect, but now, finally, I don't give two shits about your contempt. 'Cause you're at least as low as me. Or as high, brother, or as high." He puffed on the cigar, thinking. "I'm alone now, all alone. But that's fine, because I'll do it myself. I'll do it the American Way—*by your self.* Remember, Orvy, you're born alone, you die alone, and whatever you achieve you do it on your own."

"Henry?"

"What?"

"You're not born alone."

"What do you mean?"

"Nobody's born alone. There's a mother there, remember?"

"Not for me. Not me. I didn't even have one. Not one worth anything. And look at me." Henry spread his arms wide, as if about to flap them in a vain attempt to lift himself up off the porch. "Look."

Orville did look, then. What he saw surprised him. He saw the kid, the child, the child without a real mother, before he grew big enough to shame and bully and beat up the other kids. He saw the fat, lonesome child.

"So long, Henry. I'm sure you're gonna be a big success." He opened the door and took a step into the house.

"Orvy! Lemme in!"

"Sorry, I'm busy. As you said, got someone here who loves me. Night." He started to shut the door.

"One more thing!"

With Schooner, always. He waited, back turned.

"Give me something."

"What?" He turned back to face him.

"I need something from you. To remember you by. I respect you and your mom so much. Give me something."

Orville paused. "Sorry," he said, and without shutting the door he turned his back and went inside, moving down the dark hall toward the kitchen. He stopped in the kitchen doorway and glanced back. Henry was still there on the porch. Orville stood staring from the dark. He could see Henry, but Henry couldn't see him.

Henry's arms stayed up for a while longer and then flapped down to his sides. His head dropped down, too. The whole refrigerator of the man seemed to melt, defrost. He turned around and trudged down the porch steps toward the front gate and his empty house.

Do something kind, Orville thought. Break the cycle. Do something kind.

Orville looked around the kitchen.

PhwweeeeeEEEETT!!

He grabbed the birdcage and the Mexican blanket he used to cover it at night and hurried back up the hallway and out the front door.

"Henry?"

He was at the crosswalk in the middle of the square. He stopped, stood still for a moment with his back to Orville, and then turned around. "Yeah?"

"Here." Orville walked down the walk and Henry walked toward him and they met on the edge of the square. "This is for you."

Henry stared at the bird.

The bird stared at Henry.

PhwweeeeeEEEETT!!

Henry's eyes widened. He smiled. A smile, Orville sensed, not of appreciation so much as victory.

"Hold the cage by the ring at the top," Orville said. He passed it to Henry's waiting index finger. The lovebird migrated from one man's life to another's.

"What's its name?"

"Starlight."

"Starlight." He nodded and smiled. "Orvy, I don't know how to thank you."

"Just take care of it. Here, cover it up—cover it with this blanket at night. The three things that can kill it are drafts, chocolate, and avocado."

"Drafts, chocolate . . ." he seemed to cherish these words, "and avocado."

They stared at each other.

"Better get it home. Drafts, remember?"

"Drafts . . . chocolate . . ."

"Henry?"

"Yeah?"

"You're standing in a puddle."

Henry looked down. He was up to his ankles in a puddle of ice water. When he looked up he was beaming, triumphant, like a child glad to be muddy and wet. As he jumped up lightly from the puddle he called out, "Unhappy feet! Unhappy feet! Yes!"

Holding the cage high he moved quickly away, so quickly that soon, seen from a distance, he and the lovebird seemed to be riding the rising mist, a few inches off the ground.

36

"What did he want?" Miranda asked, as Orville came back into the room. She was still sitting on the bed.

"Who knows. He wanted . . . well, he wanted everything. Respect. Revenge. Wanted to beat me up, and wanted friendship. Adoration. Maybe denigration too. Kindness."

"And you gave him—?"

"Starlight."

"You didn't!"

"Nobody else wants her. He went dancing off with her through the puddles like in a film, and they both seemed happy."

She laughed. "I guess Nelda Jo will take care of her."

"If she comes back."

"If?"

"Just a feeling." He was standing in the turret, staring out the window at the air space where he'd often seen Selma. Again, it was as if he were seeing himself out there, in her place, looking in at Miranda and him, both older, taking care of a teenaged Cray who was sick with the flu in Orville's old bed.

"What?" Miranda asked, staring at him.

"What's that?"

"You drifted off."

"Oh. Yeah. I was just seeing myself—and you and Cray—in the future." She looked at him and nodded.

He glanced out the window again. Nothing, except Henry's lit-up house.

"Y'know," he said, "when I first came back, sitting in front of the TV I had the sense that while I'd been away America had turned. . . . Turned, definitely turned. But I didn't know what *to*. Now I do."

"And?"

"To Schooners. To the big disconnect."

"What does that mean?"

"I means I'm still way too bitter, that's all." He picked up the large framed photo and laid it on the floor at her feet. At the bottom was an inscription, scratched by hand with a sharp point into black, so that the letters came out silver:

20TH ANNIVERSARY
BANQUET AND BALL OF THE
FIRST STANISLAUER YOUNG MENS
BENEVOLENT ASSOCIATION
SUN. DEC. 30, 1923
AT THE LEXINGTON HALL

He got down on his hands and knees and studied it. Jews. Immigrants. A sea of faces, hundreds of them, flowing out to the horizon of a gaslit grand ballroom. In front, the faces were large, with the sharp detail those big, glass-plate cameras of the day could give. Every eye and nose, every Jazz Age hairdo, every birthmark. In the back, amid the fuzz the long exposure made of the flickering gas lamps, the faces seemed indistinguishable from one another. Almost all were seated at round tables. They were dressed to the teeth—the men in black tie, the white Vs of their shirts beneath their dark jackets making them look like a colony of penguins, and the women in grand dresses, mostly black, brocaded or silk, with oval necklines graced with gold and pearls. Flappers.

And the faces! They'd been told to "hold still." This generation of immigrant Jews, fleeing the pogroms, built low to the ground for speed, about to "hold still"? Yet most had, except for the few young children sitting on laps, who came out as blurred as the gas flames. The enforced stillness made them look stiff. The men's faces, even on this gala occasion, seemed somber or sternly ambitious, skeptical or fearful. The women seemed worried. There was only a rare hint of a held smile. Napkins were tucked into old men's shirts. Many of the young men's arms were around the young women's shoulders and necks, or vice-versa. Across the top of the photo, like a halo over the fearful, were the smears of the flames of the gas chandeliers.

Stuck in the back of the frame was an envelope addressed to him in Selma's hand.

Orville and Miranda glanced at each other.

"Forget it," he said.

"Oh, come on. She can't hurt you now."

"Wanna bet?" He opened the letter and read it out loud.

Hi, flier!

This is a photo my mother left me. It's the burial society, the Stanislauers. You'll find the plot out in Queens, where mom and pop and my sister are buried. Just ask anyone there for "Stanislauer." (Be careful of the Hassids For Hire at the gates. They say prayers for cash—Jewish, but *gonif.*) The name of their town in Poland. The one thing the Jews saved money for and wanted more than anything when they came to the New World was to have a place to be buried with people they knew, with people from their hometown. So they chipped in and held benefits like this and got the money to buy the plots. It turned social, as it does with Jews usually. Jewish holidays are everybody moaning and groaning about death and that Holocaust thing and then somebody says "Okay, let's *eat!*" So this is one of their balls.

Can you find me and Lil and Sam and Molly? Probably not. The Four Fleishers are the only ones not sitting down, standing along the right-hand wall (actually, Lil is sitting, but her new shoes made her feet hurt, and when a person's feet hurt you can always see it in their face). We all look pretty good, all things considered. Dad, the metalworker who worked on skyscrapers, had been nicknamed—because of his daring, way up high there—"The Flying Fleisher." So we called ourselves "The Four Flying Fleishers." Too bad we had no act. I'm on the left. Cute, eh? I was ten years old.

While I've got you, two things. First of all, about mice. There was a report and a warning to all about the lethal air virus created by mouse droppings. All produce and packaged stuff and even cans are subject to droppings and urine of rodents in storehouses and markets. Everything should be washed carefully because dust as well as the animals can be on most anything. Second, a question about your Buddism. Spiritual, okay. But is it *Jewish?*

Enjoy Mom

Orville and Miranda looked at each other.

"Oh boy," she said, rolling her eyes. "Watch out for those mouse droppings!"

"You can say that again."

She laughed. He heard it as music, as before.

"Which one is she?" Miranda asked, leaning closer to him.

"Here." In shadow stood Sam, short and strong. Towering over him and twice his girth was Molly. Next in line, sitting in half-shadow, with Molly's bulk and a dark patterned headband across her forehead that made her look like the last of the Jewish Mohicans, was Lil, aged eighteen. And then, against the wall on the edge of the family, stood ten-year-old Selma.

"I'll get my magnifying glass," Orville said.

With heads close together, they looked through the glass at the portrait of his mother as a girl. She was all in white. Around her lily-white swan's neck, pearls disappeared down into the oval neckline of her dress. Her arms were at her sides, and her dark hair was bobbed and captured in a white headband, a purer statement than her sister's dark one.

She had a face that took his breath away—oval, simple, elegant. Her straight nose fell from arched dark brows down to a plump ellipse of lips. There was a classic symmetry of her face—a Modigliani, like Celestina! And then the eyes. Those ten-year-old eyes, full of frailty, curiosity, intelligence. What else? They were steady. Unsteady. Sure. Unsure. Questioning. Hoping to hope and fearing to hope. They conveyed an overwhelming openness and, he thought, in their wistfulness, a precocious nostalgia.

"Amazing eyes!" Miranda said. "Such innocence there, such hope!"

"Truly. Wide open."

"Like the photo of Anne Frank."

"Yes. And like what I used to see in Amy."

"And I still do in Cray, though less and less."

"I know." He looked again. "You can almost see in her eyes that she really did have a vision then, even a dream. One time this summer, when you were away, Amy and I were talking about having a vision for our lives, and she asked me if I thought Selma's vision had died here."

"And you said?"

"I didn't. But seeing this . . ." he sighed. "If she's ten, here, she . . . yeah, she was something of a child prodigy as a pianist. She would've been playing on New York radio by then, WQXR. Smart, too. She'd already started high school, and—"

"At ten?"

"In the City, they skipped kids, then, if they were really smart. She graduated high school at thirteen, Hunter College at sixteen. She had a bright future, real bright."

"She never mentioned . . ." Miranda said. "Never played for me." She took the magnifying glass. "How beautiful she is—she almost glows!"

Orville stared at her, at this girl who was standing so shyly there, wanting only to live out her small dream, and in her slight fear he saw the bruised woman he knew. How had it happened? When had she started to float? She was so gifted. Everything was moving along nicely—Bach, Beethoven, even Debussey—a college degree in botany and then, during the Depression, she went to work at the New York State Employment Office, where she met a coworker named Solomon Rose. She married and went off to war with him in North Carolina and had children and saw Sol's limits and decided to divorce him before I was born but didn't and tagged along with him to Columbia and was a housewife and turned bitter. And then she got dizzy and was mutilated and turned again, becoming savage in private, saintly in public. A force of nature. A *gift*.

Orville had a glimpse, then, of the enormity of her wound, and of how hard she had fallen. How, broken and cornered, she had taken it out on those she loved. In that simple understanding, in seeing her this way, his anger left him. Everything changed, and there passed through him, as lightly as a breath through fog, a sense of sorrow. Tears came to his eyes. Understanding, sorrow, love—maybe they're just different words for the same thing? Understand, and you love. Love, and you understand.

Miranda put a hand on his shoulder. "What?"

"It's just so sad," he said, "so damn sad. I feel so bad for her! So much pain. And she was alone with it. There was no way in."

"For her."

"For me, for any of us. She got what she feared. She *was,* in a way, terrific, and she ended up so desperately alone." He struggled to breathe. "Except, maybe here in town, with people like you?"

"In a way. She did do wonderful things here, but yes, she was so unhappy, so unhappy in secret. I never really saw it."

"*She's* the one who should've left. Look into those eyes—do you see it?"

"What?"

"Everything! All of us! The girl's hope. How the woman ends up. She's just a child here, like Amy, Amy's age. Like Cray. Like you."

"You too."

"What happens? Why all the grief? We—all of us—we start out turning toward, and then we turn away? When does it happen? How do we, yearning to be *with,* turn away?"

The sorrow grew, edged all around with pain. He felt her hand on his cheek. He leaned his face on her leg tenderly, from the slightness of it realizing it was her bad leg, and leaning more tenderly on it, for that. "Everything. It's so sad."

She put her hand on his head, feeling the warmth there. They sat still like that, his sorrow echoing hers. This is my story too, she thought. Our story.

After awhile he raised his head to look at her. She had never seen him this way, so open, so raw. She was deeply touched. Frightened, too, about what she had come to say. She took a deep breath.

"There's something I have to make sure you understand before you leave." She looked away, unable to look him in the eye. "You know it already, in a way, but . . . Orvy, I'm so ashamed of what I did. To you, to us."

He blinked, to clear the past, to stay with her now. "You don't have to—"

"But I do. Every day, every single day, I relive it, I see it, I'm in it, the horror of it. I can't let you go without you knowing, really, *really,* how sorry I am, how awful I feel. It was so stupid, so brutal, so selfish." She pulled away from him, her fists clenched in her lap. "I thought by going away alone, in secret, I could protect myself and Cray—and ever since I've been back, trying to be with you, seeing it from your side . . . . My God!" She took a deep breath, looked down into his eyes. "You have every right to hate me."

He sat there on the floor looking up at her. The past few times with her, whenever they'd tried to talk about it, he'd felt angry, or deathly sad or even contemptuous—some feeling or other. This, now, was different. He wasn't filled with feeling, no. What came over him was an awareness—of her being so merely human. And with it, just then, he loved her. Looking at her scarlet hair, white skin, and dark-circled eyes, her strong shoulders, and hearing the music of her voice bringing back their losing each other, his heart opened to her, like a fist opens to a palm. Something greater than him, maybe something of the tattered "we" that lay between them, *moved.*

"You, Miranda . . . you're just a human being. We, you and me, we're just human beings."

She stared at him, at his light eyes so softened now that even though he was not crying you'd think they were made up wholly of tears. She understood.

"Yes," she said, "living out our little histories."

"Yes."

"Not famous."

"Not at all, no. Not even as advertised."

"Doing the car pooling, the laundry, the weeding, the animals, the protesting."

"The doctoring."

"In a town known for breakage."

They sat with each other, looking into each other's eyes, seeing each other now not so much as separate beings but each as a member of this common, frail, flawed, and ordinary part of the whole. Connected by their flaws.

He felt, then, unworthy of being loved by her. His mind flew to the moment on that winter night outside her house when he'd found himself standing alone by the river, alone in the frigid cold, bent over shivering, when his eyes caught the glow of the light in her doorway and he realized that the two people he loved most in the world were inside. A moment of gratitude, even of grace.

"You . . ." he started crying and so he blurted it out, "you've tried so hard to love me—and I you. We tried."

"Yes," she said, her eyes tearing up again, "we did."

"And it ain't easy."

"No. We did as best we could."

"Yeah."

They cried together. His face buried in her neck, hers in his. Tears wet their ears, their hair. He was leaving. It was over, and hopeless, and the hopelessness allowed them to tell their truth, like travelers holed up somewhere by chance or fate, for a time.

In that brief moment they understood that because they were parting, they could both be there. It no longer mattered that he would go and she would stay—they were held in the simple humility of who they actually were. Death was so much in the air that the future was irrelevant. They were forced into the present. With no future, there was no fear, no need to secret away, to protect. The sorrow, shared, receded.

He sighed. "I . . ." He stopped, tried again. "Don't take this the wrong way—"

"How could I now?"

"When I look at my own life, at everything I've done, the grief I've caused, well . . . *I* feel crippled too."

She found herself cherishing the moment, a kind of revelation that the past was past. "It's not how we're crippled," she said, smiling at him, "it's how we walk."

37

The next morning Penny picked them up in her brand-new beige Lincoln. Cray insisted he sit with Orville and Penny in the front seat. Miranda and Amy had the roomy back to themselves. They threw Orville's backpack and small suitcase into the trunk, which was only slightly smaller than the Chrysler's, and headed around the corner of Courthouse Square and across Fourth and started down Washington toward the train station. The day was sunny and fine, with that autumnal crispness that lets you see a long way through the bare trees and makes you notice the little puffs of breath surrounding your words and prompts you to remember cozy times around fires and under comforters in the night.

"Milt's got the Hong Kong flu," Penny said. "He was up at dawn for a meeting with Henry and went back to bed. He sends his regrets."

As they approached Third they were rocked by a tremendous explosion. It shook the ground and perturbed the shock absorbers of the Lincoln. Just ahead rose a plume of smoke. People were shouting. They drove toward it until they were stopped by a bright orange sign: DETOUR.

Officer Packy Scomparza was directing traffic. They stared.

The General Worth was gone.

"Hong Kong flu my ass!" Penny screamed. "I'll kill the sonofabitch!"

"That reeker!" screamed Amy. "That total creep!"

They stared.

The only piece of the 200-year-old hotel still standing was two stories of a part of the back wall. On the surface facing them, on the second floor, were the demarcations of two rooms painted an identical pink-and-yellow with vertical dark bands where the walls separating them had been. The bright colors of the twin rooms perched precariously above the rubble seemed to cry out to them like stranded children about to fall, or jump. What stories, in those gay colors! Everything had happened in those rooms, everything! A porcelain sink still stuck to one wall, filled with what looked like glass from a shattered mirror. Bad luck.

To all of them, it was as if they were seeing a scandalous public display of the insides of the dead.

"Unreal," said Amy.

"All too real, dear," Miranda answered sadly.

"I'll kill him," said Penny, looking around. "Where is he? And where's Henry?"

There was no sign of anyone except Jeffrey Liebowski and another member of Scomparza Demolition and Upholstery. They were sitting on two upturned soapboxes across the street in the weedy courtyard of the boarded-up Painted Lady Lounge, relaxing, having a smoke. Before them, like a portable electric organ, was the control panel for the explosives.

"It's like a person," said Cray.

"Yes, it is, hon," Miranda answered.

"And it *died*. The hotel *died*."

"It was a great old hotel," she said, her voice unsteady, "with a great old history. We'll try to remember the best of it."

"The pigs are at the trough," Orville said. He looked at his NOW watch. "We'd better go."

They barely got to the station on time. The sleek train-animal was wailing from upriver and then gliding in around the bend from the north, its red, white, and blue AMTRAK logo looking like the Stars and Stripes stretched out in a funhouse and frozen in chrome.

The engine stopped just opposite them, the rest of the train stretching way out behind.

Their good-byes were mercifully brief. Hugs, kisses, tears, more hugs, final kisses, and hands slipping out of hands, finger by finger, losing touch, and then the race toward the open doorway far down at the other end of the train where a conductor had put down the steel stairs and was beckoning.

Orville took the high step up—reminding him of a time as a boy in Bill's office he'd seen an old man diagnosed with "Train Conductor's Knee," a chronic sub-patellar tendonitis caused by conductors repeatedly stepping up abnormally high to get into the train—and then he was in.

He turned quickly left into the Pullman car, threw his suitcase and backpack onto the overhead rack, and slipped into a window seat that would allow him to wave good-bye to them as the train left. He couldn't see them from the stopped train. They were too far up the track, at the station. He waited.

And waited.

The train was not moving. He looked at his watch. Late. Time seemed stalled. No information was forthcoming.

Miranda and Cray and Amy and Penny stood there, waiting for the train to leave. Miranda's hand was on Cray's shoulder. She could feel it tremble, felt her own heart break all over again.

It's over. Bury it.

"Chilly," Penny said. "Shall we go?"

"You think anything's wrong?" Amy asked.

Orville sat there, starting to dull down, to resign himself to leaving, as he had resigned himself to so many leavings over the course of his life.

The whistle blew. The engine cleared its throat. The train rocked, ready to move.

Don't spread more suffering around.

Orville was stunned. The phrase echoed inside him.

Whatever you do, don't spread more suffering around.

The train moved.

The boy reached up for his mother's hand. Penny put her arm around Amy's shoulder, and Amy leaned into her. As the train started to ease out, tilting to stay steady around the first curve out, they all turned away and began to walk, at Miranda's pace, back to the car.

Orville jumped up from his seat and grabbed his backpack and suitcase and ran to the door. Locked. He tried the other side, the one tilting away from the town, and put his shoulder to it. It gave, opening. The train was moving and he had seen too many disasters of Columbians jumping from moving things like cars, tractors, bikes, and, yes, trains, but the choice was not a choice and he gauged the movement and jumped and seemed to fly out into thin air and hit hard rolling, and rolled up against the second set of tracks, and caught the acrid scent of creosote, the scent of that something else finally here finally now.

Looking up over the rails he could see the train vanishing around the bend. Far down the tracks the little group was moving away. They seemed beaten down, stooped over, hunched together, deadened. Penny's arm around Amy, Amy's hand in Cray's, Cray's in Miranda's—all matching her slow limp toward the peeling brick station with the sign announcing the Carribean outpost of OLU B A.

Orville jumped to his feet. "Hey! Hey!"

They couldn't hear him. He snatched up his backpack and suitcase and ran a few steps and then stopped and screamed at the top of his lungs, "Hey, I'm here!"

They heard. They turned. He saw their bodies shift as they realized, shift from hunched and hardening to softer, straighter, and the wind being against them he couldn't hear their cries but he saw Cray break free first and run full tilt toward him in that funny way he ran with his body stiff except for his hands pumping like pistons making his legs move fast, and he saw Amy start to run too with that pinwheel run of older girls and women the knees pinwheeling out because of the inward tilt of the femurs down from the widened childbearing pelvis, and then he saw Miranda hesitate a second and then she too started to run, actually run!—a lopsided galumphing run bringing to mind at that moment of all things a cowboy of his childhood Hopalong Cassidy she was actually running!—and even Penny ran too and he expected to see Selma flying low above it all but no, he'd learned in his time in the town that she wouldn't fly in the face of love, and in no time they were close enough so that their cries to each other to the new in each other could be clearly heard, as if all those present are coming back from the dead.